# THE CHILD'S WORLD OF ILLNESS

# The child's world of illness

## THE DEVELOPMENT OF HEALTH
## AND ILLNESS BEHAVIOUR

SIMON R. WILKINSON

*Consultant in Child Psychiatry*
*Ullevål Hospital, Oslo, Norway*

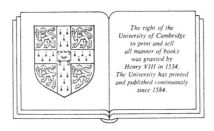

*CAMBRIDGE UNIVERSITY PRESS*
Cambridge
*New York    New Rochelle*
*Melbourne    Sydney*

CAMBRIDGE UNIVERSITY PRESS
Cambridge, New York, Melbourne, Madrid, Cape Town, Singapore, São Paulo

Cambridge University Press
The Edinburgh Building, Cambridge CB2 2RU, UK

Published in the United States of America by Cambridge University Press, New York

www.cambridge.org
Information on this title: www.cambridge.org/9780521328739

First published 1988
This digitally printed first paperback version 2006

*A catalogue record for this publication is available from the British Library*

*Library of Congress Cataloguing in Publication data*
Wilkinson, Simon. R.
The child's world of illness.
Bibliography:
Includes index.
1. Health behavior in children.   2. Sick children – Psychology.
I. Title.   [DNLM:   1. Attitude to Health – in infancy & childhood.
2. Child Behavior.   3. Child Psychology. WS 105.5.A8 W687c]
RJ47.53.W54   1988      155.4      87–26825

ISBN-13  978-0-521-32873-9 hardback
ISBN-10  0-521-32873-X hardback

ISBN-13  978-0-521-02904-9 paperback
ISBN-10  0-521-02904-X paperback

# Contents

# Acknowledgements

I would like to acknowledge a few important people and institutions which have influenced me in the course of preparing this book. They may not recognise the various roles which they have played but they have been important in the development of my thoughts.

First I would like to thank all the children and their families who participated in my research; as well as the staff at the various nursery schools and schools.

I would like to acknowledge the creative environment at the Department of Child and Family Psychiatry, Royal Hospital for Sick Children, Edinburgh, Scotland. During my time there I attended Colwyn Trevarthen's Intersubjectivity Seminars at the Department of Psychology, University of Edinburgh. These seminars played an important role in getting me to rethink established ideas. I thank Rosemary Johnson, sociologist at the University of Edinburgh, for most helpful earlier criticism.

I am indebted to Rom Harré's writings for the development of my theory. These writings have moulded my approach to the topic and played a vital part in creating the final form.

My thanks also go to the following: Sheila Gear, Ken Heap, Jostein Ingulfsen and David Stevenson.

Figs. 3.1 and 3.2 are reproduced with permission of Routledge & Kegan Paul. Figs. 2.1 and 4.1–4.4 first appeared in my MD Thesis for the University of Cambridge. Parts of chapter 4 have previously appeared in the *Journal of Family Therapy* and of chapter 8 in *Family Systems Medicine*.

# Glossary

**animism**   The belief that things which are in movement are alive and conscious.

**ecological systems**   These comprise the four variants described below (Bronfenbrenner, 1979):

**exosystem**   'One or more settings that do not involve the developing person as an active participant, but in which events occur that affect, or are affected by, what happens in the setting containing the developing person' (*op. cit.* p. 25).

**macrosystem**   'Consistencies in the form and content of lower-order systems (micro-, meso-, and exo-) that exist, or could exist, at the level of the sub-culture or the culture as a whole, along with any belief systems or ideology underlying such consistencies' (*op. cit.* p. 26).

**mesosystem**   'The interrelations among two or more settings in which the developing person actively participates' (*op. cit.* p. 25).

**microsystem**   'A pattern of activities, roles, and interpersonal relations experienced by the developing person in a given setting with particular physical and material characteristics' (*op. cit.* p. 22).

**ethogenic approach**   The ethogenic approach is the name given to a research methodology developed by Rom Harré (1977, 1979 pp. 124–8). The approach combines microsociological analysis with linguistic analysis of accounts.

**ideal speech act**   In an ideal speech act the speakers make maximal use of all their communicative competences.

**immanent justice**   The belief that an automatic justice emanates from inanimate objects.

**mathetic/pragmatic**   I use this distinction in the way developed by Halliday (1975). The child's mathetic use of language refers to its use in learning, whereas the other functions of language are subsumed under a 'pragmatic' rubric which includes the use of language both to satisfy one's own needs and to control and interact with others (*op. cit.* pp. 54–5).

**moral order**   A moral order has a characteristic form of conduct dependent on who has the rights in that setting to show respect and contempt, and give a moral commentary, together with the rituals of the setting (Harré, 1983 pp. 243–6).

**transforming experiment**   'A transforming experiment involves the systematic alteration and restructuring of existing ecological systems in ways that challenge the forms of social organization, belief systems, and lifestyles prevailing in a particular culture or subculture' (Bronfenbrenner, 1979, p. 41).

**validity types**   These comprise the three variants described below (after Bronfenbrenner, 1979 pp. 29–35):

   **developmental**   Change produced in a person's conceptions and/or activities carries over to other settings and other times.

   **ecological**   The environment experienced by subjects in a scientific investigation has the properties it is supposed or assumed to have by the investigator.

   **phenomenological**   There is a correspondence between the subject's and the investigator's view of the research situation.

# 1

# Presenting a problem

From time to time we all have difficulties knowing how to be certain that another person knows what we mean. At times this is unimportant,but when we want a response from that person we need to know that they have understood. When it comes to complaining about our own discomforts, the uncertainty of knowing whether our message has been adequately received is pressing. It becomes an acute problem when we rest in hope that those to whom we have presented our discomforts will take what we feel is appropriate action to help us feel better.

Sometimes we have opportunities to appraise beforehand relative strangers who might help us. Children like to be familiar with teachers who might have to help them in a crisis. They have their own ways of finding out whether they could rely on them in an emergency. People can visit their future general practitioner before they register with a practice, although this is seldom encouraged. It is sometimes very difficult to find answers on such a preliminary visit, as we remain uncertain which questions to ask and uncertain to what degree we can rely on the answers we receive.

Whether the potential care-giver is a parent, doctor or teacher, the aim of a child often appears to be to find out what makes a difference to that person. 'Will he react to what is important for me or will I have to adapt to his way of doing things in order to be "heard"?' 'Is it even possible for me to work out how to be heard?' At other times the whole process of presenting the problem occurs intuitively without a conscious appraisal of the care-giver, instead relying on the experience that what has occurred before is likely to occur again. This is not to suggest that there exists some basic natural 'illness behaviour' which is revealed in such emergencies but that the way of presenting the problems reflects the well-tried methods of old.

People appear to have a very wide range of ways of making public their discomforts. Children are known to cry with pain and distress, throw tantrums and literally pull their hair out. At the moment I will loosely refer to discomforts rather than illness because I wish to stress that what is conveyed is the state of the individual. I do this rather than moving on to discriminate between different forms of discomfort some of which will be interpreted as illness. The ways in which illness is deduced from children's behaviour will become clearer in the course of this book. Illness represents an *interpretation* of the child's state based on the observed behaviour. This point becomes particularly important when looking at how the states of young children are remarked on and responded to by the 'others' around them. The child's discomfort is first noted before the possible description 'illness' is applied to the child's state. With young children their states of discomfort are initially offered for public inspection rather than being presented in a direct way to another for consideration as a complaint. In a two-stage process the children are dependent both on others being observant, that is being cued in to observe their form of presenting their distress, and on these others recognising this as illness.

Mechanic (1962) introduced the term illness behaviour to account for 'the ways in which given symptoms may be differentially perceived, evaluated and acted (or not acted) upon by different kinds of persons'. He chose to use the word symptom. I interpret a symptom here as conveying something closer to an aspect of experience which has been recognised as a signal by that person. A symptom is a body 'state' which has been recognised as signalling something, whereas initially natural states of individuals need not necessarily have attached signalling properties learnt by the individual. In other words, how children have learnt to transmit their state is built onto a foundation of being with other people who noted their state before they had found significant movements or words to convey it to others. 'Symptoms' are the result of this dynamic developmental process (see also Mannoni, 1973 ch 2). It is this developmental process I hope to elucidate here.

In investigating the origins of health and illness behaviour it is necessary to go back to the perception of discomfort, back to before the time that children could overtly evaluate or act on it themselves. This would potentially involve going back to the stage when the states of young babies are 'perceived, evaluated and acted (or not acted) upon' by their parents. This is the time when the interpersonal dance is dependent on moderately accurate interpretation of the baby's state, and the baby has barely begun to develop a signalling system in response to the parent's handling (see chapter 2). Neonatal learning research suggests that some learning can occur before birth, so it will always be difficult to achieve observation of demonstrably naïve subjects. Here I am going to take up the story of the development of health and illness behaviour from the point at which children can first present and reflect on their views on illness – about 3 years old. By this age they are discriminating the state of illness from that of health. It is from this point on that it becomes possible to carry out a verbal enquiry into both the nature of a child's discomforts and how he appraises them. Much learning has already preceded this stage.

It is particularly the verbal discussion of discomforts which lies at the core of a clinical consultation. In my clinical practice as a child psychiatrist my problem in that particular form of consultation is often how to facilitate children and their parents presenting their discomforts in a way which enables them to be shared – for the meaning of them to be understood by others. We know that the meaning of his illness affects the child's response to it (Willis, Elliott & Jay, 1982). An additional but related problem involves understanding how children and parents come to attribute intention in their individual ways to what they observe each other doing and experience being done to them. I will return to these elements later, particularly in chapter 8, for the effect styles of attribution of intention can have on the development of delinquent or illness behaviour.

The research which constitutes a large proportion of what I am presenting here arose from a need to know more about how people learn to present their discomforts, how their illness behaviour evolves both before the consultation and in the consultation. The behaviour patterns established in childhood are of great significance in the causes of disease and death occurring in later life (Graham, 1985). It is through an exploration of the origin of these patterns that I believe it possible to evolve better consultation practices; and so use the drug 'doctor' (Balint, 1964; see also chapter 9) as helpfully and effectively as possible. I will here concentrate primarily on what happens prior to a consultation but in chapter 9 make some suggestions about how these results can be used to review consultation practices. It will be seen that these suggestions lead naturally to integrating health education approaches into our daily life when listening to other people's problems.

When patients come to see me, they arrive with their own set of assumptions about what is likely to happen in the consultation. I approach the patient with my own set of assumptions – assumptions which I have not always made explicit to myself, and rarely made explicit to the patient. The differing expectations that are involved in the interview may lead to a clash of perspectives in which there is little mutual understanding of the other's position (HESU, 1982 p. 80), ineffectual communication (Mayer & Timms, 1969; Burck, 1978; Lewis, 1980), and, to borrow a phrase from family therapists, no engagement. The same can happen between parents and their own children.

Usually children are brought to consultations with doctors by their parents or care-givers. The adult who brings the child often carries assumptions about the aim of consultation (Stoeckle, Zola & Davidson, 1963) built up through discussion with others in the social network prior to making the decision to consult. The decision-making involved here uses what Freidson (1960) terms 'the lay referral system', and through this cultural values are mediated. Additionally the adult has ideas about what would be helpful for the child based on an opinion of what caused the condition and the appropriate remedy. The child has his own ideas about the nature of the problem which are likely to have developed from his experiences both at home and at school with his teachers and peers. They may not necessarily be the same as those of his parents and his parents may not both share the same viewpoint. In these circumstances a clash of perspective in the surgery may be just the start of a continuing process of discussion and negotiation on return home as the different family members and even neighbours make sense of the consultation from their own viewpoints (Stimson & Webb, 1975).

A clash of perspectives can occur at the many levels mentioned above. It can occur between adult and doctor, child and doctor, child and adult, or between children when they recount their experiences to each other. My aim here is to explore the child's world, so that it is possible to build up a picture of how the child sees illness, and the causes of illness in particular. The research was organised so that I obtained a picture of the child's world when it was uninfluenced by the circumstances of acute illness or hospitalisation, aspects generally controlled by adults. Causes of illness are commonly seen as central to the consultation, in the belief that understanding the cause will explain what should happen next and how the illness could be prevented in the future (Posner, 1980; Blaxter, 1983). A clash of perspectives about the cause of illness could be at the heart of a dissatisfying and unhelpful consultation, as constructs about the causes of illness have potent social organising potential. This relates to taking responsibility for one's condition. Pill & Stott (1982) pointed out that 'readiness to accept responsibility for one's health depends partly on the views held about the aetiology of illness'. It is these views that link lay illness models with the disease models attributed to professionals and leave people to varying degrees with a sense of their own effectiveness in combating illness and preventing it in the future.

An awareness of these issues seems to have moulded the conclusion presented in the Health Education Studies Unit (England) report with regard to the educatory potential of consultations. The first conclusion of

'The Patient Project' was 'that little attention was being paid to patients' ideas and theories and that this fact was a major barrier to successful educational outcomes of consultation' (HESU, 1982 p. 80).

Much of the child's behaviour when ill is determined by others rather than being moulded by the child. The youngest children are the most constrained within the limits set by their parents. What constitutes acceptable behaviour conforms primarily to the values of others rather than those of the children themselves. This balance in the importance of the values of the adult and child can be anticipated to change throughout development. The social pressures of others push the child into what has been termed a sick role whilst his own developing autonomous sense of how one is when ill leads him to present ever more forcefully his own illness behaviour within these role constraints. Instead of concentrating on observations of the child's behaviour when ill I will therefore concentrate on the subjective element for the child – how his views on illness become established and part of his own repertoire to be called upon in future consultations. My assumption here is that these views will come to occupy an ever more important place in determining the form of the child's illness behaviour as he grows up. Nevertheless the language he has developed for sharing his discomforts has been shaped by the dynamics of the responses made to him by important others. A study of the different origins of children's views will reveal how this balance between role, a social construct, and individual behaviour evolves. It appears to be linked to the developmental dynamic between individual and social factors in enculturation and socialisation.

This emphasis poses problems of methodology as children's views are initially very labile because more of their constructs, compared with those of adults, are loosely held (Bannister & Fransella, 1980 p. 30). Different views are elicited in different circumstances and are held with varying degrees of conviction. This appears to be necessary to cope with the lack of a coherent framework into which children can fit their experiences, and leads to a state of 'mental fluidity' (Tizard & Hughes, 1984 p. 131).

The children's constructs I will be describing here were dependent to varying degrees on the contexts within which I saw them. The children were seen in everyday settings such as home or school, rather than hospital or doctors' surgeries. The emphasis was therefore on the views which a previously healthy child might bring to a consultation, rather than how these views are modified by the sickness setting. It is the factors which will potentially influence illness behaviour that I want to elucidate rather than the social pressures to occupy particular sick roles.

Through looking at how a child's views on the causality of illness change, not just with context but also with age, a developmental perspective is added which can bridge the gap between the child's views and those of the adult. The developmental perspective emphasises the mixture of biological development, individual experience, social responses to the child throughout development and the transmission to the child of cultural values in his socialisation (Piaget, 1970). Nevertheless children of the same age are at different developmental levels due to variations along these different dimensions. A study of development emphasises the processes which affect their changing views to set beside the content of those views. It can be anticipated that a wide variation in the views of different children will be found, but that the developmental processes which affect the children will have much in common. It is these shared processes which I believe it is necessary to find in order to extrapolate the results of this research to other situations.

There is a continuous reciprocal interaction between the different elements in these processes: the biological, the individual psychological and the social. At the same time as the child's state is modifying the behaviour of others towards him, he is changing in response to the way he is handled by those same people. The ways in which adults communicate with children and facilitate particular forms of their communication mould the processes of this coevolution. A similar process must occur in the gathering of their views, and a 'clash of perspectives' could well have been the outcome in this research if it had not been possible for researcher and child to adapt communication patterns to each other. The ways in which such a clash of perspectives seems to have been avoided in the research reported here suggest some pointers towards how consultations can be as productive as possible for all involved. These are observations on the process of the research and how it can mirror the consultation process, the presenting of a discomfort to another, whereas the views obtained are the content of the discussion. I will return to this in chapter 9. Throughout the following presentation of the child's world of illness this mutual reciprocity and coevolution of process and content must always be kept in mind.

I am suggesting here a communication model of how illness behaviour is built up throughout development without having presented any evidence for why I believe this to be the case. I have so far begun to point out similarities between the form of communication in the consultation process and the research method. Additionally the interpretation of what constitutes a consultation can be broadened to include a child's 'consultation' with his parents – in other words to all situations in which there is presentation of the child's discomforts and an associated expectation on his part that others will take some initiative on the basis of that 'consultation' to help him. For the youngest children that expectation is poorly developed, as that in itself is learnt on the basis of experience; but when studying verbal 3–4 year-olds it is in my view appropriate to use the term consultation. Some of the evidence for this assumption will be presented in chapter 4, 'The primary structure to the child's world of illness', where the ways in which children present their discomforts and have them evaluated by their parents are described. When consultation is seen to include what occurs with parents, similarities between processes in development, consultation with professionals and the research method become clearer. The 'processes' I refer to are the forms of communication.

Information on the development of communication is presented in chapter 2, which is the background for the intersubjective communication model I use and which links the form of communication in the consultation and the research to a developmental perspective. The fundamental principle in that presentation is that I allocate a primary role in the developmental process to intersubjectivity, rather than building up an ego psychology in which understanding is based primarily on individual qualities in the child or adult. Should this primary role of intersubjectivity be subsequently cast aside by future research then the results reported here will require a reinterpretation. Nevertheless I include a pointer in the review of the development of children's communication to illustrate how an ego psychology could develop from a primary intersubjective psychology.

Besides needing to illuminate communication processes for their effect on the *content* of children's views on illness as well as on the *form* of the consultation process, it is necessary to orientate the reader with reference to what is known so far about the nature of children's views on illness. Chapter 3 reviews some of the background research which illuminates such themes as how children view illness as being caused, and how these views are mirrored in the adult world to which they are becoming socialised. As I have described above, interpretation lies at the base of attributing the label 'illness' to particular forms of a child's behaviour. This means that adults are dependent on using categories from their own experiences and intuition to interpret the child's underlying subjective state: parents of young children use certain categories, and researchers use categories based on what is known so far about the nature of illness. I note particularly which categories from research on adults as well as children can be useful in building up an interpretative system which is coherent with the intersubjective framework I have adopted. My purpose is not to present a treatise on child development and socialisation but to provide enough details to enable connections to be made with the literature.

I have mentioned the value of exploring the child's views on illness for the way in which they can help the consultation process. The last three chapters explore some of the implications of this intersubjective communication model. In chapter 9 the consultation process is considered in more detail, especially the implications of what is presented here for facilitating consultation. In this way I aim to widen the applicability of my observations of children. I suggest that it is to these consultation processes that psychotherapy directs itself in the establishment of an (as near as possible) 'ideal discourse' (McCarthy, 1973). The ideal discourse emphasises the intersubjective element necessary for elucidating the nature of a child's discomforts, but it does nothing to help develop expectations about what forms of presentation the child might use to describe his discomforts. It is to these expectations that the results presented here are also relevant. Knowing which views are typical of different ages allows a certain degree of identification with the child's position, but it must not be forgotten that one can never be certain that one knows exactly what is going on inside another person. This degree of uncertainty appears to be necessary for establishing the 'ideal discourse' in which there is enough respect for the uniqueness of each individual.

The positive value of uncertainty becomes clearer in the example of a communication analysis of 'pretend illness' states which constitutes chapter 8. In this detailed analysis of how a particular form of illness label can be attached to a child's behaviour I apply the rules for deciding about children's behaviour as deduced from my observations and described in chapter 4. Some of the implications that can follow should parents, teachers, doctors or others have diminished communicative competences in particular areas are then considered. This study was primarily observational and I did not set out to test these implications; this testing represents a necessary second stage in the research. All the time people are dependent on observations, interpretations and the testing of these, just as parents are with their children. Gradually though we can approximate our understanding to the child's state, and I hope the results presented here are a good enough approximation to the child's world of illness to be practically useful, both in consultations and in formulating models of illness behaviour to facilitate further research.

There remains one further application of these results, which I consider very important: knowledge of developmental processes can be used to produce strategies for health education and improve preventive medicine.

Chapter 10 describes some of these potential implications of my observations for health education strategies. These strategies are dependent on communication for putting over their message in such a way that the content is understood by the target population. That population must also have some desire to make use of the information. In this sense the model presented here should be suitable for reviewing both the strategies and content of health education. Currently it adopts a teaching approach which lends itself in some degree to a classroom but hardly at all to the mass media campaigns we are familiar with. It is essential to take into account the balance between social role pressures and individual initiatives when designing helpful health education campaigns. (It is with some care that I have chosen to use the word helpful in this context rather than effective, as I hope will become clearer in chapter 10.) Illness and sickness models are the appropriate ones for health education, yet information tends to be provided according to disease models (see pp. 37–39).

It is also necessary to direct information to people in age-appropriate ways. Different age groups differentiate between information which they interpret as being directed at controlling them (social information) and 'facts' useful for them personally (personal information) using various strategies. There must be awareness of how 'facts' are digested by particular age groups and differentiated from attempts at controlling their freedom. These communication aspects are ones already emphasised by the Health Education Studies Unit: 'The best interests of health education can be served by focusing attention on communication, and within that explanation' (HESU, 1982 p. 125). Additionally, more effective communication in consultations would, I believe, lead to improved consensus on treatment strategies and better patient cooperation (see also Millstein, Adler & Irwin, 1981). Although I tend here to look at what adults can do to facilitate things for children, it must not be forgotten that communication is a two-way process. Adults have responsibility for children, doctors have responsibility for the medical consultation, and those who have that responsibility must make certain that they carry out their duties as effectively and helpfully as possible. My hopes are that the research presented here will help communication between adults and children concerning health and illness matters.

# 2

# The form of dialogue

*'The self is not so much a substance as a process in which the conversation of gestures has been internalised within an organic form.' (Mead, 1934 p. 178)*

In Chapter 1 I outlined some of the similarities between the difficulties experienced by children in learning the language of complaining, that is the ways in which they can share their discomforts with others, and the problems which a researcher can have in trying to elicit children's views on illness. Inherent in both is a form of dialogue directed at sharing the nature of someone's internal world. A consultation consists of the same sort of dialogue in which one person is trying to present a problem and another is trying to be open enough to hear what that problem is. A shared language is required.

In order to lay the basis for research methods which can be used to explore children's views and at the same time point out the sorts of communicative skills held by children, I will summarise here some of what is known about the development of children's communication. This will not be a comprehensive documentation of child development and socialisation; my intention is rather to provide a theoretical framework that can be drawn on when evaluating both what children say about illness and the research on the subject. (For those readers who have a knowledge of the development of communication this part of the chapter could be unnecessary for their understanding of the rest of this book.) In addition the research method I used to explore the child's world of illness will be described. My aim is to illustrate how my method approximates to the ways in which 'an ideal discourse' can be established and maintained, based on the results of the intersubjective psychology of development described in this section. As an ideal discourse can only ever be approximated and never achieved, it is for the reader to judge to what degree I achieved a good enough discourse with my subjects.

## An interactional framework

Children can be all things to all people. They can be thought of as mini-adults or maxi-babies. Adults have differing expectations of the same children, and different children have different expectations of the same adult. Not only that but the general forms of these expectations change over the decades along with changes in societies (Ariès, 1960). I do not wish to start here with a description of how we come to attribute differing expectations, or come to understand different things from looking at the same behaviour. These all represent developments from the earlier stages in which naïve children are responded to by others. I have already hinted, though, at the possibility that children at birth can have learnt things from their time *in utero* (*Science* News and Comments, 1984), such as recognition of their mother's voice, and so this state of naïvety is in all probability just a necessary assumption for allowing a description of how the child learns to communicate to begin from its birth.

Communication involves interaction between people, directly or indirectly, where a wide range of behaviours has potential meaning for those involved. The signals may be perceived using any of the senses, and similarly may be emitted in a variety of ways. It is the origin of a signalling system which is of interest here. As mentioned in Chapter 1 a child learns how to communicate his natural state to others. The concept of a natural state is a necessary hypothesis which represents our deduction of what lies behind the observed behaviour, to which we have attributed some meaning.

Although some people say that it is impossible not to communicate (Watzlawick, Beavin & Jackson, 1967), this is not a very helpful approach when studying the origins of children's communication. It lays emphasis on the fact that people are always searching for meaning in what they observe, whereas I wish to emphasise here the intention in the child to communicate. If one person in an interaction is not intending to communicate, and is not open to attributing meaning to what is occurring around him, then communication is not taking place even though the other interactant may be busy attributing lots of 'significant' meaning to what he perceives. The standard riposte to that argument is that 'not intending to communicate' is a particular form of communication. But children learning to communicate are subjects to whom it is inappropriate to attribute awareness of 'intention' and 'communication' without further evidence. Research into communication must pay attention to what goes on both within individuals and between individuals. The emphasis of Watzlawick *et al.* is totally on what goes on between individuals; in this way they avoid exploring the coevolution of individual and social development. When reviewing the development of communication, and especially the communication to others of the internal discomforts of illness, this understanding of what goes on within individuals and the changes over time in which biological maturation plays its role must have a more prominent place.

In order to identify all the influences affecting the child's signalling system it is important to use a conceptual framework which will reflect the multi-level nature of communication. A helpful starting-point is the terminology of Bronfenbrenner (1979), who views children as belonging to several interacting systems which all affect their development in different ways. Children live primarily within their *microsystems*, usually the worlds of school and family for school-age children. To varying degrees the children enter society at large, as represented by the stippled part of fig. 2.1. The ways children communicate to others within their microsystems also affect and are affected by how significant others in the different microsystems (e.g. class teacher and parent) relate to each other. This order of system is termed the *mesosystem* and is represented by black area in fig. 2.1. At the same time outside influences such as work demands on parents, unemployment at home or threats to teachers' jobs can bring new effects into the microsystems and affect the child indirectly. These 'outside influences' are termed by Bronfenbrenner part of the *exosystem*, and are repsented by hatching in the figure. These three different levels of system are all embedded within a particular culture or *macrosystem*.

Much research on children's communication has focussed on the very early stages, so that researchers have felt justified in limiting the number of systems included in their analyses. The younger the child the more they have felt it valid to look only at the interaction between child and care-giver, giving little attention to exosystem or macrosystem influences. Initially

Fig. 2.1. Ecological systems.

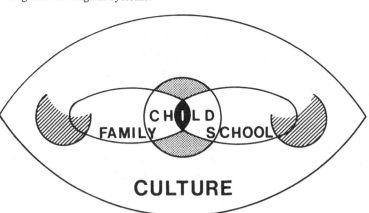

children tend to live in just one microsystem with a single primary caregiver, and so mesosystem effects can justifiably be ignored. At this stage the predominant exosystem influence has come about through the relationship between the mother and the father; the child only gradually enters the father's world, having been totally enveloped in the mother's world and only indirectly influenced by the father. In this way the child becomes a member of a family microsystem before proceeding to become a member of other microsystems, such as school, later on. The mode is one of nested systems in which each layer reflects the form of the other layers.

Fig. 2.2 shows how this can be visualised for an earlier stage of development in the family. The child is here portrayed at the stage where most of his world is shared with mother (diagonal hatching). The mother shares a good deal of her world with her husband (horizontal hatching), whereas the father has only a small part of the child's world which is unique to him (black area), otherwise sharing the child's world through his wife (cross hatching).

Fig. 2.2. The family system for an infant.

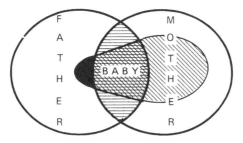

Within this systemic orientation it is most important to note the processes that occur in the interactions typical of each of the levels, rather than any static states of the individuals. The communicative processes are part of the interactants' repertoires and it is through making use of their whole range that communicative reciprocity can be maintained, with the usual testing of assumptions about each other. Communicative competence is based on successful use of this repertoire, but first the nature of the repertoire must be noted.

## Development of communicative competence

Research has begun to look at how babies interact with their mothers from immediately after birth. As early as 12 hours after birth infants are known to engage in complex turn-taking with their mothers (Condon & Sanders, 1974). This has come to be termed the 'dance' of the neonate with human speech. Initially the parents are involved in carefully fitting his or her mouth movements and accompanying sounds to the infant's pattern of facial expressions. If the fit is right the parent is rewarded by the infant prolonging and elaborating his pattern of primitive facial movements. The cue interval to elicit the parent's response is very short and the 'dance' does not appear to tire parents. It is therefore proposed that this mutual responsiveness must be at an intuitive level, rather than being a fully conscious and planned activity (Papousek & Papousek, 1983). It is regarded as critical to the enjoyment of this dance and its effectiveness that there is this short cue interval, so that parents' responses are contingent upon the infant's acts in this very special way. At the same time parental responsiveness has to be cued to the individual variability inherent in the newborn. This can be particularly hard for parents with an infant sick at birth. Subsequent interactional failure with a greater risk of child abuse appears to arise more often with premature babies (Elmer & Gregg, 1967), probably because they are less competent at turn-taking and so place greater demands than normal on their parents' communicative competences. In addition these infants' cries are often atypical, signalling unclearly their forms of discomfort (see further below). Nevertheless exosystem influences can operate effectively to the child's advantage from the early months, as the benefits of making the professionals working with these families aware of these vulnerabilities has shown (Ounstead *et al.*, 1982).

Although these first steps may appear a long way from child communication, they emphasise the basic reciprocity required in the process. This develops when parents do not have preconceived expectations of their children, but learn to 'dance' together. The human brain appears to have systems which integrate interpersonal and practical aims virtually from birth (Trevarthen, 1982). It remains hypothetical whether the problems some older children have in turn-taking in conversation have their basis in difficulties at this early stage, but clinical experience identifies many individuals who appear regularly to talk over others and miss their cues.

Exosystem influences which affect this reciprocity act indirectly and so are much harder to identify. At this very early stage mother plus child constitutes the microsystem, and father is an 'exosystem' influence on the mother. It is suspected that depressed mothers are less accurate in their responses to their babies. It may be that fathers have an important role in the genesis of this problem as puerperal depression is commoner in situations with marital conflict (Cox, Connor & Kendell, 1982) and following conflict during the pregnancy (Cullen & Connolly, 1982). Maternal depression in the first year of a child's life is particularly important as it can lead to later (aet. 4 years) significant intellectual deficits (Cogill *et al.*, 1986).

These early signals to which mothers are responding are very varied. An important one in terms of the precursors to illness behaviour is crying. Cries have many different forms which are said to be characteristic of different states of the infant, such as hunger, pain, loneliness and tiredness (Dunn, 1977). Parents use their intuition to respond differently to the different forms of crying so that the internal needs of the child are contingently responded to: crying is a potent social releaser of adult behaviour (Hinde, 1982). When the adult responses are made up of well-coordinated movements and/or quiet vocalisations to the infant, the infant is shown to learn most successfully. However after a time the individual cry patterns revert to the basic 'hunger' pattern, which appears to be why so many care-givers overemphasise a link between crying and hunger. At the same time we can see here a basis for misinterpreting infant states which could lead to misinterpretation of illness states. I am not aware of any research which has discriminated between these above states and states of illness.

Another ingredient for successful learning of pre-speech communication is the way in which a parent alters his or her speech to personalise it for easy identification by the infant. He or she will speak more slowly, at a higher pitch, in simple and repetitive patterns with exaggerated facial expressions and other movements (Papousek & Papousek, 1983). Even children as young as 4 years old will adopt this pattern when speaking to younger children.

## From competence to sharing meaning

The basis for a competence to communicate has now been established, but as yet no evidence presented that there has been communication of intended meaning from infant to mother. One aspect of the mother/infant interaction subsequently becomes the sharing of meaning in joint 'play'. Initially it is the parent who provides the context in which the messages are given meaning. Messages are dependent on the context for defining their content, such that 'message + context = meaning' (Hinde, 1982 p. 218).

Hopkins (1983) describes how the social preadaptation of infants can come about through the parent's desire to attribute meaning to the infant's productions. Through regular contingent interpretation the infant's behaviour gains meaning and subsequently interactive purpose for him. At the same time it comes to be peculiar to the social group of the care-giver. The infant can then experiment with those particular responses in communicating with that person, before extending his range further to others. These are general comments about conveying messages of all types, but it is from this basis that the specific messages about the infant's own state are conveyed to another, and how he comes to have his discomforts and illnesses labelled. It is believed that the ways in which infants signal their emotional states are similar across divergent cultures (Trevarthen, 1984). The new methods being developed to look at 'infant/care-giver' interaction in relation to differing physiological states of the infant (Miller, Hollingsworth & Sander, 1985) can be expected to help elucidate the issues involved here, particularly in regard to discrimination between different states of discomfort, states of emotion and illness.

As a way of improving orientation to each other visual cues exchanged between parent and infant are very important. They are used to set the turn-taking in 'proto-conversations'. This important element of looking at each other is also part of the mirroring process whereby the child sees the parent imitate his facial expressions. In this way he appears to develop and refine his emotional effectiveness, which from the start regulates interpersonal interaction (Trevarthen, 1984). It will be seen later how important this eye contact is when parents come to judge whether their child is ill or not. Eye contact is attributed a similarly important role in the ascertainment of the truth value of statements, such as whether a child is falsely claiming illness.

If a parent comes to be preoccupied with his own needs this mirroring usually ceases to be contingent on the child's initiatives, and he begins to reflect the child inaccurately. In this way the exosystem, for example, can come to influence the primary microsystem. These reciprocal imitations have been detailed by psychologists (see for example Trevarthen, 1974), while the potential 'pathology' of these interactions has been detailed from psychoanalytic perspectives which have also used mirroring as a central concept (Winnicott, 1967; Lacan, 1968; Mannoni, 1973). Current research suggests that this form of reciprocal interaction is required to foster an inherent emotional sensitivity and an ability to reflect on it. These sensitivities are developed early. Four-year-olds respond to their younger siblings' distress, and secondborn children as young as 14 months have attempted to comfort older siblings (Dunn, 1984 p. 23).

The relevance of these observations to the communication of illness remains to be clarified, but it appears justified at present to use the above as a model for what is necessary for communicating about subjective states of discomfort. How these can become linked to states of illness will become clearer subsequently. The problem for a researcher here is how to fulfil the requirements of valid research, which means not being preoccupied with his own needs when interacting with the children. It is necessary to develop ways of being as engaged as possible with a child while observing the effects of this engagement so that the forms of validity of the data elicited can be established. I will return later in this chapter to ways in which I tried to achieve this in my research. It is the same dilemma faced in a consultation, where asking questions minimises the desired reciprocity unless it is clear that the person asking the questions does not already know the answers and genuinely wants to find them out (Wood, 1982).

Head postures are another group of important communication signals, especially in young children (Hopkins, 1983). We are all familiar with 'cocky' and 'dejected' postures in others. These represent the labels attached to various positions; however if the previous meaning ascribed by other care-takers has been outside cultural norms our own interpretations of the child's emotions may well be misplaced and unhelpful. An example of this could be if the 'dejected' posture had been used to irritate others and hence has become attached to alternative emotional states.

Communication is most effective when cues such as pitch and tone of voice, visual eye contact and head postures are coherent in message and appropriate to the interactant's behaviour. Although duplication of a message along several channels of communication has been termed redundancy, it can enable the message to be heard clearly by the less advantaged who may not be tuned in to all the channels (Fraser & Grieve, 1979). Should conflicting cues be given – for example the verbal message 'Stay away' at the same time as non-verbal messages to 'Come close' (head nods, beckoning and a welcoming facial expression) – the effect, at least in children between 1 and 3½ years old, can be particularly upsetting (Volkmar & Siegel, 1979). The coherence of the total message is important for assessing its truth value. States of discomfort which we observe can only be safely interpreted if our own array of messages to the child is coherent.

After the above stages in which the focus of communication has been face to face the infant moves on to sharing things with the parent. First they begin to look at the same things ('co-orientation') and then share the objects that they have looked at together. Three- to four-month old infants begin to concentrate on objects which the mother's hands bring into the conversation. At the same time the infant is introducing objects into the conversation by mouthing and manipulating more of the things around him. As the object is transferred from one to the other affective interpersonal contact is regained or maintained. Herein lies a basis for game behaviour which establishes the sharing of objects and people (Winnicott, 1971; see also Goffman, 1961). Within these games voice qualities change and signals become established which facilitate discrimination between different forms of moral order to the interactions (termed metalevel signals as they determine the interpretative set to be used for understanding the communication: Batcson, 1955). These facilitate the differentiation of the peculiar values of play and alternative 'games' (See Harré (1983) for a detailed analysis of the concept of moral order. He includes a short statement about moral order which gives the key ingredients: 'In a moral order the three characteristic forms of conduct – rituals, confirmations of respect and contempt and displays of proper character and moral commentary – are permitted only to those who in this or that collective, have the right to perform them' (p. 245).) Until these characteristics of play signals are clearly established for the child he will tend only to play with the care-giver and have an associated fear of playing with strangers.

Voice quality (Laver, 1980) is the most powerful way of indicating change of intention and interpersonal affect. Changes in voice quality are also used to discriminate between an intention for joint affectionate play, and aggressive or soliciting individual play (Trevarthen & Marwick, 1982). As play and games are important ways of engaging children without entering a question-and-answer format these observations on voice quality play a critical role.

The ways in which objects become involved in different play relationships give them differing meanings and they can come to have the qualities of signs and even symbols. The child has now moved on from the stage of primary intersubjectivity to secondary intersubjectivity through a game phase (Trevarthen, 1982).

## Words

When Piaget (1926) first looked at the child's use of words and language from a developmental perspective he stressed developmental processes within the child rather than exploring the interactional elements in their conversations which I have emphasised here. It was partially his cultural perspective which led him to stress the child's egocentrism up to about the age of 7 years and the value system inherent in his stage model (Harré, 1983). In fact children can coordinate different viewpoints much earlier than this provided the tasks they are set make sense to them. (See

Donaldson (1978) for one criticism of Piaget's position, and Tizard & Hughes (1984 p. 126).) Much of the meaning of the tasks set children comes from the context, especially non-verbal gestures which at early ages override the influence of words.

Before children are able to participate in verbal conversation other competences for vocalising must have been developed. One of these is termed 'pre-speech', in which lip and tongue movements are coordinated as though in conversation but without sound. Infants adopt a specific breathing pattern and 'speak' in 3-second bursts, which happens to be equivalent to the average length of a short sentence. These productions are usually not initiated by the mothers but are a type of 'proto-conversation' developed in the infant (Trevarthen, 1974). Subsequently sound is added and in a 'proto-language' phase vocalisations succeed in getting people to do things (Halliday, 1973). Interpersonal effectiveness in the use of language appears to be based on this interactional process. The implication must be that this is essential for verbally sharing our discomforts with others.

When language is developing children have a mixture of ways of deciding how to respond to verbal messages. At times of uncertainty when they are older it may be that they adopt similar strategies. They respond with those actions which they believe to be most probably correct according to their experiences up to that time. For instance, if asked to illustrate 'the fence jumps over the horse' they will move a toy horse to jump over a toy fence. Usually this response has ceased by the age of 5 (Strohner & Nelson, 1974). Otherwise, if still uncertain how to respond, they use 'local' personal rules based on the context of that moment to interpret a task, even apparently changing the meaning of words in immediately following tasks as the context changes (Donaldson & McGarrigle, 1974). These are similar to rationalisations. In addition children like to make the easiest possible movement in response to a verbal command. So if a child is holding a red brick and is asked to put it on top of a green one, that task will be completed successfully more often than if he is asked to put the green on top of the red (Huttenlocher, Eisenberg & Strauss, 1968). These predispositions need to be included in an analysis of children's accounts of what constitutes their world of illness, as does an awareness of the forms of uncertainty prevailing for them. These processes will affect their performance when faced with questions concerning their health or discomforts.

The rate of development as regards word use varies. First-born children speak earlier, twins later, and girls develop their use of language more quickly than boys. Although the last difference has been attributed to inherent differences between the sexes, it is possible to view it as a product of the different ways care-givers communicate with children. Mothers speak more to their girls than to their boys (Moss, 1967).

The mother's personality is associated with different patterns of responding to her children and this has lasting effects (Trevarthen & Marwick, 1982). Parents also develop expectations whilst the fetus is *in utero* of how the child's personality will turn out, and these are surprisingly durable after the birth (Zeanah *et al.*, 1985). These observations emphasise that parental state and expectations from the time of conception, and most probably prior to that, can influence the form of communication which develops with the child, and hence his language and grammar for conveying his discomforts. (As yet the equivalent expectations of adoptive parents have not been researched and so interpretation of the results presented later (pp. 190–192) concerning adopted children must be interpreted with caution. Presumably the expectations of many adoptive parents are built up on the often scanty information they have received about the biological parents.)

The first words of children are signals rather than symbols. They are interpreted by the child in relation to his local knowledge of the language, his assessment of what the speaker intends, and how he understands the physical situation in which he has received the message (Donaldson, 1978). Gradually this slightly idiosyncratic interpretation of words gives way to the development of words as universals. 'Sickness' shifts from a family-based meaning to a larger social meaning. Words become abstract objects divorced from the personal relationships within which they were first understood (Piaget, 1926). It is at this stage of universals that 'egopsychology' comes into its own. Words then gain some of the properties of a child's play object; they become as it were objects with which the child plays and experiments (Cazden, 1973). Further they are chosen and put together with appropriate gestures to enable the child to adopt the roles of others, and to explore what it is like to act as though you were someone else. Taken together with blossoming creative propensities in play, the child's expressive skills are becoming refined. His ways of accounting for how he is become more diverse, and he begins to develop the skills necessary to account for why he sometimes does not function optimally, such as when ill. In addition, the possibilities for deceit arise and the parental strategies for finding out whether their child's messages are warranted must be refined.

It appears to be because of the emphasis which adults give to words, especially in schools, that children soon begin to concentrate more on verbal messages than gestures. Many symbols, as conveyed in words, are universal for particular cultures (macrosystems), but some variation arises from the particular family myths to which children are inevitably exposed and which often remain unrecognised as such. The myths of fairy tales are moderately universal and they illustrate some of the symbols children are introduced to (Bettelheim, 1976). Illness is a common theme in these stories around which myths are woven. Unfortunately in our scientific age the recognition of myths has sometimes led people to try and 'remove' them, rather than accept them as necessary organising constructs which facilitate a form of social order.

## Play

An understanding of play is essential for anyone communicating with children because that person is continually confronted with problems of knowing what meaning and value to attribute to messages from the child. The problems are the same for parents trying to understand their sick child and the researcher trying to elicit the child's facts about the world of illness.

Piaget (1946) viewed play as providing the meanings for symbols. This accords with the earlier portrayal of how words gain their meaning. Just as the child has a wish to play and make sense of the world, so he grasps powerfully after 'meaning'. Play has at times been thought of as frivolous, at others as children's 'work'. It must not be regarded as so important that it is converted into some serious and ponderous activity in which intuitive timing and fun are lost. Most children have none of these essentially moral dilemmas about play and just busy themselves with it, fluently expressing their interests and values of the moment without having to account for their actions using the moral value system of their elders.

Because of the way in which play situations can be defined by the use of metalevel signals it is possible for the child to interact in such situations without a sense of being judged, blamed or having to get it right. Nevertheless the metalevel signals of play can only be registered as truthful if the child's anxiety is sufficiently low for him to cease being preoccupied with minimising those anxieties. High anxiety often characterises the states of both children and their parents when coming for a medical consultation. It is not that the consultation should be directed at enabling children to play, but that during the appointment there needs to be an absence of a judgemental or blaming quality, which means that the consultation relationship shares some of the characteristics as a play relationship. The 'moral order' of the consultation needs to have some of the same qualities as those found in play.

Children's anxieties need to be taken care of before their communicative competences, which can usefully be built on in a consultation, can be maximised. Maximal learning has been shown to occur in the play situation of social interaction with the child's care-giver even prior to the development of language (Papousek & Papousek, 1983). An emphasis on verbal communication can make it more difficult to gain the engagement of children (Dare & Lindsey, 1979) and so the non-verbal basis to the development of children's communication must always be borne in mind.

Play is a world of metaphor. Gradually, however, the 'as if' quality of play can be lost and a new adaptation to reality fostered as the metaphor becomes one which is 'real'.

## Learning from problems

The old adage that we learn from our mistakes can be extended to include the observation that we learn more from them than from doing things correctly. This applies equally to children and the adults who have dealings with them. Children develop their communicative skills in those situations where the forms of response they get are different from those that they would otherwise have expected. The same applies to psychologists who have looked at the developing child's skills: more is learnt from refuting a hypothesis than finding more evidence which agrees with it (although the latter increases the strength of conviction with which that hypothesis can be held).

In order to study the importance of the contingency of adults' responses to the infant's initiatives Tatam (1974) carried out experiments to disrupt these using time delay in a video feedback loop. This produced marked problems with severe distress for the infants and their mothers. These observations are not dissonant with Seligman's learned helplessness model, which has been developed and modified for the human situation (Abramson, Seligman & Teasdale, 1978). In brief the thesis is that regular non-contingent responding results in a long-term effect characterised by helplessness which has many of the characteristics of depression. Perhaps a more descriptive term could be hopelessness. In such situations it is then very laborious to restore that important sense of personal effectiveness. This is one of the factors which is seen as being necessary for children to be able to act as though they have a sense of their personal 'agency' or self-efficacy (Bandura, 1977) – a state required in order for people to take responsibility for their own bodies (see Harré, 1983, for further discussion of 'agency').

Non-contingent responding may result from a variety of factors; the possibilities of it happening in puerperal depression have already been mentioned. It is hypothesised that this non-contingent responding could lead to diminished communicative competences in the child as a result of learned helplessness.

All factors which affect language development can be expected to influence the vocabulary children have available and how they use it when communicating their states of discomfort. Additional factors appeared in a survey of 3-year-olds who were followed up until they were 8 years old (Richman, Stevenson & Graham, 1982). A delay in language development was found for those 3-year-olds who came from families characterised by low maternal warmth, family tension, and with financial and housing problems. These children additionally showed pre-school behaviour problems. These factors point to roles for macrosystem, exosystem and microsystem effects in shaping children's communicative competences. Maybe it will turn out to be these factors, acting to minimise people's sense of personal efficacy, which contributed to the phenomenon described by Koos (1954) whereby those lower down the socioeconomic scale were seen as expressing increasing indifference to their symptoms of ill-health.

There is a well-established association between boys' problems with language and disorders of conduct. Rather tongue in cheek it is possible to describe conduct disorders – socially problematic behaviour – as potentially leading to 'learning from problems' in a non-verbal way rather than through verbal discussion. Verbal discussion would be unlikely to be so suitable a method of expression for these children because of their associated language problems. Nevertheless not all language problems are due to problems in responsiveness between child and care-givers. Physical factors in the child affect the child's ability to 'dance' with his mother (Trevarthen, 1985). Wolff *et al.* (1982) have shown an excess of minor signs of neurological dysfunction in their group of boys with combined language and conduct disorders. It was additionally found that the boys' neurological status predicted their language performance. It is natural to expect a variety of physical factors in both the child and adult to affect communication at all the different levels and phases mentioned so far, although at present these are poorly identified.

Although being aggressive is a very natural response, we nevertheless tend to regard the elicitation of an aggressive response as indicating that there are problems in our interactions with another. When showing our aggression to others we convey a very special message about our state of arousal. At the same time people interpret the origins of that type of response differently, and it has been shown that the nature of these expectations about the origins of that type of behaviour in children are often erroneous (Manning, Heron & Marshall, 1978; Manning & Hermann, 1981). Teachers' interpretation of aggressive behaviour in children was that they 'got away with murder at home', while the more demanding children were felt to get everything done for them at home. The children and teachers seemed stuck in their respective ways of accounting for the responses that were repeatedly being elicited. Their attributions of intention in the children were erroneous. The aggressive children were at the bottom, not the top, of the power hierarchy at home. Another sibling seemed to be preferred in the families of the demanding children. Our expectations can thus hinder us from learning from problematic episodes.

This work reminds us, that is parents, doctors and researchers, of the need to respect the mesosystem – the system whereby the worlds of school and family meet – so that realistic expectations and interpretations can be formed. If the teachers had had the benefits of a more constructive set of relationships in the mesosytem they might have used alternative ways of accounting for the children's behaviour, such as that the aggressive child had to prove that he was independent of people, and the demanding child to prove that he was lovable. In order to interpret forms of emotional response elicited when talking about illness, it is therefore clearly necessary to meet children in their different microsystems as well as to hear how these communicate with each other. Additionally it can be hypothesised that anything which would be likely to change hierarchies or attachment behaviour at home would affect both aggressive and dependency behaviour in the school or nursery. The state of illness is one such important influence. It is as well to underline here that this phenomenon of markedly different behaviour at home and school is widespread (see for example Rutter & Graham (1966) for 'disordered' behaviour), and it is to be expected provisionally that illness behaviour will differ similarly.

### The setting

So far I have placed emphasis on the forms of interaction with children and how these can lead to communicative competence and the sharing of meaning. I now wish to turn to the settings in which this development is taking place to see whether there are pointers to be observed when setting up research interviews with children, or factors to note which could help account for their views.

The fact that the micropsychological research reported here has been carried out largely within western cultures cannot immediately enable us to assume that the same developmental and communicative processes occur in other cultures. Trevarthen and colleagues' research on mother/infant interaction has been repeated in Lagos, Nigeria (Trevarthen & Marwick, 1982). The main differences they observed lay in a greater emphasis on physical social play rather than play with objects. Nevertheless development interpreted as passing through the same phases from primary to secondary intersubjectivity was seen. The chief variant was the relative quantities of some of the elements.

The structures of children's microsystems are difficult to define as there are a variety of ways of accounting for 'structure'. Here I want to consider the physical properties. These can affect the form of interaction with research subjects and how they come to construe the research situation. In this process children make assumptions about the value system required for accounting for their actions which then naturally affects the form of their response. Similar evaluations occur when children attend doctors' surgeries. It must not be forgotten that interviewing in children's homes and schools sets up expectation sets in the interviewer such that his objectivity is subject to bias. Some of the factors involved have been reviewed by Cline (1985); they can include seating arrangements, comfort of the seats, distance between different groups of seats and how space is divided up.

The above represent some of the microstructural details, whereas the grosser differences between the important constituents of school and home environments have been researched in more detail. For children the school rules which set limits for their interactions with other pupils are closely linked to the physical structure of the school buildings. Certain building structures, for example, 'imply' certain safety rules. The different settings of school classroom, playground and home are associated with very different forms of communication with children. These differences are exaggerated by social class differences (Tizard & Hughes, 1984).

No standard relationship is noted between how children talk at home and at school, so a researcher cannot deduce from seeing a child in one setting how he might be able to communicate in the other. In order to maximise the information obtained from the children in my sample all of them were seen both at home and at school. Provisionally it can be assumed that information which children might convey about their illness states will differ according to whether they are seen at home, school or in hospital – but any clear pattern to the nature of these differences is unlikely to be found.

One additional important result from the research of Tizard & Hughes

(1984) into the differences between home and school focussed on how the way in which questions were asked of children affected the elaboration of their replies. These observations have clear implications for an enquiry into children's views. The least productive questions were those asked by the teachers as a form of 'testing' to see whether the child knew something. These only became interesting if presented as part of an organised game with the child. The staff who asked most questions in nursery schools received the least elaborate answers from the children and were themselves asked the fewest questions by the children (Wood, McMahon & Cranston, 1980). The children's curiosity was most obvious at home, where the moral order of that environment was more facilitating. These observations will be considered again when looking at the consultation process in chapter 9. Again the researcher faces a paradoxical problem, for in order to be effective in eliciting the children's views he is dissuaded from asking directly about them. This dilemma is shared especially by the teachers and possibly to a lesser degree by the parents, by virtue of the differing moral orders inherent in the different situations. There appears to be the foundation here for a criticism of studies of children based on questionnaires, as they will reveal minimal information relative to the children's total views.

The moral order found in the playground is different yet again. The form of communication developed here reflects yet other value systems. These have not always been the same as they are today. A school inspector's report from 1840 in Scotland (Paterson, 1986) makes clear some of the origins of the thinking developed by the authorities in relation to the placing of schools:

> Spatially, one way of securing a school's exemplary status as a purveyor of a healthy and morally correct way of life, as well as ensuring its accessibility to the population, was the stipulation by the Minutes that the school had to be in a central location which was free from the dangers of moral and physical pollution.

We shall have cause to return to this value system, based on what was then regarded as pollution, in establishing the moral order for the setting for education. They went on to say about playgrounds that:

> in the absence of a school playground, the street becomes the resort of the children after school hours, . . . they meet with vicious men and women, and with children of their own age, who have been corrupted by vicious parents, or other bad example, or even children trained to desperate courses by thieves.

Although the aim was for the extension of the moral order of the classroom into the playground, there is no evidence that this was successful. Thus for a long time there has been recognition of the effects of establishing particular moral orders, as these influence value systems about the nature of what is healthy or dangerous. It is this structure which will be seen later to play a role in setting up particular forms of dialogue for accounting for 'illness' states and hence to exert an influence on the child's world of illness.

It is noteworthy that the rules evolved in the playground today nevertheless appear to prepare children for the adult culture in which they are growing up, as amongst other things they learn similar kinds of negotiating skills (Sluckin, 1981). It then becomes important to be aware of the playground games which can have an impact on children's developing views on illness. The languages of these games introduce them to ways of accounting for their states in situations outside the playground. The moral values of their play with illness themes are transferred to their interactions with the adults in their microsystems.

## Children's games

British children's games have been catalogued by the Opies (Opie & Opie, 1969). One of the important illness themes in games is the nature of the transfer of 'it', and ways of preventing 'it' having any influence on you. It is asking too much immediately to equate the concepts involved with what adults understand by contagion, but the rules of games such as 'Hospital Touch', 'Body Tick', 'Flea Bite', 'Doctor Touch', 'French Touch' and 'Dreaded Lurgy' (*op. cit.* p. 75) provide clear models for the transmission of something undesirable, and the names illustrate the links which children make with the world of illness. These games and other variants also introduce children to the idea of there possibly being things they can do to protect themselves. For example children write 'PAL' (Protection Against Lurgy) on the skin to prevent the 'Dreaded Lurgy' being passed on to them by touch. Another strategy is to remain in a safe territory in the playground, adopt a safe posture, or touch something protective, as for example in 'Touchwood', 'Off-ground He' and 'Tom Tiddler's Ground' (*op. cit.* pp. 78, 81 and 84). In some games no preventive strategies are allowed; these very clearly have names associated with illness, such as 'Germs', 'The Plague', 'Fever' and 'Lodgers' (in the last the person who is 'it' 'lodges' fleas) (*op. cit.* p. 77). The particular forms of dialogue developed in games are important for the development of the skills of negotiation. An interesting perspective would be gained by comparing in different cultures the form of 'contagion' games and the nature of the protective strategies allowed. I would provisionally expect that the rules revealed in these games would be coherent with the ways in which illness states are viewed in that society.

Through knowing the child's world from the child's perspective his system of meanings becomes clearer and communication is fostered. Having presented sufficient background on these communication aspects to facilitate understanding of how children develop their chosen points of view, and how they come to be left with particular illness vocabularies and grammars, I will now briefly describe how this view of communication with young children led to the particular research approach I adopted.

### From forms of dialogue to a research method

At various points in the preceding presentation of research into the form of developing communication the conditions required for successful interaction have been highlighted. At times the difficulties presented can be experienced as almost paradoxical, such as the need to interact spontaneously and at the same time to be aware of the effects of one's interventions/responses. An interactive process has been described which is influenced by the respective states and communicative competences of all family members. It is also dependent on the setting and especially on what is perceived to be the moral order of that setting. What happens early on in this developmental process is felt to influence that which comes later, but not in any regular fashion as there are so many variables which play their part. The process can be seen as one of coevolution in which the family system evolves in parallel with the development of the child, and in conjunction with the development of the child's relations with other important people in his world such as school teachers. Emphasis has been laid on the role of decision-making rules which reflect the value systems of those who use them in introducing the child to the value systems of his caregivers. In this process the ways in which the child is handled come to present him with ways of understanding his world and accounting for his various states, be these states of illness, naughtiness or health. (We need to note that one is seldom called upon to account for a state of health unless the prevailing local norm is temporarily illness.) As the child accounts for his behaviour he adopts that system of values which is deduced to be most coherent with the moral order of the group to whom he is accounting for his behaviour in that particular setting.

In order to find out the nature of the child's world of illness one is not free simply to ask about it. It is not morally neutral to ask questions, and as we have seen questions can be singularly unproductive in eliciting information from children. Story-telling time is most productive for eliciting children's curiosity – a technique long used in teaching.

To take account of these observations a superficially unorthodox approach must be adopted, but one that has much in common with the ethogenic approach described by Harré (1977, 1979). The research method I adopted will be described briefly in order to explain how I obtained my observations (for a fuller description see Wilkinson, 1984). There are pointers here to consultation techniques, as well as to understanding the difficulties faced by parents when deciding whether their child is ill. I do not wish to suggest that the details of my research method should be repeated in other settings, but rather that some of the principles can be used for eliciting as nearly as possible children's ideal communicative competences. Both these topics will be discussed further in subsequent chapters.

The requirements for obtaining as much information from the children as possible were that they felt at ease with me and that I established a relationship in which they wished to share their knowledge. I needed to maximise their communicative competences and so approach as near as possible to an 'ideal speech act'. It is to these elements of the research process that psychotherapeutic skills (here distinguished from theory) are directed, skills which become necessary in order to maximise the sharing of information in consultations generally. The aim was to find out the maximal range of the children's views, not to investigate what proportion held particular views or how tenaciously they held them. The children were not preoccupied with the stresses of a current illness, but could instead elaborate their views as they had developed over the years.

At the same time, to be able to interpret this information it was necessary to see the children in some of their different worlds in order to have knowledge about the decision-making in these different places and how the different places shared knowledge about the children's illness state – i.e. how the mesosystem functioned in relation to illness/health themes. The 'worlds' chosen were home and nursery school or school. At the same time children were seen from pairs of schools at each age as their views are dependent on the ways curricula are tackled (Williams, 1977). In this way a picture of the child's world of illness and how it is constructed can be created, based upon an understanding of the communication processes necessary to develop a language for conveying states of discomfort.

The techniques required for facilitating communication with children of different ages will of necessity differ, and at the same time details must be modified for each child so that the 'dance' can be both established and maintained. The stages to my enquiry and the methods used are outlined below.

### Nursery school sample

I saw eight children (four boys and four girls) from each of two Education Department nurseries in Edinburgh, Scotland. The age range at the time of the end of my contact with the children was 3 years 1 month to 5 years (mean 4 years 2 months). The children were first acquainted with me as a regular visitor to the nursery before the study began. This was necessary because men who entered the nursery were approached by the children with the assumption that they must either be someone else's father or the local policeman, who occasionally visited without his uniform as part of his community relations exercise. These assumptions were very durable, and one girl thought I was another child's father for two months.

I subsequently saw the children twice in the nursery in same-sex and mixed-sex pairings largely of their own choice. I joined with the children in making up a story about a child who did not feel like getting up in the morning. The rest of the family downstairs were then discussing the child, trying to decide what 'might be up' with him or her. The details were constructed by the children and it was essential that each time some novel ingredients were included so that it became *their* story. Everytime the theme chosen by them was illness (and never malingering). These stories were tape-recorded and transcribed. In order to facilitate entry to the child's way of accounting to other children, the discussion was at times directed to getting the children to explain themselves to each other if there was anything unclear. In this form of enquiry the questioning used must not push too far towards the child's basic assumptions, because the engagement with the child in the interview is maintained through the belief that some part of his world and yours is shared; the 'taken for granted' world (Berger & Luckmann, 1966) can only be gently probed without threatening the basic engagement. This always puts some limit to the depth of enquiry possible.

In order to establish the seriousness with which the children held their views and to discriminate the serious views from those stated primarily to elicit reaction, I then played them back the tape-recordings and recorded them listening and spontaneously commenting on their earlier comments (a particularly difficult form of recording to transcribe).

Meetings were then held for each child together with all those living in the family home, in which the family decision-making rules concerning illness, past experiences of illness, accidents, acquaintance with 'health'/'illness' personnel etc. were explored. (For details of the themes see appendix 1.) A particular point was made of asking about 'half-ill' states, as these force people to account for their decision-making more clearly. The form of questioning of the family group was also arranged so as to maximise information about the family's way of accounting for things to each other, through requesting that each family member checked with the others that they understood what was meant. This also meant that the ways in which things were explained for 3–4-year-olds became clear. The method was similar to one described in greater detail for use in family therapy (Selvini-Palazzoli *et al.*, 1980a).

*Primary and secondary school children (age 8 and 13 years)*

The basic organisation of this part of my sample was the same as for the nursery school samples above. The younger children consisted of two randomly allocated groups each of four boys and four girls from two Edinburgh Education Department primary schools (age range 7 years 10 months to 8 years 10 months; mean 8 years 5 months). In order to establish the sense of genuine enquiry into their views in a way which also left them feeling supported I saw them initially in groups of eight at school (see appendix 2 for themes covered in these group discussions). The aim of these group discussions was again to facilitate explanation and accounting by child to child rather than by child to me. After a series of such meetings with the children I saw them individually. Story-telling was not appropriate for this age group and instead the open-ended questionnaire which they had filled out individually at the end of one of the group meetings (see appendix 3) was used. Its aim was both to provide a provisional picture of their world of illness and to act as a focus for a discussion in which the child accounted for the views he had put forward. In addition one task not so dependent on words was used (Wilkinson, 1985). In principle this was a development of *Kinetic Family Drawings* (Burns & Kaufmann, 1971) in which one drawing of the child's family is compared with another in which a family member is ill. In both drawings all family members must be portrayed doing something. This task facilitated entry to the child's world of illness without words being so important for establishing contact.

The subsequent family interviews followed a similar form to that used with the nursery school sample. Throughout the study all group, family and individual meetings were tape-recorded and transcribed.

The parents of four 8-year-old girls from one school refused permission for their daughters to participate, as did the parents of one girl from the other school. None of the parents of the boys refused. Although I did not explore this in detail, the reasons given by the parents suggested a wish on their part to protect their daughters from having to discuss illness.

The basic form of the secondary school sample was similar again: two groups, two schools and a total of 16 children (age range 12 years 11 months to 13 years 10 months; mean 13 years 5 months). Similar group and open-ended questionnaire strategies were used. Appendix 3 identifies the questions brought in additionally for this age group. The drawing task and family interviews followed the same form to that used with the 8-year olds.

My methods of approaching the children, and establishing relationships with them, their teachers and families, were aimed at maximising the information obtained yet at the same time checking its validity. The collective picture to emerge from the discussions in pairs (nursery schools) and groups (primary and secondary schools) represented more than the sum of individual points of view. The children's worlds of illness necessarily evolved throughout my enquiry.

It was not possible to make links between the children's different ways of accounting for their states and their subsequent illness behaviour, or ways parents and teachers allocated the sick role to the children. The physical concomitants of the varying disease processes encountered in childhood would be expected to limit the children's illness 'vocabularies' in varying ways and to varying degrees. In the same manner the changing states of the parents will alter their perceptive skills when noting their child's 'messages', as well as their cognitive sets which will mould their conceptualisations of the child's condition based on those messages. Further exploration of these even more complicated issues awaits future research.

# 3

# What has gone before: some
# background information

In the preceding chapter I presented a brief overview of the development
of a child's capacities for dialogue and the communicative competences
which appear to be the basis for this. The form of dialogue we establish
sets the limits to the sort of information we can obtain, be that in a
consultation, research or finding out whether our children are ill. The
complementary aspect of dialogue is its content, and it is this that I will
concentrate on here. In the previous chapter the developmental model
proposed was one of coevolution of the child and the systems within which
he develops. It is a similar relationship which I believe exists between the
form of a dialogue and its content. Certain views can only be presented
in certain fora. The moral orders of different settings facilitate the presentation of some types of information and hinder others. The content also
plays its part in signalling what sort of moral order pertains, as does the
form of dialogue used. Thus caution is necessary in interpreting the research
presented here on what is known about children's views on illness, as the
settings in which these views are elicited were seldom analysed at the same
time.

I have used the phrase 'some background information' in the chapter
title because I want to point out some additional similarities between the
positions of the researcher, parent and doctor in a consultation. All of us
approach a new situation with a degree of uncertainty which we try and
minimise through applying as much 'background information' as possible.
It is our background which leads us necessarily to approach a new situation
with a range of expectations about what is likely to happen. The totally
strange situation where no assumptions can be brought to bear is extremely
threatening. I am here presenting the background information I had when
I started to explore the child's world of illness.

The dominant framework for research into children's views has been
that of Piaget, but the usefulness of results obtained using his framework
is questionable on the basis of what is now known about the development
of dialogue (see previous chapter). It is necessary to record the conceptual
framework used because it will have played its part in creating the data

analysed. Where these concepts are coherent with the others I introduce here from sociology and medical anthropology I adhere to them for the further analysis of children's accounts. The categories chosen for analysis of the children's accounts reflect the values found elsewhere in the culture as potential accounting variables which are intelligible and potentially warranted. The ways in which childhood is conceptualised affect what is permitted here (Ariès, 1960).

The validity of our background information is something which should always concern us. It seems a human tendency to treat as general facts things which are in fact dependent on their particular social context for their replicability, without acknowledging that limit. Bronfenbrenner (1979) provides a language for describing different forms of validity which will be of help later when looking at how we clarify the nature of our observations and, especially, evaluate research which has not always accounted for these different forms of validity:

> *Ecological validity* refers to the extent to which the environment experienced by the subjects in a scientific investigation has the properties it is supposed or assumed to have by the investigator (*op. cit.*, p. 29). This is recognised to be an ideal goal to be 'pursued, approached, but never achieved'.
>
> *Phenomenological validity* is 'the correspondence between the subject's and the investigator's view of the research situation' (*op. cit.*, p. 33).
>
> *Developmental validity* has the following criteria: 'To demonstrate that human development has occurred, it is necessary to establish that a change produced in the person's conceptions and/or activities carries over to other settings and other times' (*op. cit.*, p. 35).

These concepts need to be borne in mind when considering the implications of the research I will recount below. It is also possible for the reader to 'translate' the terms to ones which all parents struggle with when trying to work out the relevance of the messages they are getting from their sick children, especially when the messages apparently differ from those given to others outside the intimate family.

## The pragmatic and the mathetic

Before proceeding further to the adult and the child's world of illness there is one last link in the developmental process which I will present here. The problem which I have so far avoided is how children begin to signal that their communication is not just to maintain the interactional 'dance' within which they were learning about meaning, but is directed to the establishment of the factual nature of things – the mathetic (see below). The responses of adults to the infant's actions sets the effectiveness of those actions for eliciting particular responses. The child grows up with the experience that his behaviour, including his language, is functional in the sense of affecting personal interactions. Following on from this first phase which I had mentioned earlier, the child then begins to discriminate between two different types of function to communication.

Halliday (1975) showed how at about 19 months an infant could initiate interactions in two different ways depending on which of two response forms he was wanting. The infant did this through using two different tonal patterns: a rising tone was associated with utterances which were instrumental or regulatory in function, whereas a falling tone was used for all those that were personal or heuristic, i.e. those which did not necessarily require a response from another person (*op. cit.* p. 53). Our voice patterns potentially reveal which sort of function is our current priority. For adults these two functional components of speech, usually here termed the interpersonal and the ideational, can be present in every utterance at the same time. The clues to our adult priorities have become lost as our tonal patterns have become mixed. For children of about 2 years old it appears that utterances are concretely either one or the other, and hence Halliday felt it appropriate to use different words to describe these functions. The function analogous to the interpersonal he termed the pragmatic and the one analogous to the ideational he called the mathetic. The pragmatic is associated with the processes of human interaction, the mathetic with the content. I will refer further to these distinctions later.

The ways in which these two elements of the language are intertwined are well summarised by Halliday:

> Since they [the ideational and interpersonal components of the semantic system] are not just aspects of the use of language, but are at the basis of the system itself, every actual instance of linguistic interaction has meaning not only in particular but also in general, as an expression of the social system and of the child's place in it – in other words it is related to the context of culture as well as to the context of the situation. This explains how in the course of learning language a child is also all the time learning *through* language; how the microsemiotic exchanges of family and peer group life contain within themselves indices of the most pervasive semiotic patterns of the culture. (*op. cit.* pp. 80–1)

It is noteworthy that a dilemma in research is how to approach the child's views in line with his mathetic use of language. The problem is how to maintain the engagement with the child using adult interpersonal uses of language whilst at the same time facilitating the complementary function of language. It is likely that a more refined analysis of voice patterns will help to discriminate between these different forms of message so that more reliable research methods can be developed. At present adults interacting with children must rely on intuition to help with the discrimination.

At about the age of 2 years children are also developing their sense of self (Kagan, 1982). They are able to stand 'apart' from the interactions and begin to view themselves as though they were objects to themselves, i.e. to be reflective (see also fig. 9.1, p. 235). This enables the child to view his words and what he means by them in isolation from the individual interaction he is involved in. He has acquired the capacity to reflect on things, including his body states such as in illness. He must have a sense of self before he can distinguish his illness states. He has moved on from primary intersubjectivity to secondary intersubjectivity (Trevarthen, 1980).

This distinction between the pragmatic and the mathetic is particularly helpful for an analysis of children's views on illness, because it highlights two components to the development of their views. They are likely to develop a language for complaining about their discomforts based on the effectiveness of that language in altering their relation with another, whereas their knowledge about illness and the nature of discomforts can come to be expressed in a different language with a different grammar. Giving people more information about illnesses is not associated with them altering their ways of managing their illness (see chapter 9).

The 'causes' of illness have a very special place in how people come to construe their illness because 'causes' are integral to notions of functional relations. There will be causal explanations which are associated with pragmatic/interpersonal factors and those associated with the mathetic/ideational. The nature of these associations will reflect the ways in which the different sorts of message have been recognised and differentially responded to by the children's care-givers. Causes are important in linking disease models to illness models and so are particularly important in communication between professionals, who are said to use a predominantly disease model, and lay people, who tend to use an illness model (see below). Illness is experienced whereas disease is observed.

At present it is only necessary to note the above distinctions, which I will be returning to when interpreting the likely modes of development of children's views on illness. At the same time I note that there is a specific developmental change which has occurred between the first two age groups in my sample. When children are about 6 years old they begin to appreciate that messages can simultaneously have more than one meaning.

## Sickness, illness and disease

Most readers are probably aware of the distincion that has been created between illness and disease by researchers in this field, but for clarity I will analyse some elements of it here. Some languages have only one word for sickness, illness and disease – for example '*sykdom*' in Norwegian – which emphasises that it is researchers' needs which have subdivided the meanings rather than social usage.

Social construction of part of the concept of illness (see below) seems to be agreed, but some people attribute a power to define illness to particular groups in society. There have been some sociologists (for examples see Wright & Treacher, 1982) who have seen illness roles as being defined by health professionals, and believe that this has come to be a means of controlling the people by a professional elite, especially in the United States (Freidson, 1970). Those viewpoints minimise the importance of physical and psychological states of the individual, ignoring 'hypothesised' pathology of the individual (disease states), and emphasise the influence of powerful social groups for deciding the norms of health. In this sense they are describing rather *sickness*, the social dimension to the illness experience which Twaddle (1981) defines as 'the ability to meet obligations of group living. It is the result of being defined by others as "unhealthy". It generally results from having one's failure to meet social obligations defined by others as the result of disease or illness'. Not everyone discriminates sickness from illness and disease, but joining Twaddle in using sickness for the social dimension attached to a special 'person–illness' unit enables the separation of the social, psychological and physiological aspects to the processes underlying 'discomforts'. It must be noted, though, that this specific use of sickness does not necessarily correspond to popular use but is one encouraged by Berkanovic's (1972) analysis of the sick role which highlighted the ways it differed from illness behaviour.

Within the medical profession the distinction between illness and disease has assumed greater significance (Campbell, Scadding & Roberts, 1979). I will here follow the distinction of Feinstein (1967, pp. 24f). I use illness to describe the sum of the clinical manifestations of a disease. Illness is separate from disease as it does not include the internal pathology observ-

able by microbiologists, biochemists and pathologists, but limits itself to
the clinical state including the elements of subjective discomfort. These
are the aspects of disease which can be communicated to others by the
patient, or observed by untrained others. Illness is closer to dis-ease than
disease in the way I use the terms here. The subjective distress and the
significance of dis-ease signs will be moulded through the responses of
others around the ill person, minimising or elaborating the complaint;
hence this usage incorporates some degrees of social construction of the
concept of illness. It does not produce an absolute definition of illness but
points out the way in which '*illness* is the way the sick person, his family,
and his social network perceive, label, explain, valuate, and respond to
disease' (Kleinman, 1978).

Symptoms are central to illness and usually come to be negotiated with
others as the ill person reacts to change in his state. The meaning of the
symptoms rises from a dialectic between the current negotiations and the
individual's previous experience of negotiating his states of discomfort
with important others. It is to this negotiation that the child turns the
communicative competences at his disposal at different phases of development. How far he gets in this negotiation will depend on the degree to
which it assumes the properties of an 'ideal speech act'.

The distinction between pragmatic and mathetic can be used to suggest
that the relation between illness and disease involves a similar difference.
If illness and disease become confused it can lead to the state of affairs
described by Friedson (1970), but by just having the one word (*sykdom*)
available does not mean that Norwegians, amongst others, confuse the
different usages. It is necessary, therefore, to look more closely at the
relationship between states of illness and disease in order to understand
the nature of the arguments put forward by some sociologists. The developmental perspective allows one to see how this lack of clarity arises and this
will be presented in chapters 4–7.

Logically it should be possible to present clarification of what people
understand by health beside the above, but this has proved a more difficult
task. The discussion of these issues has been ably reviewed and comprehensively integrated by Stacey (1980). Suffice it to say at present that discussion
focuses on both state definitions such as that used by the World Health
Organization ('Health is a state of complete physical, mental and social
well-being, not merely the absence of disease or infirmity' – or the more
natural modification suggested by Gillon (1986) of 'adequate or sufficient . . . well-being' instead of 'complete . . . well-being') and the definition of health as a 'relationship' (Jago, 1975) i.e. emphasising the dynamic

intersubjective element in the social. Again the potential value of the mathetic/pragmatic distinction which relates to the state-fact and dynamic-interactional qualities recurs.

## The adult world of illness and its causality

The views of adults on illness need to be considered for their part in setting up the framework as well as for the models of causality they introduce to the children and towards which the children's views are socialised. Nevertheless it has already been seen that the correspondence between these worlds is imperfect. There appears to be no research describing how adults account for illness and its causes to children in order to cast direct light on the forms of the associations between the views of the adults in a culture and their children. Instead the concepts which appear to be widespread in the adult worlds must first be differentiated before looking further at the ways in which they are reflected in the worlds of the children.

Because I am here looking for concepts rather than examining data, we need to be aware that we choose the concepts for their potential to organise the data – for their explanatory power. This is exactly the same sort of process carried out by lay people (and described by Blaxter (1983) for middle-aged working class women in Aberdeen) when they try to make sense of all that has happened to them. They are extracting representations useful in accounting for both the child's and the adult's world of illness, just as researchers and consultants must also do.

*Exogenous and endogenous causes: external and internal loci of control*

In the Western world the majority of causes of illness appear to be attributed by lay people to things outside the self, such as germs. These are termed exogenous causes and form part of the 'germ theory' of illness. There is a gradual increase in another theory, the 'immune theory' which as presently formulated in lay terms also seems to avoid any imputing of responsibility for the immune response to the agency of the self. In contrast in other areas of the world endogenous causes predominate. An example of the latter would be 'theft of one's soul' in Mid-Asia. It may appear confusing to a Westerner to describe this as an endogenous cause because he would typically ask the question 'Who stole it?'; in this way the framework is converted to one with which he is more familiar. In contrast the most important aspect for the individual in that culture is that *he* lost a part of himself. Clearly the form of questioning is able to convert one model to the other and vice versa. The meaning of the cause is not sufficient to enable one to say from which type of culture it comes unless it is linked to the individual's understanding of his position in that culture at the same time. It has been suggested that the Western tendency to emphasise exogenous causes arises from a desire to attribute good things to the self and bad things to factors outside the self (Heider, 1958; Farr, 1977). Similarly 'Everything friendly is initially referred to the "me"; everything hostile to the alien "not me"' (Becker, 1971, p. 31).

It is possible that what is being recounted here is an end point in socialisation, as Gottschalk (1976) has shown how 'overt hostility outwards', attributing the bad to the other, is more the position of the adult than the child in the United States. More specifically in connection with views about the causes of illness the 'references to the weather being bad, dangerous, unpleasant, or otherwise negative . . . increased with grade'.

In case it should be felt that these non-Western endogenous models have no special importance for us, I will here quote from the Dundee Courier (Scotland) of 5 March 1983, where the dialogue reported in dialect illustrates the ways in which we may facilitate an 'endogenous' model:

> 'Eh think eh'm takin' the measles; ach it's nothin' – Eh took the measles afore, aince'. 'Ye dinna get tae tak the measles again, stupit!' 'Eh'll tak the measles again if eh like, an' you shut up. Anyway it wuz mibby the chicken-pox, an' you never took that, did ye, hah!' 'Ah, but eh took the mumps, though, an hoo did you no', like meh cousins an' a'body?' At which the wee sister complains, 'Hoo dae eh never get tae tak' nothin'?' 'Ach you took a sair belly on Sunday, didn't ye?' 'But eh never wahnted that! An' ye wudna even gie me the mumps, but a'body else, though!' At which Mum seems to come to a decision to accept symptoms of her own – 'Eh'm takin' an affy headache wi' you's anes' cerry-on!'

Blaxter's (1983) research from further up the Scottish coast at Aberdeen also refers to the widespread use of the term 'taking' an illness in that community.

Herzlich (1973) used the two categories, exogenous and endogenous, extensively when she examined French urban and rural adult views on illness. She recognised an inherent difficulty in their use because clearly an individual has a part to play in creating the world in which he lives and vice versa. Aside from this paradox, the resolution of which appears to require the abolition of the two categories as independent, it is useful to use these concepts as people do appear to vary in the extent to which they perceive themselves as able to affect their environment or be affected by it. Exogenous causes were found to be most important in the groups who felt powerless in the face of their environment, either 'having to' live in the town or 'having to' live in the country. These groups came from the less educated sections of society who perceived their whole environment and way of life as unhealthy. They had few clear ideas about what it was in their environment that caused their illnesses apart from the lack of choice to alter the air they breathed, food they ate or place they lived in. They were also more susceptible to a variety of diseases (McKinlay, 1981). Their *way of life* was perceived as constraining and all illness arose from it (see Blaxter, 1983, for a similar view on the role of poverty). Pill & Stott (1985) found similar views on life style in Wales: 'The women in our sample could recognise the relevance of life style choices for illness prevention and still not hold any strong belief in the possiblity of their actions affecting outcome', being constrained by their life style, rather than in control of it.

By way of contrast, historically the way of life in Britain had been seen as a cause only of chronic illnesses, through personal activities such as too too much of the 'gratifying pleasures of smoking, over-eating, drunkenness, sloth and masturbation' (Taylor, 1979). Here way of life was associated with endogenous rather than exogenous factors. It is important to note a distinction between attributing illness to personal activities when these are your own compared with accounting for why others are afflicted. In the latter situation they are almost 'exogenous' causes because they lie outside the person doing the accounting for the affliction. A recent example of the same phenomenon is reported by Eiser, Patterson & Tripp (1984) for 11–13-year-olds in England. Significantly more of those who did not have diabetes attributed the cause of diabetes to eating too much sugar, whereas the diabetic children were more likely than healthy children to believe that diabetes 'just happens'. Chance happens to us, others are negligent – a conclusion in line with Blaxter's observations.

The degrees to which people feel that they can control their environment or feel controlled by it, have been approached by psychologists using the framework of 'locus of control'. If people feel able to master many aspects of their environment, they are said to have an internal locus of control. Alternatively if the environment controls the person he is described as having an external locus of control. This framework provides a bridge between the adults' concepts of illness explored by Herzlich and some work done with children.

It has been shown that children with a more pronounced internal locus of control recognise more internal indicators of illness from the age of 8 years. They respond to more of the cues coming from inside their bodies

(Neuhauser *et al.*, 1978). This did not alter their expectations about the probability of becoming ill (Gochman, 1971*b*). It appears that the pattern of parental nurture at home alters the locus of control orientation in children (Levenson, 1973; Carlson, 1984). This picture could be explained by children having a strong sense of their own agency through effective pragmatic strategies for communication, whereas their knowledge of expectations is linked to the mathetic mode. The concepts of locus of control, learned helplessness and self-efficacy have many overlapping facets which make discrimination difficult, and clarity in what is being measured is often lacking.

I have already suggested that certain cultures foster expectations that the causes of illness will be predominantly either exogeneous or endogenous. At the same time individuals within a culture develop a range of loci of control. If adults reinforce the child's tentative attempts to master his own environment or identify his inner sensations, then the child is likely to develop an internal locus of control. It may be this effect that accounts for why people with a more pronounced internal locus of control show evidence of a greater desire to seek out health information (Wallston & Wallston, 1978). At the same time other life style factors, further education and active religious involvement (regardless of persuasion) have been found to be associated with increased behaviour consistent with an internal locus of control in a group of Welsh women; these factors could be mediating or facilitating the effect (Pill & Stott, 1985). In contrast, if the child's attempts at being effective in this way are negated by those around him he is likely to develop a sense of helplessness (Abramson *et al.*, 1978) and ultimately hopelessness. His sense of self-efficacy and mastery becomes severely impaired, although his searching for information, his mathetic motive, remains initially intact. This 'learned helplessness' model has been used to represent depression, and it is worth recording that exaggerated illness behaviour, associated perhaps with some of the premises of illness as a liberator (see below), has been regarded as one factor of importance for monitoring childhood depression (Kolvin, Berney & Bhate, 1984). What is clear is that health beliefs are enmeshed with the psychological dynamics of the person and that locus of control factors appear to play a mediating role (Harris, Linn & Pollack, 1984). Although the language is different these concepts are not new, being very similar to those developed much earlier by Adler (Lefcourt, 1966).

It appears as though the pairs of concepts of internal/external locus of control and endogenous/exogenous causality reflect similar phenomena occurring at the level of both the individual and the group. This provides for interplay between the two, so that if there is a change in the number of individuals with pronounced internal locus of control this will affect the cultural norm and vice versa.

As a development from these concepts Herzlich hypothesised three modes of being ill. Illness can be a *liberator* for those who feel constrained by what they perceive as the imposition of social rules in their environment, because it can come to free them from some of these expectations. For example 'A really serious illness is like a first love affair' is a statement from someone with an 'illness as a liberator' orientation. In contrast those who are very aware of their own role in actively creating and controlling their environment will find their ability to do this curtailed by illness and come to perceive illness as *destructive*. The third mode has been translated (from the French) as 'illness as an *occupation*'. In this state the ill person is not overwhelmed by either the advantages or disadvantages of illness but instead follows the approved social role of letting himself be ill and at the same time actively cooperating to get himself better. This third mode is mainly defined by the resulting sick role behaviour, whereas the first two leave others to deduce the expected form of sick role preferred and proferred – reflecting the dual direction of the forces in role creation (for further discussion of illness behaviour and the sick role as earlier constructed see Kasl & Cobb, 1966).

Williams (1981) has analysed the apparent premises to the states of 'illness as destroyer' and 'illness as an occupation' as described in Herzlich's work (1973 p. 105f and p. 119f), and I include these tables here (tables 3.1 and 3.2). They show the logical consequences of holding these premises which illustrate the nature of these forms of illness.

Comparisons can now be drawn to the situation of children who perceive themselves as controlled by their parents in such a way that they may find a liberating role through illness as it alters their parents' responses to them. Reduced punishment of the ill child within the family has been reported (Burton, 1975). In contrast other children may find the curtailment of their activities frustrating and see illness as destructive. We can for the moment imagine them becoming angry at their parents for limiting their activities and attributing the 'cause' of their illness to their parents as their discomforts reside in the frustrating nature of their parents' responses.

The way of life is seen as a *cause* of illness by most of those in Herzlich's sample, rather than as setting their level of *vulnerability* to illness. Although the frequency of this response could reflect the slight bourgeois bias in her sample (but see also Pill & Stott, 1985), it is the nature of the phenomenon rather than its origins I wish to highlight here. Vulnerability is conceptualised from the contrasting pole of their personal resistances to illness, following the predominant Western pattern of attributing the 'good' aspect of resistance to infection to the self. The individual's health arises predominantly endogenously, and is revealed through resistances to infection. Resistance to infection is not inevitable. Blaxter's (1983) working class sample thought rather that certain diseases ran in families and that one was born vulnerable.

It is useful to include here some of the views on health which Herzlich elicited, as these relate to the views on illness mentioned above. The simplest of these views was that health was the absence of illness. This can be interpreted as being based on an individual's predominant sense of an external locus of control, where temporarily the external influence of illness is not acting. It was this view of health that Blaxter & Paterson (1982a) described so succinctly for their working class mothers in Aberdeen

Table 3.1. *Logical representation of 'illness as destroyer' (after Williams, 1981)*

Each consequence depends on the premises (or on the consequences which in turn have become premises) which are numbered on its right-hand side

**General premises**
1   If I am active then I am not ill
2   If I am myself then I am active
3   I have something to offer if, and only if, I am active
4   If I do not have something to offer, then I can not repay help
5   If I accept help, either I repay help, or else I am a child
6   I need a medical diagnosis if, and only if, I am ill
7   I act ill if, and only if, I am ill
8   If 'I' am 'dead' then I have nothing to fear from death
9   If I have nothing to fear from death then the doctor can do as he likes

**Definition of the situation**
10   I am active

10   I am ill and I must accept or refuse help

**Consequences**
11   I do not need a medical diagnosis   10/1/6

11   I am not myself 'I' am 'dead'   10/1/2

12   I do not act ill   10/1/7

12   I do not have something to offer   10/1/3

13   I cannot repay help   10/12/4

14   I refuse help or I am a child   10/13/5

15   I have nothing to fear from death   10/11/8

26   The doctor can do what he likes   10/15/9

as 'being able to decline the role of "sickness"'. Health was essentially a moral category. 'Illness was . . . giving in to diseases' (Blaxter, 1983). The second of Herzlich's categories was one in which health was viewed as a capital asset, built up throughout childhood from that with which the child was endowed at birth. I relate this belief to the effect of having a predominant internal locus of control where the individual perceives himself as being responsible for building up this asset. Her third category was of health as a dynamic process whereby an individual feels himself to be in equilibrium with his environment. This view appears to represent a balance between the influences of an internal and an external locus, which mirrors my interpretation of the concept of 'illness as an occupation'.

As already mentioned the distinction between exogenous and endogenous causes of illness or resistance to illness is not absolute. In addition it is

Table 3.2. *Logical representation of 'illness as an occupation' (after Williams, 1981)*

Each consequence depends on the premises (or on the consequences which in turn have become premises) which are numbered on its right-hand side

**General premises**

1   If I am myself then I am active
2   I have something to offer if, and only if, I am active
3   If I do not have something to offer, I can not repay help
4   If I accept help, either I repay help, or else I am a child
5   If I am healthy then I am strong
6   If I am strong then I am active
7   If I am ill, I fight and fight well
8   If I fight well, I cut losses and develop any resources I can find
9   If I fight, I am active
10   If I do not demand explanations, I do not find out what I am fighting
11   If I do not find out what I am fighting I do not fight well

**Definition of the situation**

12   I am ill and I must accept or refuse help

**Assumptions consistent with the premises**

13   I am myself
14   I can repay help

**Consequences**

15   I have something to offer   12/7/9/2
16   I can avoid being a child   12/14/4
17   I cut losses and develop resources   12/7/8
18   I demand explanations   12/7/11/10

necessary to mention a growing belief that mental conflicts can generate illness in adults. This belief also finds expression in 11-year-old children in the United States, who used 'psychophysiologic' explanations of illness (see below); Bibace & Walsh (1980) regarded this as 'the most mature understanding of illness' found in the children they saw, indirectly stating as it did the predominant value system of 'mature' American adults. This endogenous cause is believed by some sociologists to be fostered culturally by the way in which psychoanalysts concentrate on internal processes, and the status of psychoanalysis in the culture (see Moscovici (1961) in Harré (1979) for how psychoanalytic concepts have been taken up in France). This view seems to reflect an ignorance of the aims of psychoanalysis to help an individual gain an equilibrium between his part in creating a situation and the role of others in putting him in that situation, i.e. a balance between endogenous and exogenous factors. In contrast Harré (1983) has interpreted the primacy of psychological explanations in the West as following industrialisation. The development of psychoanalysis, cults of the individual and ego-psychologies can be accounted for as reactions to the social processes occurring at the same time as industrialisation.

Nevertheless the medical profession as a whole appears to have been preoccupied with internal factors, although it is largely the exogenous factors (exemplified by the removal of the handle to the Broad Street pump to 'treat' a nineteenth-century cholera epidemic in London) which have had the greatest effect on public health. By concentrating on way of life and exogenous factors doctors would have to enter the political arena to a greater extent.

The medical preference for internal factors is seen by some as an attempt to increase the individual's sense of responsibility for 'endogenous causes' of his illness (Berkanovic, 1972; Zola, 1973). These efforts appear to be resisted by some because they increase an individual's sense of guilt about his illness. The need to resist complements a feeling of being attacked by a powerful profession; this is a view taken much further by some sociologists (see for example Zola, 1972). A continued emphasis on exogenous causes, such as germs, enables individuals to remain relatively guilt-free (Stoetzel in Herzlich, 1973 p. 49) and yet allot 'blame' (Blaxter, 1983). At the same time Blaxter's sample paradoxically favours 'mind over matter maxims for management of illness . . . [and] . . . psychological explanations for the cause of disease'. In this way a coherent framework of exogenous and endogenous factors is produced which, as will be seen, fits with the world adults introduce to children. The results are consistent with those of Pill & Stott (1982) where the two main reasons for illness given by the Welsh mothers in their sample were 'germs, bugs, viruses, infections' and 'being "rundown"'. As Herzlich (1973 p. 38) summarised, 'it is society which, through the way of life, brings illness; at the same time it is society which demands that the individual should be healthy! . . . Therein lies the paradox of society: it demands from the individual what it refuses him'. It is this relation of the individual and society which Blaxter's (1983) sample formulates in its own comprehensive way with its complicated multifactorial model of illness which in many ways mirrors the detail of current medical models.

### Naturalistic and personalistic systems: events and agents

The concepts which Herzlich has used based on the accounts provided by her respondents give little idea of how people account for the agency of the causes of illness. The ways in which children distinguish between agents such as germs and 'events' which preceded the illness will be discussed later. Their distinction is the same as one which Foster (1976) used in accounting for the range of views he came across in adults from various cultures. He noted that adults tend to seek an answer to the question 'Why has this illness affected me at this point in time?' This was the same question which Balint (1964) stressed in his efforts to help general practitioners understand their patients' problems.

Just as Herzlich exaggerated the dichotomy between the two categories of exogenous and endogenous, so Foster has used the non-exclusive categories of naturalistic and personalistic. He hypothesises that when adults search for the meaning of their illness, which they do by focussing especially on the cause, they are trying to minimise their anxieties about it (see also, for example, Blaxter, 1983). They then tend to adopt predominantly one or the other system of explanation depending on the culture in which they live. Although communities have their dominant approach, not all individuals within that culture will use it – just as was seen earlier with the range of loci of control modes in communities.

The *naturalistic approach* involves the individual attributing the cause of his illness to particular events or natural states which preceded the illness:

Naturalistic systems explain illness in impersonal systemic terms. Disease is thought to stem, not from the machinations of an angry being, but rather from such *natural forces or conditions* as cold, heat, wind, dampness, and, above all, by an upset in the balance of the basic body elements . . . . health conforms to an *equilibrium* model. (Foster, 1976; italics in original)

Measles in a man in Hong Kong is said to follow intercourse with a woman during the ritually prohibited period of 100 days after childbirth (Loudon, 1976 p. 42) – a transgression against the prevailing moral order. In some South African communities it is believed that if a child becomes ill when his father is away from home the mother has been unfaithful. Where this approach predominates the same moral order tends to occur with respect to misfortunes and accidents. In some of these cultures these states are not differentiated and a common word denotes all three; for example *wola* in New Guinea covers all undesired states including illness (Lewis, 1976 p. 53).

In this system the individual makes his own diagnosis about the cause of his illness by retracing his steps over the preceding day and choosing the events which his cultural values dictate as the most likely precipitant of that illness. In Scotland similar observations have been made that 'the cause of illness can be the event which caused the patient to perceive the disease or admit to it' (Blaxter, 1983). It appears to be based on that process reported by Piaget (Piaget & Inhelder, 1966) for children where a causal connection is assumed between two events happening close together. The difference here is that the event immediately preceding illness is not felt necessarily to be the cause unless it is one of the events which is culturally determined as a sufficient cause for that illness. The naturalistic approach is a refinement of a natural classificatory scheme of children, which in all probability reflects the way in which we expect accounts of things from our children. What is lacking at present is a developmental anthropology which has explored this socialisation.

A naturalistic approach is especially conducive to the development of health rituals, so that behaviours particularly dangerous for health are proscribed. A degree of social order is then maintained through the sharing of a common value system of desirable and proscribed behaviours. Douglas (1966) has looked at social responses to what communities define as dirt, often interpreted as being that which signifies disorder, and charted the ways in which order becomes established. I will not repeat the details of her classic study here but only point out that religious rituals have been particularly significant.

Lest naturalistic approaches are thought to be 'non-Western', it is as well to cite the example of 'fresh air', which has been a powerful organising concept around which middle class health behaviour crystallised from the 1850s onwards (Davidoff, 1976). What has been understood as fresh air has varied over the years. It is currently often proferred as an explanation to children for why they should or should not do certain things. Whether this is perceived as rationalisation for the children, or subtly controlling them, depends on where the locus of control is allocated. The concept has a very long history dating back at least to the miasmic theories of contagion of the 1600s (Taylor, 1979). The mephitis in cemeteries and surrounding areas associated with the mass burial practices current at the time set up a widespread association between foul air and death (Ariès, 1977). So long as the individual feels able to alter his environment rather than being constrained by his way of life, his beliefs in the benefits of fresh air enable him to prevent illness for himself. Besides these important locus of control factors health must also be salient for him (Gochman, 1971a).

Our nursing traditions have been much influenced by Florence Nightingale's writings. Her *Notes on Nursing* (1860 p. 72) describes the importance of fresh air and its effects on children:

> To revert to children. They are much more susceptible than grown people to all noxious influences. They are affected by the same things, but much more quickly and seriously, viz., by want of fresh air, of proper warmth, want of cleanliness in house, clothes, beding or body, by startling noises, improper food, or want of punctuality, by dulness and by want of light, by too much or too little covering in bed, or when up, by want of the spirit of management generally in those in charge of them.
>
> That which, however, above all, is known to injure children seriously is foul air, and most seriously at night. Keeping the rooms where they sleep tight shut up, is destruction to them.

It will be seen that several of these viewpoints are reflected in the world of children today when the construction of the child's world of illness is discussed in chapter 4.

There is a corollary to this 'naturalistic' organisation which is that the patient will already have made the diagnosis from his reflections on the preceding events so that when he approaches a healer it is solely for cure and not for diagnosis. If this value system predominates and someone else presumes to make the diagnosis this is tantamount to claiming magical powers, as otherwise there exists no way this other could have monitored the individual's previous movements. This view is also currently found in Scotland where women are recorded as resenting 'it when doctors attempted to impose such explanations upon them [e.g. stress]. Such theories of cause were acceptable only when they were based on the detailed knowledge which they themselves had of the interrelations between life events and symptoms' (Blaxter, 1983).

In contrast in the predominantly *personalistic system* the healer is approached in order to divine the nature of the agent causing the illness, and, through giving a name to it, provide a diagnosis (the basis of reification). Campbell *et al.* (1979) described it in Canada in this way, that 'To the layman a disease seems to be a living agency that causes illness'; or alternatively 'disease is "it", separated from the body and imposed upon it' (Blaxter, 1983). Classically in this system curing is regarded as the more minor role and tends to be delegated to an aide.

In the personalistic system the healer is allocated a role in diagnosis. He finds out which 'agent' has affected the individual, how it did it, and whether any agent which normally protected the individual had withdrawn its support. Although germs are the agents we most commonly think of and fear in the West (see for example, Blaxter, 1983), they are the most recent of a long tradition. Previously there have been supernatural powers, existing as 'real monsters', which invaded people to cause illness. 'Sins' have been conceptualised as concrete objects which roamed around autonomously and afflicted people, or could even be acting on behalf of particular deities (Taylor, 1979). These views may appear fanciful now that the power of the religious community has waned and in ways adapted to the more dominant scientific ethic. There appear to be few attempts at religious exorcism currently, although reports of exorcisms seem to be appearing in the British newspapers more often. In other non-Western countries, however, healers diagnose various spirits, such as dead ancestors, which have entered a person and they then instruct curers on how to effect their removal.

Relics of these thoughts are still found in our children! In Britain parents still on occasion attribute the cause of their illness to their children, albeit usually to their high spirits rather than to any ethereal quality (Newson & Newson, 1976 p. 391). Although adults may not perceive this as a direct attribution of causality the children have a tendency to attach their own alternative meanings – at least provisionally.

## Children's views on the causality of illness
### The Piagetian framework

Most of the background research on children's views on illness has looked at whether the developmental changes in children's views on the causality of illness have followed the sequences to be expected from using Piaget's framework. Piaget's model of development is one in which the child goes through sequential stages in which the skills developed at one stage prepare the child for the next. In the first stage, the *sensori-motor stage*, the young infant understands his environment mainly in terms of his own bodily senses and movement. The transition to the second stage, *preoperational thinking*, is believed to occur usually in 2-year-old children. These children are developing a sense of self, language and symbolic functions. Thus so far Piaget's framework is congruent with the data presented earlier on the child's development. He goes on to add that children of this age and up to about 7 years old think in idiosyncratic and egocentric ways. It is useful to note that, together with Inhelder, he felt that the latter 'term has often been misunderstood, although we always insisted on its epistemological meaning (difficulty in understanding differences in points of view between the speakers and therefore in decentration) rather than on its popular or "moral" meaning' (Piaget & Inhelder, 1966 p. 118). Although it has been implied that egocentrism is a quality in the child, Piaget has also said that 'Childish egocentrism, far from being social, always goes hand in hand with adult constraint' (Piaget, 1932 p. 57). It is this intersubjective dimension associated with a form of moral order to which particular attention must be paid here, in order to avoid getting too immersed in the ideas of ego-psychology where egocentrism tends to be attributed solely to the child's developmental 'stage'.

At about 7 years of age children begin to move into a stage of *concrete operational thinking*, where they start to use classification and 'adult type' causal thinking, but usually limiting this to present concrete objects or specific experiences. Then over a 2-year period, between the ages of 11 and 12 years in Piaget's community, they go through a transitional stage before they reach a stage of *formal operational thinking*. This last stage is characterised by children having an ability to conceive of possibilites and abstractions separate from their immediate reality (Piaget, 1926).

Besides these stages Piaget had some other important observations about concept development in children. He concluded that concepts developed in conflict situations. For example if parents disagreed about an illness state in a child, the child would be in a conflict situation if his relations with them were moderately similar. Additionally Piaget believed that abstract concepts developed first, becoming more specific later, and at the same time harder to transfer to new situations. It can be anticipated that children's early viewpoints will not be very specific. As pointed out earlier they will tend to have loose rather than tight constructs. Piaget noted that the development of language tended to send the level of concept formation back to the preceding stage. Although working with concepts of non-conservation of area, he did find that these concepts were built up from concepts of conservation. If this is translated to an illness/health dimension, the common-sense observation is anticipated that concepts of illness follow from non-conservation of health.

### Nursery school age children (3–4 years)

There appear to have been few studies of young children. Rather than looking at how these studies have portrayed the apparent stages in the development of children's views it is necessary to describe the form and content of their views without imposing the Piagetian framework within which the results were analysed. In order to interpret the results for their form of validity it would be necessary to know more about the setting within which the views were obtained. Instead I must present only the main concepts, the form of the validity of the interpretation of the results waiting until later. For ease of comparison I include descriptions of how the original researchers have linked these stages to those of Piaget.

Bibace & Walsh (1980) studied 4-year-old children's views on causality of illness in the United States. The children were unable to explain the manner in which events co-occurring with illness might have caused the illness, but the 'more mature' children (i.e. those having views closer to those of particular adult members of that society) were beginning to use concepts of contagion. That is they believed that the cause of illness was located in objects or people which were proximate to but not touching the child. The link between the object and the illness was accounted for in terms of 'mere proximity' or magic. Using Piaget's terminology the majority of these children used phenomenism to explain illness (see Piaget & Inhelder (1966) for elaboration of their use of terms). They were introduced to a model of exogenous causes in a predominantly personalistic system.

### Primary school age children (5–11 years)

There have been many more researchers from different cultures who have looked at the views of illness held by children of the age group 5–11 years. Again I will try to emphasise the concepts used in interpreting the data which have been found to have most explanatory potential.

Bibace & Walsh (1980) went on to study 7-year-olds and their explanations of illness. They categorised their responses predominantly using the ideas of 'contamination' and 'internalization'. They used contamination in the sense that the cause of the illness was viewed as a person, object, or action external to the child which has an aspect or quality that is 'bad' or 'harmful' for the body. The effect is then transmitted through contact. A further explanation would involve the idea that the harm came to be associated with a particular moral order established in connection with those things which could contaminate. Internalisation is somewhat similar except that the contact comes internally after swallowing or inhaling. This is clearly compatible with the exogenous/personalistic system exemplified by the younger children's responses.

By the time the children in their study area were 11 years old (and as they believed in Piaget's stage of formal operations) they appeared to be using a concept of cause built up on their ideas about the physiology of the body, the body's structure and functioning or malfunctioning. In addition some were allowing of explanations involving a person's thoughts and feelings which had somehow predisposed people to illness through affecting the body's functioning. This they termed a 'psychophysiologic' explanation. Perrin & Gerrity (1981) had noticed that between the ages of 10 and 11 years children shifted from believing that all illnesses were caused by 'the mere presence of germs' (an example of that which could contaminate, using Bibace & Walsh's classification) to having an understanding that there are multiple causes of illness and that the body can have its own resistance. These results taken together provisionally suggest that developing awareness of their own body's functioning plays an important role at this age in the United States, but from the ways in which the research is presented it is not possible to establish any correlations with school curricula changes at this age or other influences. The 'good' aspect, the resistance to infection, is here attributed to the self as would be expected, but there is also a hint that people's own thoughts and feelings may predispose them to illness, reflecting hints of some old moral teachings perhaps.

Carandang *et al.* (1979), also working in the United States, kept more closely to comparing the children's views to what they expected from rigidly following a Piagetian framework. The part of their sample with a mean age of 11 years 6 months had similar views to those mentioned above, but described them by using different language. An example they quote makes the differences clear. They stress that the children's views are tied to concrete events with only the beginnings of some generalisations – because of the following example amongst others:

If it's somebody you're around with and when he breathes out, you take in the air that he breathes out. Or it's just the germs that he's got. The germs are in the air. They get in your clothes and, later, they get on you.

This illustrates the possible muddles resulting from sticking rigidly to a given framework of interpretation. Using the earlier categories of Bibace & Walsh, the above would seem to be an example of a 7-year-old's use of internalisation and contamination, which they interpreted as being coherent with the earlier concrete operational stage; Carandang *et al.*, though, interpret it as belonging to a stage of transitional operational thought.

Interpretation alters with the framework of the research, expectations and the moral orders of the setting in which the researchers operate and account for their observations. Different moral orders in the research situation have facilitated children's communicative competences in different ways, but this can only be a partial explanation of these different ways of interpreting children's views on illness. Unfortunately the results as presented do not allow a clear testing of their ecological and phenomenological validity.

In summary, children of this age in the United States appear to be moving from believing that contamination by or internalisation of agents such as germs causes illness to psychophysiological concepts. How this relates to the moral order at home, school or in the research situation is unclear. The concepts are coherent with the adult concepts described earlier.

### *Secondary school age children (12–18 years)*

According to Piagetian theory children of 12–18 years would be expected to be developing more general and abstract ideas about the nature of illness – an ability to go beyond specific events. This does not reveal, though, how socialisation towards particular cultural norms is proceeding. Carandang *et al.* (1979) note an example which they interpreted as fitting this category of Piaget for the causes of illness.

> Being around other people. Not getting the right nutrition or sleep. Not wearing the right clothes at winter. If you cough or sneeze without covering your mouth, the germs float in the air and the other person breathes the germs; your body tries to fight the germs and that's what makes you feel bad.

As will be seen it gives more clues to the social values the children are assimilating.

Note that the children have included ideas of sleep, nutrition and clothing as being potentially protective, i.e. personal strategies for resistance to infection. They are aware of what one might forget to do which could make one more vulnerable – the possibilities for breaking the social rules. The other comments about germs fit with the earlier idea of internalisation, and suggest a well-ordered progression through an exogenous/personalistic system in the United States.

### *The effects of family illness*

The disease which appears to have been most studied for its effect on the siblings of ill children is diabetes, and so I will draw some examples from this condition to illustrate a few points; but it is unclear how representative it is of other conditions, or how culturally bound the reactions are.

The study of Carandang *et al.* (1979) went on to look at how the children's views of illness at particular ages were modified if there was diabetes in a sibling. With the necessary caveat that they were imposing the Piagetian framework onto all their observations, they interpreted their results as showing that children who had a diabetic sibling tended to function at one developmental level 'behind'. For example those functioning otherwise at a level of formal operations functioned at a transitional stage in relation to illness. They suggested that the effect could have been mitigated through the effect of the stress of the illness on the whole family's way of communicating about illness. It is known that sibling illness ranks as one of the most stressful life events for children (Coddington, 1972); as well as it being concluded by Crain, Sussman & Weil (1966) that of all the family members the siblings of childhood diabetics bear the greatest burden of stress. Generally, though, it is visible handicap which is reported to have a greater negative effect on siblings' psychological coping than illnesses which are less obvious (Bruvik *et al.*, 1986). In her review of coping in the face of illness Shapiro (1983) concluded that siblings particularly at risk for maladaptive responses were undergoing other concurrent stresses, had poor relationships with parents and/or with the ill child, poor support systems, and limited communication skills.

An alternative explanation could come from illness behaviour modelling. Siblings of diabetic boys had been found to have somatic complaints four times as often as controls, a form of complaining associated with younger age groups. This specific form of complaining was felt to be related to the fact that the diabetic siblings tended to have several somatic complaints, rather than it being a general function of having an ill sibling (Ferrari, 1984) or the effect of stress on the family's communication style. Nevertheless family functioning has been shown to be correlated with the self-reported stress felt by the diabetic child, the sibling and the mother (Caldwell & Pickert, 1985). It must not be forgotten that of all family members siblings can expect to live the longest with the chronically ill.

Diabetes seems to have a particular effect on family functioning as mothers of diabetics attending hospital have been shown to be more often anxious and depressed than other mothers of children attending hospital (Wolff, 1981 p. 76).

The hypothesis of Carandang *et al.*, (1979) that stress had altered the family's way of communicating about illness receives some support from the research of Brodie (1974), who surveyed the views of 6–10-year-old schoolchildren in the United States. Those children with a high level of general anxiety, regardless of their age, responded more often as though their illness was a punishment for which they were personally responsible. In this way the older anxious children's views could be interpreted as congruent with the more moralistic judgements of younger ages, or alternatively that the effect of the moral order and how people cope with it becomes more pronounced when they are anxious.

There may well be a cultural effect here. Zola (1975) reported how 17–19-year-olds in the United States would communicate about illness to a child under 5 years of age. The results showed that they used a lot of morally loaded words. When Stacey (1980) expected to replicate this with British students she was unsuccessful, and notes that mentions of morality in the responses have declined annually. This is one of the few longitudinal perspectives I have found.

As children's states of health at the time of the research are not generally noted in the literature on children's views it is difficult to interpret the results as presented. The provisional conclusion from the research referred to above must be that the views obtained are dependent on the child's state and the context, which is not surprising but nevertheless not accorded its due importance. The conclusion of Carandang *et al.* was in line with the thesis here that the form of communication about illness must be attended to. They ended with further questions for future research, which can also be important to note in consultations and when exploring developmental influences: 'Who initiates family discussions of illness; at what cognitive level are illness discussions carried on; and how do the tone and frequency of family discussions affect children's conceptualisations of illness?' As far as I know, there has been no linking of these ways of looking at developmental factors, to the frameworks of exogenous/endogenous and naturalistic/personalistic systems.

It is necessary to be cautious in assuming that diabetic children will necessarily function developmentally at a different cognitive level from children not suffering from a chronic illness. Eiser *et al.* (1984) in England found only one significant difference between healthy and diabetic children (samples in age groups 6–10, 11–13 and 14+ years) in their definitions of health and their knowledge of the causes of various illnesses. This was limited specifically to knowledge of the causes of diabetes in the oldest age group. The variability in the beliefs diabetic children have about their illness and its causes can most easily be explained by suggesting that it depends to a large degree on the ways in which people have responded to them rather than it being inherent in the 'diabetes' or their phase of development. These authors were not looking at illness behaviour though, but instead concentrated on the children's factual information, the mathetic elements, which are relatively independent of the form of communication about the ill child. As will be seen in chapter 10, increased knowledge does not tend to change illness behaviour or coping (Kalnins & Love, 1982).

When the children whose views are elicited are themselves ill the family dynamic is shifted. Relative experiences of illness become important and these effects change with the age of the child. For example Campbell (1975) found that illness experience in children less than 9½ years which was greater than the recent illness experience of the parents, was associated with them holding less sophisticated concepts than their peers. In contrast children over 9½ years in this situation had a greater sophistication in their illness concepts. (There is a much greater literature on the topics of ill and hospitalised children, but only the above example will be included here as the theme of this book is not the effects of hospitalisation.)

Again Brodie (1974) provides a clue to the interpretation of this result as she had additionally found that ill children had similar views on illness to the highly anxious ones. It could be that anxiety influences the younger children's concepts to make them less sophisticated, whereas children older than 9½ years have developed more effective strategies to cope with the anxieties engendered and so could learn from their experience. In Brodie's sample it was only major illness which had this effect; experience of illness involving up to five consecutive days off school in the preceding five months did not in any way alter the child's perception of illness.

Ferrari (1984) looked at the psychosocial effects of chronic illness in boys on their siblings. This approach emphasises the pragmatic effects on behaviour of diabetes in a male sibling rather than its effect on their views about diabetes – a mathetic element. He emphasises the importance of recording the length of time that the siblings have had together since the diagnosis of diabetes, as the longer the time since diagnosis the lower the level of behaviour problems and the higher the self-esteem in the sibling. Although he used a different framework from the researchers quoted above, Ferrari found that children functioned better who had mothers with a supportive social network and marriage partner. These factors are known to mitigate against the effects of stress, improve the interactional 'dance' and affect illness behaviour (see McKinlay (1981) and Hammer (1983) for detailed descriptions of social network effects).

We see here a complicated pattern of interaction between the child's maturity and state of anxiety which apparently affects his interpretation and the influence of family illness. It appears as though the forms of illness with which the child has come into contact can act as models for illness-like behaviour as well as sensitising the child's care-givers. The effects on family communication about illness, both the form and the content, seem variable from the variety of responses reported.

Besides the observations here about the interactions between the child's state and illness in other family members, there is also a complementary interaction observed between parental state and child 'illness', or more accurately the research reports the allocating of the sick role to the child by the parent, or the place of sickness in family life. For example Mechanic (1964) in the United States illustrated the way in which mothers under stress tended to report more illness symptomatology both for themselves and for their children, and were more likely to consult their doctors. An interesting relationship was noted by Howie & Bigg (1980) from Aberdeen, where they found in a general practice sample that children were brought to their GPs more often when mothers who were otherwise taking antidepressants were not taking them. This observation fits with the report by Wolkind (1985) that children of depressed mothers were taken more often to their GPs and had more frequent hospital admissions than others. As noted above mothers of children with diabetes tend to be more depressed than other mothers of children in hospital.

I will not try to unravel causal relations from the wide-ranging research in this area, as my aim is to highlight the interactions between states of the individual, be those of anxiety or illness for example, and their being either allocated or willing to allocate a sick role, or to show illness behaviour. There is an inherent intertwining of psychological and physical factors in a tight social matrix which makes accounting for the origins of children's illness behaviour difficult. This is something which has already been anticipated from the previous discussion of the development of how children learn to signal their discomforts to others.

### *The effects of family views on illness*

When researchers have tried to establish correlations between the views of children and others they have never pointed out a one to one relationship. Instead the views of groups of children correspond at a general level to the views of their mothers taken as a group. But there is no correspondence between the views of specific children and their mothers or fathers (see for example Mechanic, 1964; Cambell, 1975; Blaxter & Paterson, 1982*a,b*).

Although the consultation behaviour of children is generally dependent on the behaviour of their guardians, one study in the United States tried to find out what sorts of consultation behaviour the children would show independently of adult guidance in a school setting. In that situation the children (aged from 5 to 12 years) showed the consultation patterns of their parents (Lewis *et al.*, 1977). (Other factors from this study associated with consultation behaviour will be discussed in chapter 9.) As Campbell (1975) points out, family influences appear at the stage of translation of the concepts of illness into sick-role behaviour. Older boys with mothers with better than average education were more likely to reject the characteristic passivity and dependence of classical sick role and see themselves as stoic and unemotional in the face of illness. It would take further research to see whether their premises about illness corresponded to those of 'illness as destroyer' (table 3.1).

These two superficially conflicting results fit in with the distinction between the mathetic (the children's factual information) and the pragmatic (related to the way in which views are shared). The ways in which we communicate about our states are crucial for determining the ways in which we act in relation to them, apparently regardless of our own views on illness at this age.

*Germs: causal agents versus natural justice*

Contagion is used widely by 7–9-year-olds to explain things. It has already been described indirectly in connection with contamination and internalisation. It occurs as a general element in children's games for this age group (see chapter 2). The dramatic ailments of childhood are still the contagious diseases. Whether children's uses of contagion will alter with altered frequencies of infections in childhood remains to be seen. Children have described how they view infections getting from one person to another (Nagy, 1951, 1953). They described germs, drawing them frequently as though they were primitive insects, acting as the agents to convey or become the illness. They conceived of a single germ ('bacillus' was the word used by Nagy's Hungarian children) causing all sorts of illness. Only by the age of 11 years (in 1947–8 when this research was carried out in Budapest, Hungary, and in 1949 in a comparative group in Bristol, England) were children beginning to be aware that different diseases had special germs. Children of this age were described as still believing that all diseases were caused by organisms of some sort, making no reference to organic and functional diseases or dietary deficiencies. There was a predominant idea that if a germ entered the body that person automatically became ill to a predetermined degree, with no concept of the body's degrees of resistance to infection.

Ideas change over time and in different cultures. Kister & Patterson

(1980) in the United States showed how children between the ages of 4 years 8 months and 9½ years used 'immanent justice' explanations of illness, and did this more frequently than for either misfortune or accidents. Immanent justice describes the belief that a form of natural justice can emanate from inanimate objects. It appears as a special form of animism which tinges objects with the power to mete out justice just as significant adults have previously done to them. It was hypothesised that the more widespread this concept the less would be the need for children to use the concept of chance, and hence the more ordered their world. It has been recorded as a belief of children in relation to illness for a long time (Langford, 1948). The use of explanations involving immanent justice decreased in Kister & Patterson's older age groups in association with a better understanding of contagion. At the same time their use of contagion began to be more differentiated as it ceased being used to account for the cause of all discomforts including that resulting from accidents, as had been the case previously. This differentiation corresponds to that described by Bibace & Walsh (1980) and Perrin & Gerrity (1981).

One way of interpreting these results is that the pragmatic mode dominates in the younger children, contagion reflecting the development of the mathetic mode as the child begins to generalise from the phenomenism of earlier years. The difficulty in eliciting their knowledge of contagion or contamination at the earlier ages is likely to be a function of the research method and situation.

Contagion facilitates the belief that agents such as germs can transmit illness. As will be seen subsequently the roles of agents as illness transmitters is widespread, but there also exist for children other events which have occurred prior to the illness which can become associated with the illness and viewed as its cause. This is the same phenomenon reported above in Scottish women. The immanent justice explanations fit more into this category and reflect the moral order of the pre-illness situation. In addition the role of the food eaten, part of the pre-illness situation, is important in some communities for establishing health (see Rashkis, 1965; Eiser, Patterson & Eiser, 1983) or being correlated with the presence of illness. Current views of children in Glasgow are that you are more likely to get ill because of eating too much than because of germs (Mackie, 1980). Views on how the causes of illness are accounted for in one community over time would be illuminating for understanding the links between agents and prior events as illness precipitators, but I know of no such research. We have now come back to conceptualisations which are the same as those described for adult subjects: the potential origins of naturalistic and personalistic systems in the ways in which we socialise our children and they try to make sense of the world in which they are socialised.

## Summary

The preceding chapter described how children learn to communicate. Here we have seen how these communication skills which they have developed are moulded in the course of their socialisation so that the functional consequences of their special languages are formed through the variety of ways in which they have been effective. In this communication they also learn about the larger world they inhabit, and discriminate facts about that world.

Causes of illness occupy a central place in how people make sense of the world of illness. They are important organising constructs used in accounting for how people are and will be. What children understand by causality appears at first sight to be different from the understanding of most adults. The evidence so far suggests that the basis of their understanding is rooted in their early lives, their communicative competences and effectiveness as people.

I have pointed out various categories which can be useful for the analysis which follows. Two key categories have been used in analysing the adult worlds of illness, the worlds into which children are socialised and help create in that same transactional process. The first of these was a dimension related to the placing of the locus of control, and to what degree that was external or internal, and this was itself related to whether causes were seen as residing primarily outside the person or inside, i.e. exogenous versus endogenous causes. The second category was the distinction between naturalistic and personalistic health/illness systems which represented a way in which societies have been classified.

In addition I have shown here how these ways of being have a basis in the individual's development, so that these ways of functioning represent influences both of the society on the individual and the individual on the society. It is because of these reciprocal impacts that I have given them a key place here before using these concepts in the chapters that follow.

Yet at the same time these categories describe a world of illness which is problematic for children. Children come into contact with a variety of social groups which can have institutionalised different value systems along the dimensions of exogenous/endogenous causes and naturalistic/personalistic systems. As these exist side by side the confusing world to which children are introduced can be sensed. The children experience conflicting expectations of the healer as well as of the self. For example, how much are they expected to be responsible for their own diagnoses? At the same time there are varying notions about how much of the cause of an illness should be attributed to one's environment or one's own nature. If the illness is seen as being due to one's own nature, there are differing expectations about what can be done about it and to what degree one is responsible for one's own health and treatment.

As the naturalistic and personalistic systems appear to operate under different assumptions it will be impossible to integrate them coherently without questioning the assumptions on which they are based. As the two exist side by side children are exposed to elements of both at different times and in different places. Piaget has termed the child as 'assimilating' new ideas into an established framework, but these systems of explanation cannot be assimilated and this will push the child to 'accommodate' to a new framework of explanation of his illness (Piaget & Inhelder, 1966 p. 6). Critical sociologists would perhaps describe it as a legitimation crisis.

One of the processes of legitimation involves the adoption of the system which is most coherent with the particular society's dominant values. This could, for example, be the cause of illness favoured by the religious authorities, as opposed to the medical, or a judicious mixture of the two. The mode of operation of the healers and the form of approach to them will then be guided by the prevailing social forces. As the social forces acting on the healers may be different from those acting on the clients, both groups coming from differently institutionalised social groups (Berger & Luckmann, 1966), the dissonance generated naturally may be amplified.

The expectation which the research recounted generates is that causality will differ for different cultural groups and at different points in time. Children are confronted by a potentially confusing range of views which will become greater as their social circle expands. The resolution of their confusion will be bound up with the dominant value system of the larger social group in which their views develop. Their place within the hierarchy of that social group is likely to be correlated with the degree to which they perceive themselves as able to determine their own way of life, and hence whether their illness will be perceived as freeing or destructive. Those who feel trapped by their way of life at the bottom of the social hierarchy are likely to see that as the 'cause' of their illness.

# 4

# The primary structure to the child's world of illness

*'A child . . . has to locate his experience in a framework of social explanations and rules.' (Herzlich, 1973 p. 1)*

It is now time to describe the framework to the child's world, the primary structure. It was this which shaped and was shaped by the children I observed. It is a framework of overt and covert rules and regulations built up on functional myths which these families found necessary for ordering their daily lives. These myths represent the ways in which they have found it necessary to account for the unknown, especially as encountered in their dealings with illness in their children. As already mentioned no disrespect for these myths is implied by calling them such; instead I am wanting to emphasise their historical social construction.

The family rules presented here represent my deductions to account for the ways in which the elicited views and described behaviour are linked together into a coherent whole. They are of necessity rather intangible (Ford, 1983), and I have not tried to alter the framework in order to test the forces binding it, or the relationship of the framework to the elicited views of the children. This represents the next stage in what would have to be a long-term project, and is what Bronfenbrenner (1979 p. 41) would term a 'transforming experiment'.

## The family and the nursery school age child

I will first present the family decision-making processes for common illnesses in 3- and 4-year-old children before moving on to present how these change over the years. I will base these chiefly on my own observations from Edinburgh.

One of the critical developmental tasks at this age was for the children to establish a wider social network. Previously the majority had been at home with their mothers. They were only now experiencing a rapid expansion of their contacts to include the staff and other pupils at nursery school, as well as extended neighbourhood contacts. In Edinburgh there was a particularly high provision of nursery school places, with 85% of all children in the age range 3–4 years attending nursery (45% of total placements were private provision).

The children in the sample had spent most of their time within their families of origin; by chance no children who were fostered or living in children's homes were included. The decisions made about their various states of illness, tiredness and hunger, for example, had previously been largely made by a select group of people who often shared similar points of view. The children were now venturing out into strange and exciting new territories where people explained things in a variety of new ways, and made decisions about them according to a wider range of variables. Confusion could rule if it were not for very powerful efforts by the children, to identify what was nevertheless similar and to make sense of their expanding universe. Children of this age were only just beginning to make sense of the particular explanations and rules of the nursery school as they related to illness and health matters. The confusions which they experienced and how they attempted to integrate them reveal some of the powerful effects which construct the child's hermeneutic system. Just as children's language develops capacities in two modes – the mathetic mode for the gathering or conveying of information as facts, and the pragmatic mode for regulating interpersonal interactions – so I will show that adults appear to give their children these two forms as a framework when deciding whether their child is ill.

### 'What's the matter?': the parental observation

In spite of verbal enquiries of their children the parents did not expect them to, and the majority of nursery school age children could not, tell them about their illness in words. The parents had to interpret a variety of clues in order to gather information about their child's state. They then typically checked their observations in a number of follow-up strategies. The initial stages are characterised by uncertainty; the child is not ill or well in the parent's eyes until further confirmatory steps are taken.

The first clues depended on the parents noticing a change in the child's routine. The child who was normally quick to get up and dress in the morning became more reluctant. The child who normally had a good-sized breakfast took only a small one. There were the children who stopped talking as much as usual. The child who usually explored away from the parents became more clingy. All of these changes can have a variety of interpretations, and Rutter (1980) lists some of them which are appropriate for clingy children: 'tired, hungry, unwell, in pain, or feeling cold . . . fear, anxiety, rebuffs or rejection' (p. 272). These include a mixture of physical and psychological states. Observations from the United States (Mattsson & Weisberg, 1970) have suggested that the clingy response has usually ceased by the time children are 3 years old. Children of this age were seen as being more self-contained and undemanding when ill, tending to rest quietly – but interestingly going through a clingy and demanding phase in convalescence. This was definitely not the general impression in the present sample, but it remains unclear whether this is a cultural difference, historical or related to the fact that the American sample was upper class. In the American sample the degree of clingyness was associated only with the age of the child and not the child's sex or type of illness.

Clearly a pattern would have to be established before any divergence from it could be discriminated. Graham (1984 p. 187) points out that poverty limits a family's flexibility in its routines. Once inflexibility is established there is a family need for diminished responsiveness to these changes in the children. Inflexibility also arises as a family style in other situations, but the struggles of poverty add extra stringencies. None of the families whom I met were so disorganised that changes in routine did not stand out. I got no impression of children elaborating those signs which they knew their parents looked out for at this age, although on learning-theory principles a moulding of the children's illness behaviour in a social learning process would be expected.

Besides noting changes in behaviour, parents were alerted to the possibility of illness when the child's mood changed. Although mood states in children are deduced and labelled by the parents after they have observed small changes in a child's manner, I have concentrated on the labels attached by the parents rather than the interpretative process involved and how they came to choose those particular labels for their child's behaviour. This labelling process reflects the vocabulary available to the parents, their expectations of what is possible in certain circumstances or what it is necessary to watch out for. It probably reflects the way they themselves have had their own similar behaviour labelled previously and their culturally accepted relevant points of view, but I did not particularly explore this dimension. The labels which the parents used for the child's mood changes which alerted them to the possibilities of illness included the children becoming grumpy, listless, tearful, annoyed, irritable, miserable, 'not herself' and having tempers. During this initial orientation of the parents towards the change in the child's state they remain uncertain whether this moodiness reflects a 'bad child', an upset child or an ill child. The words used to describe the mood states could fit all three categories.

In addition to evaluating the child's behaviour and mood state the parents were trying to assess the child's physical appearance. They noted particularly changes in the child's colour, whether he was paler or more flushed; and they tried to interpret from his appearance whether he had a raised temperature. They attempted to confirm the latter by looking especially at the child's eyes and by feeling the forehead, or rather accounted for a change in the eyes or eye contact as being due to fever. The 'look' in a baby's eyes has been reported (Spencer (1980) in Graham, 1984 p. 157) as an important diagnostic sign of illness by parents of younger children, and it may be that the mother's responses are building on this earlier decision-making strategy. This *feel* to the child, when it coincides with what the child comes to feel, provides a facilitative basis to the folk models of colds and fevers described by Helman (1978), which are based on subjective rather than objective evidence of temperature changes. Temperatures were not taken with thermometers in any of these families, except in one which took it solely after they had decided to call the doctor so that they could inform him on his arrival. This lack of recourse to a thermometer is perhaps a peculiarly British phenomenon in the West (personal observations in Norway, Hansson (1985) from Denmark, and personal reports from the United States), and is one that British doctors have encouraged parents to alter. Parents are unconvinced that there is more to be gained from knowing the degree of temperature than increased worry; it is enough that there is a temperature. The 2-year-olds reported by Mattsson & Weisberg (1970) from the United States would seem to appreciate the British parent's point of view:

> The 2 year olds seemed equally bewildered about the alleged helpful effects of unpleasant medicines and temperature taking. No immediate relief followed despite the mother's assurances. The young child's emotional distress was thus intensified by their difficulty in distinguishing between discomfort from within due to illness, and discomfort imposed on them from outside, for the sake of cure.

It is sufficient to note here that the parental method of accounting for the use of, in this case, the anal thermometer creates additional confusions for the child. Medication will be discussed later.

### The child's offering

These 3- to 4-year-old children appeared to take little initiative in cueing their parents in to their condition. With the youngest children this included the everyday changes as found with tiredness, in addition to illness. For example, one mother reported: 'He never says he's tired, therefore we say he looks tired and lead him off [to bed]'. Nevertheless one must be cautious in attributing a lack of intention on the part of the children to communicate about their state, as what I am presently reporting here is what has been reported by the parents. An ethological analysis could have revealed a rudimentary signalling system which neither child nor parent was yet fully aware of, or able to reflect on. The children's language is moulded into the shape of the parents' language, through the parents' continual assumptions about the children's signalling competences for sharing their states. The parents' responses to the child's changing state and naming of it help him communicate about it. The immediate assumption is that this parental strategy can only be effective so long as the parental perceptions are accurate. It appears that effectiveness is rather dependent on the child having his state labelled similarly by the important adults around him. The word he learns to describe his state then enters his vocabulary for further use in similar situations to those where it was applied (see Schacter & Singer (1962) for details of the parallel process for emotional states).

But the child is already aware that labels are given not just to provide factual information, the mathetic, but also for their pragmatic effects. An alternative way of making the above labelling strategy intelligible is to allocate it to the pragmatic mode – an easy confusion for a child to make as the modes are less distinct in adult speech. In this mode leading the child off to bed could be regarded as a form of parental control legitimated on the basis of the child's health needs over which the parents establish themselves as the rightful deciders. When parental responses to the child's state are being established they will naturally get their interpretation of the child's state wrong on occasion. It is to be expected that the child will be more prone to account for the parents' misplaced labelling in terms of the function that label is felt to have for justifying the further action, its pragmatic effect, rather than by giving them additional information about his state. Although I am in one way referring to children as though they had available a comprehensive research methodology, what I am trying to highlight is a cognitive learning process based on their experience of their parents' accounting for their varying states. The potential confusions which can arise will lead to alternative reactions to parental use of descriptions of body states, with alternative emotional reactions to the perceived degree of control. The mathetic mode introduces the idea of body states being facts, elevated to a reified status through the way in which they are talked about and perceived as being acted upon.

These young children were able to take some part in a dialogue with their parents about their condition when asked. Their typical complaint was one of soreness, after the parents had taken the initiative to ask 'What's the matter?' Mattsson & Weisberg (1970) found that 70% of 2-year-olds could verbalise their pain and discomfort to some extent. The form to the adults' questioning forces them to construct logically consistent accounts (Tizard & Hughes, 1984). Nevertheless some questions do not expect answers, such as that prevalent greeting 'How are you?', which does not really expect that one says anything about one's state. There were a few signs that the children regarded some adults' curiosity about 'What's the matter?' as lying in the same category, as it never led to anything.

In contrast to views in medical practice that soreness in children this age cannot be localised by them, these parents believed that their children specifically directed them to the source of their discomfort, pointing to sore ears, chest, head or tummy. The other description given besides soreness was 'not well', with no localisation of the feeling of discomfort. It is interesting to conjecture on the choice of the term soreness, which is a description that could cover the outcome of illness or accident, and so could be seen as ideal for any intermediate state of health, regardless of origin, prior to definitive labelling by the parents. In this sense it has some similarities with the use of the word *wola* (see p. 48), which is used to cover both accidents and illness in New Guinea. The children's choice of 'not well' is in line with Gillon's (1986) comments on health being an *adequate* state of well-being; the child is here registering his well-being as no longer adequate.

### Arriving at a decision

The parents differed markedly in their responses to the children's offerings towards making a decision about whether or not they were ill. Two extremes were encountered with all shades of opinion in between. They ranged from, 'Don't think children lie', and 'hasn't got to the stage of kiddology yet', to a belief that you cannot believe anything a child says or '[he] . . . just says sore something if he doesn't want to do something'. The parents, like scientists, are preoccupied with the validity of what they hear, often to a greater extent than with the validity of what they observe. Very early on interplay is encountered between the parents' decision-making about deceit and the child's tentative offerings about his internal state. The parents' moral set of values about this plays an important role in creating the moral order to the world of illness (see chapter 8 for further discussion of this).

Parents did entertain other possibilities, as in the case of two children who volunteered complaints of sore ears on a regular basis. The parents accounted for this as 'She complains of sore ears as a game' in one case, and 'She uses the sore ears if she's embarrassed' in the other. At this age this was the parents' perspective and was not reflected in an ability of the child to discuss her 'pretences'.

This variety of responses to the child could either confirm the child's ability to use words to describe his internal state accurately, or hinder his ability ever to put his internal state effectively into words, potentially leading to a sense of frustration. These hypotheses would require a different form of study for testing.

## *Parental pragmatic decision-making*

When parents remain uncertain about the presence of illness their whole decision-making process shifts ground. They appear to base their decision about how to respond to the child on the likely consequences of erring on one side or the other. They change from evaluating the child's state according to mathetic principles – deciding whether he is ill or pretending, naughty or distressed – to an examination of the functional consequences of the child being ill. They appear to ask themselves if it really matters whether he is ill or not. In other words what are the consequences of them getting the evaluation of the child's state 'wrong'. These consequences follow from their expectations of the correct ways to respond to illness, society's evaluation of them as caring parents, as well as what can follow for their child depending on their understanding of the different microsystems in which he participates. These represent decisions in the pragmatic mode.

Similar changes in the parents' decision-making become apparent for the children in a superficially similar situation. The parents could have come to the decision that the child was 'under the weather', a common expression for a 'half-ill' state which is neither well nor warrants the full benefits obtained by an ill person. This is a decision in the mathetic mode, but the consequences of coming to that decision are different from those pertaining with either an illness or a diagnosis that the child is healthy. In this state there are no regular ways of responding; instead pragmatic considerations determine what should happen next, depending on the parents' understanding of the child's world. In this situation, though, the child could have had his state definitively labelled by his parents and he is made aware of both mathetic and pragmatic considerations in the ways his state is labelled and responded to.

In the situation described above the child can easily come to confuse the mathetic and the pragmatic and deduce that he is ill from the parental responses, that is he makes a mathetic evaluation based on his parents' pragmatic considerations. His 'state' is then determined on the basis of his parents' understanding of how his microsystems function, the consequences for the child, rather than an evaluation of him as a person.

There is not really such a clear distinction between these two positions as I am suggesting, as a tendency to use the label 'under the weather' rather than ill can be determined by a knowledge of how the child's illness would otherwise disrupt the parental routines.

These difficulties are illustrated mainly with the decisions about whether the child is well enough to go to nursery or not. This change in routine is very important for the majority of children, although this importance was not always acknowledged by the parents. The decision to keep the child at home breaks important attachments for the child on an illness rationale. Nevertheless, a mother found nothing incongruous in saying 'Nurseries are not important so we keep him at home if in doubt'. On analysing the premises for this position it was rather that the moral order concerned with keeping a child away from a nursery school is very different from that involved with keeping a child away from school. Although those apparently moral considerations are playing a role in the parents' evaluation of appropriate action in the circumstances, the child's understanding of his internal states and appropriate responses to them are being established.

Instead of erring in the direction of 'stay at home', alternative conclusions were reached in four other families: These were three families in which both parents worked and one single-parent family where the mother worked. In these families all the children were sent to nursery if there was any doubt. The advantage to the parents was the child's attendance at nursery. Two typical comments were: 'If he stands up he goes to school' and 'They've always gone to nursery as I work – and they weren't ill'. The latter response seemed to reflect the mother's feeling that she had erred in the right direction as the child was not subsequently labelled as ill by the nursery staff. These decisions are not without strong moral pressures in some communities about what 'mothers are there for', and so there are strong pressures on these parents, and especially the mothers, to get the decision 'right' rather than to evaluate what could be in the child's and family's best interests, and most helpful for the child's further development with recognition of the role the decision plays in the formation of early attitudes to appropriate illness behaviour. The effects this family structure and decision-making could have on the relation between the nursery, the parents and the child will be discussed later.

Other research has suggested that if the mother feels guilty about working she might overcompensate by encouraging dependent behaviour in her children, with the result that they will be more likely to remain at home when 'under the weather' (Hoffman, 1974). In this case the mother's moral code determines the child's illness behaviour, or more correctly the child's behaviour which he comes to equate with illness behaviour, and incorporates in his growing set of expectations for those circumstances.

Amongst older hospitalised children (6–12 years) Campbell (1978) noted a weak association between the longer time the mother was at work and a lesser degree of emotional reaction to illness amongst the children. This was independent of age and sex of these American children, and maternal educational level or paternal socioeconomic status. There was no association between the hours worked by the mother and willingness of the child to reject the sick role.

In one other family a similar strategy was adopted of virtually always sending the child to nursery, but what was important for the child's developing understanding about illness was that the action was accounted for in a totally different way. It seemed to reflect a sort of military pathos: 'There's nothing you can do about illness anyway so you just keep going.' There was no point for this family in giving up and retiring from active service, but at the same time there was no sense of the child being introduced to potentially effective healing strategies – helplessness without hopelessness.

### The role of doctors

The previous section described some of the strategies adopted at times of uncertainty. It might well have been expected that a third strategy of consultation with professionals would also have been employed. Instead this strategy was markedly absent at this phase in the family life cycle in families where the children had not experienced major illness. When the children had been younger the parents described using doctors in different ways, viewing it that 'when your child is so tiny you don't want to mess about'. Acceptable caring in the society insists that this is the 'right' response at that age. Mothers tend to consult doctors more often with their first babies if they have had previous experience with looking after other babies (Pattison, Drinkwater & Downham, 1982); it is as though they have already learnt the acceptability of consulting doctors about babies. Campion & Gabriel (1985) found that this only applied to first babies, and interpreted this as being due to the mothers learning from experience and having reduced their uncertainty. The comments of the mothers in my group about doctors tended to convey the premise that doctors could and almost should give the definitive answer on the young child's condition.

As the children got older the more common illnesses were portrayed as relatively less dangerous, and the families believed that they should manage more on their own. The parents did not wish to be seen as fussing too much. This same behaviour was found in other parts of Scotland (Macaskill & Macdonald, 1982 p. 70). Mothers do not wish to define their children as unhealthy as this is seen as reflecting on their mothering skills (Blaxter & Paterson, 1982a). Although parents expressed a wish to be able to phone a doctor for a discussion and opinion they felt discouraged from doing this as 'they only want to know if your child is really ill'. The doctor is thought to expect the diagnosis in terms of seriousness and possibly also in name to have been made beforehand by the family.

I see this picture as leading to referrals being determined by a breakdown in family coping, rather than as an integrated part of the diagnostic and healing procedures (see Shapiro (1983) for further discussion of family coping styles in the face of illness, and Hammer (1983) for the different ways social networks influence this process). The set of expectations described here fits in with the descriptions of consultations in predominantly naturalistic systems which are firstly for treatment; other networks are supposed to have helped address the carer's uncertainties beforehand. The role of the breakdown in coping which could have precipitated the referral is not addressed in treatment. The timing of the referral is then linked by the doctor to the child's condition rather than the condition of the child's support network. Yet Yudkin's (1961) research on mothers bringing children with coughs to consultations made it quite clear that the predominant factor determining the timing was the mother's condition and associated intentions, rather than the child's symptoms. These observations suggest that a critical change necessary for a more comprehensive preventive medicine is to open up the use of doctors in the parental decision-making phase. The implications this will have on various responsibilities and the influences of stresses in the families on consultation behaviour will be discussed in chapter 9.

Regardless of the degree of accuracy of the parents' diagnoses a form of relationship with the family is encouraged which through force of local myth* forces the family's reliance on their own resources. The myth has an added effect in that it discourages testing of the myth, a process dependent on discussion which is said to be taboo. This all adds to the develop-

* I prefer that description here as the parents who reported these views had not necessarily tested them directly with their doctors but instead reported and acted on what they had heard locally. I do not want to imply that these views were a reflection of the doctors' intentions, but they had been elevated to the status of facts about the local doctors. It is probable that these views

ment which does not allow the melding of lay and medical systems of decision-making, instead becoming one of the ways in which a boundary is maintained between the two systems such that it could maintain clashes of perspective.

Although friends often act in an advisory capacity for people who are uncertain about what to do, they tend to advise that medical help be sought (Calnan, 1983). Where the differences between the doctor's culture and the parents' culture are minimal consultation is more common (Freidson, 1961). These are likely to be situations in which expectations of a consultation are similar on both sides, and there are similar processes for accounting for illness in the macrosystem – there is a shared conceptual framework. There appear to be advantages if this shared framework can come to include the expectation that it will lead to facilitation of home nursing. Shrand (1965) reported mothers as having greater satisfaction and confidence, and their children coming to 'love mother more', after home nursing. The mother's participation in the care of her child, her 'required helpfulness' in contrast to 'learned helplessness', facilitates resolution of any sense of guilt (Shapiro, 1983) and would seem to restore to the mother a sense of effectiveness which otherwise could be jeopardised.

The above describes the role of the doctor in terms of the parental expectations and uses of consultation with nursery school age children. It must not be forgotten that the children's expectations are very different. I come to their views in the subsequent chapters, my main aim here being to establish the structure which is shaping and being shaped by the children. In contrast the children are waiting, for example, for the stethoscope to be laid on to 'see if I'm happy' (Steward & Regalbuto, 1975) or, as I found on occasion, to take away their germs and make them better. The first possibility is an interesting one which reminds us of the constant interaction of mood states with illness states in parents and children which must not be lost sight of when interpreting the ways in which microsystem functioning could lead to such intertwining (see chapter 8).

### The family and the nursery school

As the majority of episodes of illness were minor and not brought to the attention of the doctor, it was not possible to check on the degree of consensus between the parental and medical decision-making. Pattison *et*

were based in fact as Bloor & Horrobin (1975) have shown that they were inherent in the typical expectations of a group of doctors from Aberdeen for appropriate patient behaviour. Nevertheless it is not appropriate to impose untestable stereotypes onto all doctor–patient relations, although they establish the set of initial expectations.

*al.* (1982) have shown in Newcastle that mothers' diagnoses of illness in
their first babies were confirmed by the medical profession, and I have
no reason to doubt the descriptions of minor illness offered to me. The
particularly interesting episodes to have investigated further would have
been those where the children were 'under the weather'.

It was possible to check on whether any of the children were perceived
by the nursery staff as being sent to nursery more frequently than expected
when ill. Was there a group whom they felt was being sent inappropriately
to nursery? I specifically checked on the four children mentioned above
who had parents out at work and who went to nursery 'if they could stand'.
The nurseries saw them as always healthy. They never had to contact these
parents to collect their children because of illness. From discussion with
the nursery school teachers and nursery nurses it did not appear that this
represented either a protective response from them towards children who
might otherwise be 'neglected' at home or a case of the female staff being
protective of other working women. It was not as if these children of dual
career families were prematurely expected to be able to fend for themselves
– a conclusion that was also arrived at by Carlson (1984). The nursery
staff recounted a different group of children whom they felt were sent to
the nursery when ill (here using the nursery point of view on illness), but
I was not in a position to discern particular characteristics of the decision-
making processes in these families.

One difficulty with interpreting these impressions is to know how important these observations are. Clearly a specific research hypothesis would
be required to elucidate what goes on with children who are sent to nursery
only to be returned home later that morning as being ill. The impression
of the staff was that this was a clearly defined group of children, and I
suggest this for an important future project.

At present I believe that the hypothesis which suggests itself is dependent
on the above observations. These children must have an illness vocabulary
which is coherent with that of the staff at the nursery. It is therefore likely
that they have a similar cultural background. It appears initially unlikely
that one circumscribed group of children becomes ill more often than
others during nursery hours. This suggests that circumstances are eliciting
their language for presenting their internal discomforts, and that the language available to them is the illness language which they share with staff
and parents. They are dependent on using a vocabulary which makes a
difference to the staff, and which obtains the rewarding response – here
hypothesised as being reunited with the family. As the children's language
for sharing forms of stress is initially more rudimentary and open to more

misinterpretations I believe that what is happening here is that a language of distress is being wrongly labelled but with the 'right' results in that the stress is alleviated. The problem comes through the building up of a pattern which can have other consequences later. Alternative hypotheses are required if the nursery staff noted illness behaviour as soon as the child arrived.

It will be seen later with the older children how the relation between school and parents plays its part in this interpretative process going on in the school microsystem which affects the emotional climate of how the child is returned to the family. This emotional climate sets some of the moral tone to these evaluations of the child's state. Just as mothers are said to feel free from any criticism of their mothering capabilities when an infection is the cause of the child's trouble, the above hypothesis I present for testing would be facilitated in settings where teachers were vulnerable to criticism of their ability to care for their children and support them under stress.

Although the above is a working hypothesis it is uncertain yet whether it is warranted. One way in which the nursery staff accounted for the situation was that the parents of these children lacked a knowledge about the demands made on the children in the nursery. There seemed to be a lack of recognition that it was impossible to devote individual attention to a child at nursery in a way which should be possible at home. It was seen as though the parents hoped that the child would get 'ideal' parenting at the nursery, possibly being reticent about their own abilities at home or acknowledging the limits of their abilities. The relations between the nursery staff and the parents, the mesosystem, then affected how these children were responded to. If the relationship was poor, the ill children tended to elicit the staff's frustration and annoyance to the potential detriment of the support required by the children in their illnesses.

These preliminary results give the impression that children who are tentatively kept at home just in case they are ill could begin to equate more signs with significant illness than those who are sent to the nursery 'if they could stand'. As appropriate illness behaviour is moulded through the parents' responses the child may eventually be seen by others outside the family as more often ill.

Although the parents recognised that they had to take the initiative in deciding whether their child was ill, they still lived with some fear that they would have made a 'mistake' and sent their child to nursery ill. The teachers were often seen as experts in this field who would be quite critical of parents who got it wrong. Besides these feelings which could make parental decision-making more burdensome, it was also becoming more difficult because of a change in the outlook of the 4-year-olds who had established longer-term relations with people at the nursery. These children valued their contacts at the nursery very highly and were often extremely reluctant to stay at home, so much so that, 'It's very difficult to find out if she's ill before she goes to nursery as she doesn't want to tell you'. For parents who give special prominence to verbal messages from their children this could become a major problem.

The growth in the importance of the child's own separate social world and her ability to keep aspects of herself secret and pretend, characterise the 8-year-old primary school children to a greater extent. There were only occasional hints of this with the 3–4-year-old children.

### *Implications for the child*

It has been seen that the parents tried to decide whether their children were ill through checking whether all their observations were coherent in order to warrant their decision that the child was ill. If they remained uncertain pragmatic considerations crystallised the decision. For the child the distinction between a pragmatically grounded decision and one made on the basis of parental certainty that the child was ill was not immediately possible. The children appeared to function on the premise that all dimensions were important if they were to be seen as ill. Not attending nursery was as important as the not feeling hungry, looking pale and feeling lethargic, even if the parents said that attendance at the nursery was not important. This latter view of a minority of parents seemed to reflect a parental view that the children's relationships formed there were not very important or that the child would not notice a short disruption to them. In addition they reacted to the fact that the child was not involved in 'work' at nursery and hence there would be no educational delay in the event of them not attending.

It is the children's emphasis on the value of their relationships and how they interpret their disruption dependent on the happenings in their primary microsystems which leads to the following proposition about the nature of illness for nursery school age children. At the same time this sort of proposition must be expected from the basic assumptions made about the prime place of intersubjectivity in the child's reality. The prime place of intersubjectivity is coherent with the observation that the state of the eye contact is important from the parents' point of view when making their evaluation of the child's state. Other elements for the child are the sense of constancy of his personal state, and the attachments to his carers and friends. Once his capacity for reflection has developed these give him his basis from which he can say he is healthy. Deviations from this basis are then included in the illness proposition.

*Proposition*

*Illness:* Something counts as illness if it affects an important dimension to the child's relation with a significant other person and is labelled as illness.

At this age the children appeared to be limited to noting things which changed the qualities of their relations, rather than being able to observe illness in another because of its effect on a relationship of that person with a third person. The range of significant people involved nursery school staff, their peers and family members. An example illustrates some of the reasons for suggesting this proposition. One child was certain that his father was not ill when he had a slipped disc and was laid up in bed at home. The reason lay in the lack of disruption to the child's normal relation with his father who still read him his regular bedtime story which was the important dimension to their relation for the child. The fact that he could not go to work did not alter this child's perception.

Apple (1960) looked at how laymen define illness and concluded that they base their decision on the way in which the change in their condition interferes with their usual activities. For the children I observed that change which was most important to them was their relationship with people important to them. With adolescents it has been suggested that the best way of engaging them in health/illness matters is through looking with them at how their condition affects their activities and relationships (Millstein *et al.*, 1981).

These children did not see themselves as ill when they had colds, apparently because the colds did not prevent them going to nursery, or make any difference to their routines involving the people important to them. An exception illustrates the illness proposition especially clearly. Within the nursery, but not my sample, was one boy who had a baby sister with an immune deficiency disorder. It was very important for him not to catch a cold as he would then need to be isolated from her. For him colds were serious illnesses. By the time the children are 8 years old colds have become one of the most valuable illnesses which open up several possibilites for renegotiating their position in relation to friend and foe alike.

Not being able to go out to play was one of the cardinal features of illness, but the telling feature for the children was that they then missed

their contacts with their friends. It was this parental strategy which under-
lined the seriousness of grey states of half-illness. Interestingly this observation has been made use of in a 'Get Well Soon' card where the recipient
is encouraged to get well because the sender says 'I don't have anyone to
play with' (Camden Graphics Ltd).

The above proposition about illness fits with descriptions of children
this age being in a world of social symbiosis (Harré, 1977), in which their
attachment needs predominate (Bowlby, 1969). If the prosposition proves
warranted it lends particular importance to the parental decision to disrupt
the child's routine of attending the nursery and being separated from
significant people there on an overtly illness rationale. The social explanations and rules then appear to be the ones which guide the parents' decision-
making and imposition of appropriate illness behaviour on the child. The
children are brought up with the beliefs that ill people are short on appetite,
lethargic, pale and unable to maintain relationships with friends, and these
are reflected in their beliefs about what is important when pretending
illness (see table 8.1, p. 180).

These beliefs must also be set in the context of the dominant form of
illness experienced by the children of this age. The illnesses are largely
the common infectious illnesses of childhood and also vomiting and diarrhoea. My sample of 16 included 7 children who had had measles, 7 who
had had whooping cough and 2 who had had mumps. As the children's
social network has rapidly expanded at this age with the move to nursery
school, there are then two reasons for the greater awareness of illness at
this time; the first is the larger social group from whom the illness can be
caught with potential for an increase in personal illness frequency, the
second is the increased number of important relations which can be disrupted because of illness so that illness becomes more salient for the child.

Kalnins & Love's (1982) review reported children's views on health
which appear coherent with these views on illness proposed here: 'The
available data suggest that children at all ages conceptualise health as a
state arising from the observation of a series of practices or rules including
eating proper food, getting exercise, and keeping clean', with eating taking
precedence. These practices form the substance of chapters 6 and 7.

### The child's illness and the parental roles

Parental decision-making can be predominantly in either the mathetic or
pragmatic modes, which introduces the child to these worlds of social
explanation. The child is also introduced to another framework at this
age. The decisions and responses to an ill child are usually made by more

than one person, and where relevant I have referred to parents. In this sample the parents discussed together whether the child was ill, a decision which often was taken in the early morning or evening when both parents were together. Through the form of their discussion the social explanations and rules about illness were elaborated. In this way the children became more aware of the nature of illness, which ceased to be an all or none state but one with various shades of 'under the weather' being evaluated by the parents. In many other families the decision is left to the mothers (Mayall, 1986).

It is already known that for couples with 'traditional conjugal relationships', where there is unequal power in decision-making, there tends to be poorer health and health behaviour regardless of whether it is a matriarchal or patriarchal power system (Pratt, 1972). Shapiro's (1983) review points out that 'good adjustment to illness is found in families in which (a) there is a clear separation of the generations, (b) a satisfying of each other's emotional and psychological needs, (c) flexibility within roles, (d) toleration for individuation and (e) communication which is direct and consistent, and tends to confirm the self esteem of the other'.

Unequal expertise and power in decision-making about illness was most clear in two of my families where the mothers were nurses. In these households the fathers felt that they had no expertise about illness matters. Here illness was never discussed but pronounced upon by the female health expert. These mothers had a different style of consulting the doctor. They described consulting when their children were over their illness, but before they sent them back to the nursery, with the intention of getting the doctor to confirm that the child was healthy. The aim of this seemed to be to pre-empt discussion with the school staff about whether the child was well enough to return or not. A long-term follow-up would be required to find out how these children subsequently handled illness in themselves and others, and whether it differed significantly from those children who had been exposed to more detailed discussion and debate about their half-illness states. The latter parents seemed to be more open in discussing their uncertainties about the child's state, something which can have its own advantages (see chapter 8). The strategies of the nurses excluded the child being exposed to discussion about his state in alternative settings and so the strategy was particularly powerful.

I do not believe that this strategy is a reflection of nurses but of unequal expertise and some uncertainty about that expertise being respected, or of being open to respect the lay expertise of others. It is likely that the same problems would arise with other health workers, but the problems would perhaps be greatest when it came to respect for doctors' expertise.

In 4 of the 16 families the parents felt that they had equal expertise on health matters, but in the others the mothers were perceived by the adults in the family as the health experts although this was not always so clear from the child's point of view, or as categorical as in the nurses' families. Some children seemed aware of the ways in which conjugal power hierarchies can operate as illustrated in this comment: 'Daddy tells Mummy to get up and come through [in the night]'. Further exploration of the child's view elicited that the father was seen as having the knowledge which was then passed on to the mother as though she was the father's agent. The parents were flabbergasted at the child's description of how they were perceived when he told them this in a family interview. Through illness children learn about respective sex role behaviour, as well as imposing their views of what constitutes appropriate sex role behaviour in accounting for the adults' behaviour. By the time that they are at nursery school children already have established sexual stereotypes for their peers (Kuhn, Nash & Brucken, 1978) and this includes what care roles are felt appropriate for whom and who should play doctor.

Other mothers did bow to perceived male expertise in the treatment of accidents. One mother said 'I'm sort of probably a little bit sort of calmer with illness. I think F. flaps a bit when I wouldn't. And in an emergency F. would be better than me 'cos I'm inclined to get paralysed'. Here an emergency was equated with an accident or a sudden crisis in the illness. The men felt themselves experts with accidents for a variety of reasons including a First Aid course with the Territorial Army and familiarity with rugger injuries. What was common to these situations where they had learnt their skills was that they were particularly male settings associated with 'tough man' pursuits.

This pattern of women being perceived as the experts with illness and taking over its management, whilst men manage the accidents, is similar to the sex roles identified in many non-Western cultures where women provide the *care* required during illness whilst men *cure* the injuries (Loudon, 1976 p. 27). This difference has been stereotyped here in the sex roles of nurses compared with doctors, a sex role typing which also occurred in the children's play in the nurseries.

From these elements in the social framework it can be seen that the children's illnesses have functional effects on family relations through exaggerating differences in the parents and their perceived knowledge about illness and accidents. At the same time the children are introduced to role models about how to respond as a male or female to illness. An additional effect on illness in either parent is that it disrupts established sex role patterns. When the ill person is the mother who has always made the food and father must do it for the first time, children of this age can be rather concerned, finding the change in routine either mildly disturbing or a 'joke'.

## Developmental changes in the family microsystem

There remains the question of whether the processes described above continue to characterise decision-making about children throughout childhood. Although the best strategy for testing the durability of particular frameworks would have been to follow one family over several years this option was not open to me. Instead I saw families with 8- and 13-year-old children in order to see whether there were any characteristic shifts through these ten years of family life cycle. This perspective provided additional information about further social influences moulding the child's illness framework, but it is more difficult at the present time to say much about the connections between the different age groups. There are intelligible ways of accounting for the changes but alternative research strategies will have to be adopted to see whether they are warranted.

In order to advance the analysis of the processes giving rise to a particular social order around illness it would be necessary to follow these children through to adulthood and examine their decision-making as parents. I have not included here the origin of these parents' views on illness or any description of their childhood illness experiences. The concept of the parents' views as having a clear origin is perhaps misleading as it would be expected that reminiscences of what had occurred for them when managing their children's illnesses had been coloured by their own previous experiences and in turn have modified their children's experiences. The parents' subsequent experiences will have flavoured their recall; their children will have indirectly shaped their parents' recall of their histories.

### *Drawing up boundaries through illness*

With the youngest children I relied primarily on the parents for the description of the family structure. Observations of the children's responses and views have been included in order to highlight the coherence of the account. With the older children it is possible to obtain their own reflections on the family structure as moulded by illness to set beside the parents' descriptions and my observations. These reflections include their perceptions of the functional potentials of illness. The way in which the children's views on this dimension were obtained was through the use of a special non-verbal technique, 'Drawing up Boundaries' (Wilkinson, 1985), devised specifically for this research.

In principle I had asked children to draw their families according to the guidelines of Burns & Kaufman (1971) for Kinetic Family Drawings (KFD). They were asked to 'Draw a picture of everyone in your family, including you, doing something. Try to draw whole people, not cartoons or stick people. Remember, make everyone doing something – some kind of action.' The action element stresses the connections between the family members, so that when the children were asked to do a subsequent drawing with the modification that one person was ill, I was in a position to deduce the functional effects of illness on the relations between the family members (see Wilkinson (1985) for a discussion of the interpretation and validity of this information). This functional relatedness is a part of the family structure which has evolved over the intervening years (Minuchin, 1974). I will now illustrate the sorts of functional potential that illness can have through an analysis of two sets of drawings done by 8-year-old boys. The views of the children on illness, representing the mathetic, follow in the subsequent chapters, but they must be interpreted together with an understanding of the pragmatic effects as illustrated here. The following account is therefore a description of these drawings, the children's own accounts and my interpretations. My aim has been to elucidate the pragmatic potentials of illness through the eyes of the children. It is expected that these potentials reflect and create the ways in which the primary structure has evolved.

In the first drawing using the standard KFD instructions (fig. 4.1) there is no clear compartmentalisation around the three family members but there is little coherence to their activities. The top figure was described as mother 'doing the dusting'. Father is the next figure and is much smaller, portrayed 'on his way out to play the cello'. In the drawing the boy, 'John', is at the bottom of the picture doing something apart from his parents. All figures were drawn very lightly and this accounts for their poor reproduction. Rather than interpret all the elements here I will move on to the comparison with the drawing of the family 'with one member ill', as it is the change which tells us about the pragmatic effects. The categories which I used for analysing the drawings are found in Wilkinson (1985).

The pattern of relations is markedly different in fig. 4.2. The three people in this family reverted to closely involved dyadic relationships when one person was ill. These alliances were sharply demarcated, the compartments being sharply defined through the use of ruled lines. In contrast to the first drawing the top people are John and his father, with father described as actively involved in caring. This contrasts with father's min-

Fig. 4.1. John's Kinetic Family Drawing.

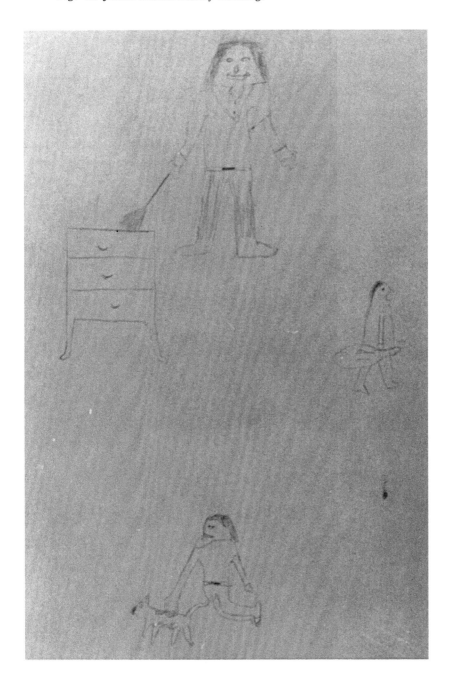

Fig. 4.2. John's drawing of the family in illness.

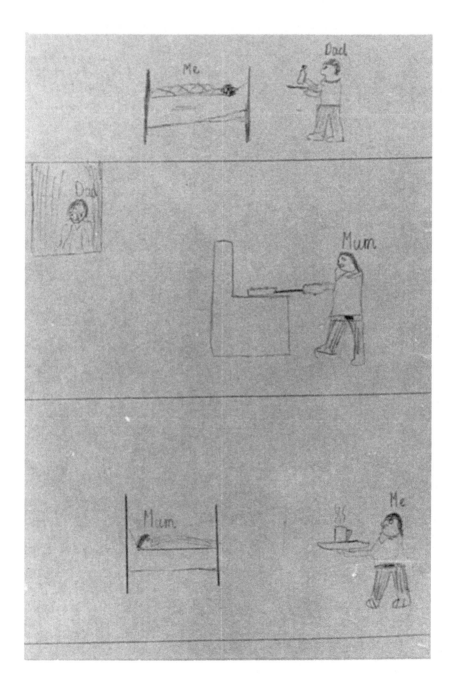

imal presence in the first picture and his disengagement from the other family members. In fig. 4.2 John's relationship to his mother is in mirror form to that usually encountered in health as John is described as caring for his mother rather than vice versa. The instruction was to do a drawing involving one person being ill, yet here everyone had to have their 'turn'. Father's turn is different from that of the other family members. The drawing shows him without legs, which I interpret as making it impossible for him to be 'leaving' the family as he was described as doing in the first drawing. Father appears framed and not in a position to lie down and receive care from his wife, who although 'preparing food for him' seems to be ambivalent about it, the cooker reflecting a form of barrier between them.

Taken together this pair of drawings shows one way in which alliances, which are otherwise absent, can be created by illness. Shapiro's (1983) review also described how illness could have a 'beneficial' effect on family function in just this sort of family situation. Father's position was on the outskirts of the healthy family (and was confirmed in the family interview section of the research which followed this phase with the children alone). Illness can be seen to have had a potential role of keeping him more involved, but solely for the child. The parents appear disengaged and illness with its especial demands on caring was not sufficient to alter this pattern. These drawings enabled the child to talk about the effects of illness on relationships without him first having to find words to describe the different effects. I do not wish to suggest that illness always has the same effect, but rather to open up some considerations of how it can play its part in loosening up established ways of relating. Illness represents a challenge to established practices which we develop for living together; it makes demands on our role flexibility and sensitivity to each other. Children have their own impressions of these effects and it is important to approach their viewpoints and so respect their experiences. John's drawings represent part of his range of experience of the pragmatic effects of illness as confirmed in the further discussion with him and his family.

Another pair of drawings (figs. 4.3 and 4.4) illustrates a different kind of effect of illness on family relationships. There appear to be countless variations on the themes revealed here. In consultations and in meeting children it is most important that no assumptions are made in advance as to what sort of effect illness will have in that child's family; instead efforts must be made to find out. The family structure existing prior to the onset of illness will set the scene for the possibilities open to the family members for reorganising in the face of illness.

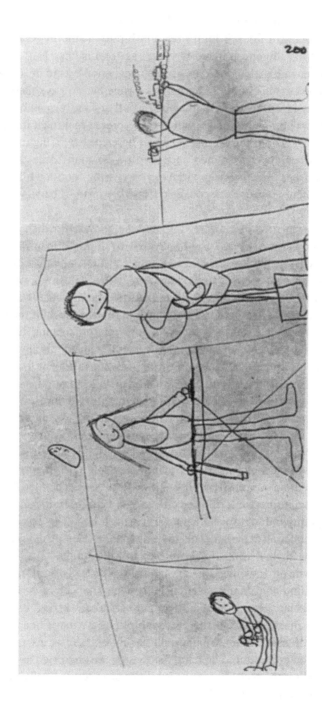

Fig. 4.3. David's Kinetic Family Drawing.

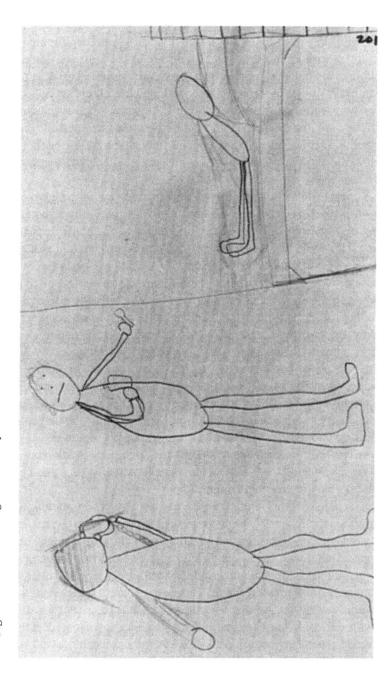

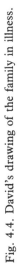

Fig. 4.4. David's drawing of the family in illness.

In this second pair of drawings the different impact of illness must be anticipated when it is seen that the initial family structure in health is different (fig. 4.3). The first drawing of the family is highly compartmentalised with drawn-up boundaries, but nevertheless the family members are in touch with each other – the parents are in the centre of things and the children are more peripheral. The parents are described as 'doing their own things'. Mother is ironing; father is 'digging with his spade'. These figures were equally firmly drawn, and the relative sizes suggest equal significance for the child of mother and father. The one person whom I interpret as keeping his emotions hidden, revealing only his back, is the boy who did the drawing, 'David'. His younger sister plays contentedly in her own way.

The impact of illness alters the whole structure. David is now the sole focus of the parents' activities. He appears to have established a boundary around his own compartment. This is interpreted as potentially controlling too much intrusion by his parents or protecting them from him as his own particular form of quarantine boundary. It was not possible in the further discussion to be quite clear about how he saw the space he had created. His younger sister is excluded from this picture, which I interpret as a way of re-creating in illness the initial family threesome where he returns to being the sole preoccupation of the parents. The parents appear to become united in their task to make him better, with no boundary drawn between them, as mother rings to the doctor and father comes with medicine. Both roles were described with equal importance and linked together through the medical advice given over the telephone. The parental emotions have changed. In the drawing their smiling faces have disappeared, and mother's face is not even shown. David meanwhile appears faceless, reflecting an avoidance of his own emotions. Additionally his arms are not included, possibly being David's way of saying that he had no hand to play in creating his illness.

Interpretations of this kind may appear to be of uncertain validity. When trying to see the effects of illness from the child's position there is much greater reliance on interpretation of non-verbal clues than might be the case with adults, who have a good command of verbal ways of describing their discomforts and whose descriptions additionally appear trustworthy. The interpretations presented here use the experience of others in interpreting children's drawings so that hypotheses can be further tested in discussion with the child. The aim is to provide some idea of what sorts of things children in general are preoccupied with and some of the 'hows' and 'whys' about these. The interpretative stage is always central for all who wish to know as nearly as possible the internal state of another, or to know the child's own views on how illness affects him.

These two examples of drawings by 8-year-olds give a glimpse of some of the data which had to be fitted into the individual interviews, open-ended questionnaires and family interviews. They show some of the children's perspectives on family boundaries as part of family structure and how these can be altered in illness. I will now briefly return to the social context which has framed these views, that of the adult's views on illness. I will do this in general terms as I am not here trying to elucidate details of the connections between children's views and those of their parents, rather the general social and developmental influences.

It will be recalled that Herzlich (1973) formulated three types of illness experience which she labelled as illness being 'destructive', 'liberating' or an 'occupation'. She had been using the individual's own perspective on his illness and did not have the benefit of an objective developmental history in order to interpret the origin of these views. Looking again at the examples of drawings given here they could be categorised according to the same schema. In this way potential origins of the adult positions can be postulated for future research testing.

In discussion with John it became clear that the altered boundaries in illness emphasised the pain of the lack of care between the parents. This was less prominent when they were healthy. The closeness which illness generated for him and his mother on the one hand, and himself and his father on the other, could have been perceived warmly and as being potentially liberating for John in his apparent isolation as presented in the first drawing. However at this age and time it was not interpreted as such by him. John perceived the loss or 'destruction' of the tentative relations between the three moderately independent people, as portrayed in the first drawing, as relatively more important. This was in spite of the way in which the coherence of the three figures can appear minimal to an outside observer. John's understanding of the sick role could therefore be described as an early stage of one sort of 'destructive' view of illness.

I checked with David how he saw the effects of his illness. In further discussion he described the advantages in having his parents to himself. He described his parents as more together in the illness situation. In other words the advantages came from the alterations in alliances and boundaries. Emotional pain was blanked out as indicated by the 'blank' faces in the drawing. The importance of emotions could have got him to categorise the situation as 'destructive'. Instead it was the altered alliances which proved to be the more salient for him. In contrast to John, David's views on the 'uses' of illness could be interpreted as a precursor to the adult 'liberating' view of illness. This could only persist if family structure continued to alter in a way which David continued to perceive as 'liberating'. At the same time it has been at the expense of the emotional component to the illness experience, which has been submerged. These interpretations which emphasise the importance of effects of illness on relationships fit with the proposition of illness presented earlier.

Throughout development the family would be expected to have to alter in different ways in the face of illness in order to have the same effect on David's perceptions of the changes consequent on illness. Whether these boys will feel the same way about their experiences of illness in the future is a different question demanding a different form of enquiry. For the 8-year-olds in general, themes of illness as destructive or liberating appeared; additionally some showed more ambivalent relations to illness where the advantages and disadvantages were more finely balanced. The evaluations were not simple and they could only be made knowing the child's value system and family structure, as well as how things were going at school etc.

When looking at the drawings of the 13-year-olds the same functional effects of illness are described by the children and observed in their drawings. The nature of the analysis meant that it was not straightforward to exclude or include the presence of illness as an occupation as this reflects a process over the course of the illness, a refined attitude which could not easily be expressed through a discussion of alliances and boundaries at the onset of illness. Illness as an occupation reflects more the development of personal responsibility in the face of illness and this was neither excluded nor confirmed through the form of enquiry I used.

In conclusion these drawings have shown ways in which the family decison-making and responses to ill children have led to definite changes in family functioning in the face of illness. These changes can only be appreciated in detail through knowing the child's world of illness from the child's perspective. Traces of the experiences of illness as a destroyer or liberator are found in both 8-year-old and 13-year-old children.

*Impact of verbal development*

The major change in family explanations and decision-making about illness as children get older is the increased verbal contribution from the child. Although the child's ability to name his discomforts is built up within the framework already described, his use of that ability rapidly alters the functioning of that framework. Once the child had mastered the words for communicating about his body states, including illness states, the parents described their role altering substantially: 'It's hard to remember before she could actually tell you because that's a very difficult stage, when you can't tell what's wrong with them. But now she can say whether it's an ear or a tummy or a throat' (mother of an 8-year-old). The changed role was associated with a change in parental strategies for diagnosing their children's discomforts. The children now play a much more active part in reducing their parents' uncertainty about their condition. This depends on parental trust in the child's accurate use of his initially limited vocabulary, as well as the parents' abilities to discriminate states of exaggerated or pretended soreness.

Some parents recognise that one of their coping mechanisms is a need to rely on their children being 'well enough' in order for the adults to cope with their own worries. One mother of an 8-year-old, who had had a previous child die through a cot death said, 'We err on the side of not believing him rather than worrying too much'. This was when the child complained verbally of discomforts which could well have been labelled as illness. The predominant aim here was for the parents to cope with the major worries raised through illness in their child, linked in their minds with the death of their previous child. They recognised their coping strategy as one of denying illness, or as it could be alternatively interpreted, as refusing the sick role to their child. An alternative strategy would have been to be sensitised to the slightest indications of illness in the child. The outcome of different parental strategies of this type for children's subsequent communication about their illnesses remains unknown.

Children by the age of 8 years are adept at playing roles and adopting the position of others. They experiment with this in the sphere of illness and illustrate in this way their beliefs about some of the most salient dimensions used in their families to decide on illness. They described for me the ways in which they might sit in front of an electric fire to make themselves flushed and appear to have an overwarm forehead, eat soap to make themselves sick, or go to the toilet and pretend to have vomited. These special factors tended to be superimposed on the changes in routine which their parents still emphasised as indicators of illness, such as the child being slow to get up in the morning or having a reduced appetite. By this age the children were able to control these behaviours and consciously adopt roles – but not always very successfully. Sometimes the parents' old strategies were still effective, as one boy described who had been deliberately slow in getting up. When subsequently faced with breakfast he recounted how he 'had to . . . eat if see others eating and I'm hungry'.

Generally, though, the parents are adopting new strategies to work out how much they can trust what their children are saying, and if there are degrees of pretending or exaggerating. The question of trust in the child's message seemed to be either very central or peripheral in the families I met. It was my impression that some parents appeared never to believe what the child said, relying instead on the non-verbal strategies which they had adopted when the child was younger. This approach would seem to have the potential for exaggerating the functional element in that non-verbal behaviour which could then become the child's predominant mode for expressing his frustration at not being understood verbally. Hence illness behaviour would become associated with frustration. The situation is analogous to that found in learnt helplessness (Abramson *et al.*, 1978), where the helplessness in this case centres on the verbal behaviour and only non-verbal behaviour is seen as effective. These individuals would have no vocabulary in the usual verbal sense for conveying their internal states. This hypothesis is discussed further in chapter 8.

### *The child's words*

So far the primary structure of the child's world of illness has been presented. In particular I have highlighted the functional qualities of illness, through illness being reacted to as though it was a message for other family members or other people in the child's microsystem. Illness has become associated with a particular value system, moral order and way of negotiating status. Illness behaviour appears to have a role in altering the structure of microsystems. These pragmatic aspects complement ways in which parents are trying to make definitive judgements about the presence or absence of illness or its type – the mathetic. The two aspects become intimately bound together, especially if the psychological discomforts are given as much prominence as the physical (see chapter 8).

Out of this mesh of intertwined messages the child has begun to establish a secondary structure concerning illness. He has changed from being predominantly a responder to the decisions and care of others to having a more durable value system of his own which comes out in a variety of different settings. It is this secondary structure which I will present in the following chapters, but provisionally I will describe here the words which the children have laid claim to as these reflect the culture which I have been describing.

The children used a variety of words for their body states. Some children were 'ill', others 'not well', 'not feeling well', 'sick' (which included feeling ill, vomiting and feeling as though one was going to vomit) or 'off colour'.

The most popular phrases for both the 8-year-olds and the 13-year-olds were 'not well' and 'not feeling well'. A particularly confusing word was 'poorly', which was used rarely and then only in three families who attributed its use to their English connections. When I enquired of a Scottish 4-year-old if he knew the word, he described the family being poorly 'only on Thursday evening' – pay day was Friday. A few children described getting 'bad feelings'; here a developing moral order about the rights and wrongs of illness was making itself felt, as 'bad' was used to reflect more than discomfort. One family pointed out that the adults in their household were 'ill', but the child was 'not very well'. Apparently they were attempting to decrease the anxiety in the child by allying the child's state with the intermediate states of tiredness and soreness rather than a definitive state of illness. Children are aware of the importance of this sort of game to keep the meaning of illness hidden and begin to adopt it themselves, describing for me how they sometimes kept what they thought of as illness secret from their parents so that the parents would not worry.

Although the children of 8 years and over felt competent in the use of these words they nevertheless were short of a precise vocabulary to explain the nuances of their condition which had given rise to their evaluation that they were not well. I was interested in finding out how they knew other people were ill also, i.e. to what degree were they able to use either the decision-making strategies which had been used with them earlier or other resources. The findings provide a degree of validity for the preceding interpretations of my observations. Additionally they show the child's ability to reflect on his situation. Once he has established a degree of secondary structure, he employs further strategies to elaborate on this basic form. If at the same time he is placed in, to him, incomprehensible situations it will tax his ability to integrate all the disparate elements within his basic framework. It was this sort of dilemma which Piaget described as potentially leading the child to revise his basic assumptions so that he accommodated to the new information, whereas normally it could be assimilated into his basic framework (Piaget & Inhelder, 1966). Assimilating to the basic framework has also been termed first-order change, while accommodating I see as analogous to second-order change (Watzlawick, Weakland & Fisch, 1974).

The 8-year-olds had some difficulty telling me how they knew they were ailing, commenting 'I don't know how to describe it. There are no words for it', or 'It's hard to find the word how you'd know you were sick'. They were able to discern a change in their internal state, but needed words to describe it more accurately than just 'not well'. Some descriptions were quite poetic: 'I felt as though I had no bones in me'. The visible illnesses such as those with spots and rashes were a different problem as any change which was superficial was quickly noticed. That change seemed to become the discomfort rather than the discomfort being associated with the state of being. In these cases the internal state was only indirectly labelled through linkage to the superficial but dramatic skin changes. Although the skin could itch terribly, that was a more localised discomfort.

The exanthemata had a special role in the child's development of illness concepts as there was very rarely any parental disagreement about the child's condition, in contrast to when the child described his own internal discomfort as that was unverifiable and relatively independent of external signs. Words could be used definitively about exanthemata without any trace of doubt. The conditions for optimal learning were present. The child's state of discomfort which arose before the rash enabled him to confirm his own suspicions about his malady even if the parents had not been receptive enough initially.

The 13-year-olds were less dependent on parental responsiveness to their altered condition as their increasingly important peer network of relationships provided them with a frequently florid vocabulary to describe their internal states. As the peer network and the parents had different ways of establishing the veracity of the 'complaint' and of respecting it, the alternative moral orders facilitated different forms of illness behaviour; when tried out in the other moral order they were often singularly unsuccessful, but this did not prevent many attempts at incorporating the adolescent illness behaviour in the family. It appeared as though they had especial needs for renegotiating their status in their peer milieu because their growing network of friends was in constant flux. Changed body states seemed to be used often, and both necessitated and facilitated the development of their florid vocabulary. At this point they made it clear that they did not share all their more vulgar expressions with me and I cannot exemplify their range, but have chosen to describe it as florid to convey the quality they wished to emphasise which set it apart from the language used at home.

The children had difficulties in recognising others as definitely ill. The most common response from the 8-year-olds was that they only knew when their parents were ill when they were told. It appeared that they had suspicions before this, though were uncertain to what degree they could rely on them. These suspicions seemed to arise when there was an alteration in the family routines, such as going to bed early, not getting up on time or moving the child to a separate room so that the adult could get some quiet. Particularly potent was a feeling that there was not the same degree of closeness with the adult. Here are found very clear parallels to the categories used with these children earlier. The changes in routines are important at one level but underlying this is the feeling that family rituals (Wolin & Bennet, 1984) can also be disrupted due to changes in the states of the family members. It takes a more serious illness to disrupt a ritual than it does a routine, with a more profound effect on the child.

The 13-year-olds were attempting to discriminate alternative causes for the alterations in family structure described as important by the 8-year-olds. They were drawing distinctions between parental illness, moodiness or cussedness. They both recognised and had a language to share with others the parental mood changes they observed. They entertained the possibility that a parent who was shouting at them more than usual could be ill. In this situation the personal vehemence was dissipated if the outburst was attributed to illness. Here the pragmatic effect of the anger disappeared because the child relabelled the meaning of the behaviour through assessing it predominantly within the mathetic mode. Because these children were older they were more familiar with parents using decision-making strategies and discussing their uncertainties about younger siblings. Hence they were influenced by two different perspectives on these processes; as direct interactants in their earlier childhood and as observers of the interaction of their parents and sibling, or teacher and pupil. I have no comments on the relative importance of these different elements from my observations, but note them for the complexity involved in accounting for the older children's views on illness and their illness behaviour. Perhaps some of the factors are here which play a role in the phenomenon whereby 'people do not ascribe their own sickness to moral transgressions, but they use these concepts in describing each other' (Cosminsky, 1977). I view it that this perspective is facilitated by being an observer of the ways in which others are socialised through the use of health/illness rationales.

## The schools and nursery schools

### Decision-making

The nursery and school worlds seem to introduce the children to alternative systems of explanation, rules and routines (see also Tizard & Hughes, 1984). When the routines are different the factors which make a difference to these routines must of necessity be different, and so the child's experiences are expanded. The primary and secondary schools had two parallel microsystems operating simultaneously: the world of the playground and the world of the classroom. At nursery the distinction was not pronounced as the people who organised the indoor time organised the outdoor time also and were equally present and active in both settings. Prout (1986) suggests that 'one of the most important modes by which children are integrated into cultural assumptions about sickness are located in the daily routines of the school around sickness absence and the teachers' and other pupils' responses to children's claims of sickness'. He sees this as part of the hidden school curriculum. I will not refer further to the world of the playground as some of the literature was referred to earlier and I did not observe the children in their play setting. By so doing I do not want to minimise the potential importance of what happens there.

Within the nursery school the decisions about health and illness are not as compartmentalised as in primary and secondary school where the function of the school welfare assistant, colloquially referred to as the school nurse, is carried out by the normal nursery school staff. The staff of nursery schools in Edinburgh have had a mixture of trainings, including those for teachers and nursery nurses. The decisions about illness in the 3–4-year-olds are made definitively by the people the children are with all the time, rather than the function being delegated to a welfare assistant.

Gender typing is seen to play its role in establishing expectations about the validity of illness claims in the older children. In the nursery gender typing was generally evident in the tendency for the girls to adopt nurses' roles, but it had not extended to expectations about the children's own illness claims. As an aside, it has been found in Edinburgh that if male nurses visit the nurseries the boys happily play the nurses' roles (personal communication: Craiglockhart project, 1978). Otherwise it is noted from the United States (Andersen (1977) in Garvey, 1984 p. 205) that these roles are played out with an apparent full understanding of the respective places in the social hierarchy of doctors and nurses, and of the hierarchical nature of the doctor–parent relationship in a consultation over a child. The hierarchical position of doctors over their patients and families seems from this to be established very early, at least in America. From Bristol in England it has recently been reported that children as young as 2 years old on an oncology ward had a similar grasp of the ward's social structure (Kendrick *et al.*, 1986). As it is known that hierarchical forms of relationship hinder the establishment of as near as possible 'ideal speech acts' (McCarthy, 1973) and thus reduce the likelihood that intimate information will be shared, research into how these beliefs are constructed in such young children has important bearings on facilitating consultative behaviour. Whether the children have developed this knowledge from personal experience, nursery school literature, parents' expressed views or from the multitude of other possible clues they meet daily is yet unknown. Maybe male nurses and female doctors could have informal discussions with children and their parents in order to introduce more facilitative beliefs as an early measure of preventive medicine!

The 8- and 13-year-old children who were thought to be ill were typically sent from the classroom to the welfare assistant after the teacher had been alerted to their condition. Although I did not observe this stage it has been reported from England (Prout, 1986) that children need to make at least three approaches to the teacher before getting to see the school secretary (there fulfilling the role of the welfare assistant). The first responses of the teacher were to suggest waiting to see how things developed, followed by getting the pupil to sit quietly and then finally sitting apart from the others as though he were half in and half out of the class. The latter two suggestions enabled the teacher to continue with the class routines and at the same time to isolate the child from any functional advantages of being sick for that set of class relationships and then evaluate any remaining illness behaviour. This strategy could not distinguish functional effects of the illness behaviour for the relation between the child and its parents. This preliminary stage in the classroom typically took between 15 and 30 minutes before the pupil was sent further to the school secretary. The school culture's gender typifications affected the ease with which children proceeded through this half-sick phase.

Once the child came to the welfare assistant, she was left to decide on the nature of the child's discomfort and to devise a plan of action. The welfare assistant in contrast to the nursery school staff does not have immediately available to her information on all the preceding events which lead up to the presenting of the complaint to the teacher. In addition she is usually not familiar with the child's home background (in contrast to the school secretary described by Prout). The child in these circumstances bridges the two microsystems of classroom and sickroom, which are bound to have less than perfect communication and hence the possibilities for misunderstandings.

Overall the welfare assistants' strategies were very similar to those of the parents. They saw it as one of their tasks to distinguish 'pretend' illness, which they did through noting any pattern in the child's attendance at the sick bay. They were assisted here by referring to a detailed log of the children's attendances. If the pattern suggested that the child was avoiding a particular lesson she then discussed that observation with the guidance teacher who would explore any educational difficulties which might have arisen in that lesson. Psychological connections were made to the pupils' claims on the sick role. These welfare assistants, like the parents, rarely used thermometers, instead relying on the child's appearance. Instead Prout's school secretary found it useful to quantify – to measure the temperature rather than rely on the quality of the signs from the child – in order to tackle the problem of too many children exaggerating illness. This is the same strategy used by the parents mentioned above. The welfare assistants' situation meant that they were unable to test the child's functioning in other situations, such as how they ate, played, got up, etc. This could account for why the children had to be pretty persistent in their presentation of their problem in order to emphasise its importance. Prout noted that only for conditions with clear visible signs or where the symptoms were compatible with illnesses which were going around was it possible to bypass these strategies.

Those working in schools have limited responses to ill children as they must follow the guidelines of the local education department which tend to specify clearly the situations where parents should be contacted and take over from the teacher or welfare assistant. They are not allowed to issue medicines. The guidelines mean that the available responses are to call the child's parents to collect the child, return the child to the class, or keep the child in the sick room for a limited period. Cups of tea seemed to be provided as the main 'treatment'. Responsibility for treatment is seen as remaining with the parents, but labelling of the problem rests with the welfare assistant. This arrangement of shared responsibility is in fact ambiguous and seen by some as a potentially troublesome zone of the parent/teacher relationship:

> one in which teachers could make no special claim for professional dominance over parents but which nevertheless constituted an aspect of their declared concern for the general 'welfare' of the child 'as a whole', a concern which suffused the pedagogical theory of the school. Teachers were also aware that responding to children's health problems in school could be seen as part of their *in loco parentis* responsibility and the possibility that they might be criticised by parents and held to account for their responses. (Prout, 1986)

I will return briefly to the distinction introduced by medical anthropologists between naturalistic and personalitic medical systems. In these two models the roles of healer and carer in relation to the diagnosis of illness differ. According to which of these models is predominant in the families involved, confusion can be expected to arise here due to the blurring of who is actually caring for the child when they are in which microsystem. If the child's microsystem is primarily school and the diagnosis is made there and then presented to the parents who are responsible for treatment, the model reflects that found in naturalistic medical systems. If the child's system is primarily that of home and the diagnosis is made by one who is believed to be an expert, the welfare assistant, and she is perceived as delegating the treatment to the parents, it reflects a personalistic medical system. As will be seen subsequently, children are continually introduced to elements of both types of system and it appears unhelpful to maintain clear distinctions between them. Due to the place of allocated expertise, and adult and child expectations based on cultural precedents, confusion can be expected to arise here and with it the potential for misunderstanding and conflict.

Depending on the parents' reactions to the welfare assistants' decision-making, the functioning of the mesosystem between school and home would be influenced. These responses would lead to further characterisation of the parents by the school, who would thus develop their way of accounting for the behaviour of the child and his family. This interaction has the quality of a reciprocal transactional process which can mutually run down the respect for all parties concerned, or escalate it, depending on the fit of their alternative perspectives. Prout (1986) describes the health care provided at home as a potent characteriser in the eyes of a child's primary school teachers of the mothering available (see also Graham, 1984). This construction of the resources of families and especially mothers, based on exosystem functioning, then alters the subsequent accounting for further presentations of discomfort by the child. The characteristics of mothers which were used were their 'minor incompetence', 'overprotectiveness', 'sensibleness' or 'emotional neglect' of their children. The overprotective mothers were said to have 'wet' children. Overprotectiveness was used to describe mothers who do not go out to work 'who revel in their children's illnesses . . . anxious mothers'. But as the research of Manning *et al.* (1978) illustrated (overprotectiveness was one of their accounting variables, as with the teachers in Prout's sample), the attributions and accounts of children made in order to understand their intention may be quite misplaced. The accounts can facilitate the establishment of forms of responding which maintain the behaviour being accounted for, such as with the 'wet' children described by Prout. This analogy with Manning *et al.*'s research gains more credence as it was noted that the parental accounting for the teacher's response, that of acknowledging their child's illness behaviour, was because of lax discipline in the primary school.

There are different ways in which this 'wetness' of girls has been characterised. Ullian (1984) describes the way in which American society construes female attributes. She believes that this can lead to young girls believing that they are physically vulnerable, and that society expects them to view themselves as 'fragile and defenseless'. Although that analysis does not attempt to distinguish the origins of the elements in that construction, Anastas & Reinherz (1984) do provide evidence that the cognitive difficulties of boys and girls are responded to differently in American schools. It may be that the emotional factors in girls' presentations of their discomforts are overemphasised at the expense of problems having a cognitive origin.

The children in Edinburgh were particularly aware by the age of 13 years of different responses in class to the boys or girls who complained of illness to the teacher. There was general agreement amongst the pupils that the boys were seen as 'using' illness more often than the girls. The teachers' responses were seen as denying the boys' discomforts more often than the girls', as the teachers appeared to believe the boys were more often pretending or exaggerating. This contrasts with the 'wet' girls described above by Prout at primary school. Boys were there seen as being 'least wet' and so more likely to have their bids for the sick role acknowledged as valid. The girls who were seen as least wet were those who participated in most sports. As will be seen in chapter 6, the dirt accumulated by boys in their sport is seen not as a danger to their health but as a sign of their toughness, and even became associated with health, as sport became associated with health. Provisionally it appears as though there has been a shift between primary school and secondary school in the gender typing responses, but this will need further investigation. My data do not allow me to check whether boys were more often introduced to rather pragmatic definitions of illness within their own families, or why teachers were seen as avoiding relabelling the boys' responses as being partially due to psychological discomforts as some of the parents seemed to do. Would the male pupil environment 'allow' them to respond to such a relabelling if proffered? These processes seem to depend partly on the ways in which the adults construe the child's difficulties, which are in dynamic interaction with the ways in which the peer group construes each other's difficulties.

*Nursery school literature*

The decision-making at school is only one aspect of the school structure. At the nursery schools it was possible to get an overview of the literature available to the children for their own browsing, as posters on the walls, songs for song time or for use by the teachers. This represents another part of the framework within which the children are forming their concepts about illness. Although I gained some similar information from the primary and secondary schools I will not refer to it further as it was in no way comprehensive enough to draw any valid conclusions from.

Both nursery schools had a liberal supply of books which contained illness themes. The stories were frequently read aloud when they were pertinent to a particular child's condition. For example, *Meg has the Mumps*, was read during story time when one child was absent from the group with mumps. Many of these tales were overtly or covertly moralistic, introducing the children to the necessary steps to take in the face of illness, such as that parents should call the doctor *quickly*. The doctor was then expected to give a prescription, which again had to be collected speedily using a variety of fantastic methods. Interestingly, in 1979–80, prescriptions were required for all the common viral conditions of childhood. Outside story time the children browsed through the pictures in these books in the story corner on their own. It was not unusual for some of the children to be able to read a few of them.

On the walls of the nurseries were several health education posters. Many of these had a high verbal content and appeared to be directed to the visiting parents. The themes covered included the advantages of brushing one's teeth (such as in a picture of the Incredible Hulk saying 'Grr even Hulk hates teeth that turn into ugly monsters', and in another play on television characters which read '"Time for bed", said Zebedee. "Brush your teeth" says Florence'), the fun of washing thoroughly, Superman extolling the gains to be had from not smoking and the dangers of poisonous plants. For the children the posters appeared as decorations often picking up on their favourite television characters, but the content appeared otherwise to be lost on them.

The same themes which occurred in the books also occurred in one of the songs about a nursery school age child who was ill.

*What constitutes a tasty morsel, and the dental health week*

The only official attempt to educate the nursery school children about health matters came through dental health weeks. These are arranged for all children in Edinburgh attending any form of pre-school provision. The children are shown how to brush their teeth over a week of intensive effort from the community dental health team. In addition they are introduced to the idea that certain foods are good for their teeth whereas sweet things need to be avoided. The Tanzanian posters advertising the value of eating sugar ('Sugar makes you more of a man') would be anathema for 3–4-year-olds here. Links are made, even at this early age, by the dental health team between the food eaten and the encouragement which certain foods give to 'bacteria' or 'germs' on the teeth. Observations from England (Eiser *et al.*, 1983) suggest that the knowledge these Edinburgh children developed about the role of bacteria is subject to local factors such as the dental health week, as in the English subjects this knowledge was not evident until the children were 8 years old.

The dental health team's regular interventions have led to an alteration in the kind of food prepared within the nursery for play time. They have switched to making savoury things such as cheese straws and oatcakes and the baking of fresh bread, in contrast to the previous sweeter diet. The changeover has not been complete as the staff at one nursery thought that it would be nice for the children if they could still make something sweet once a week. Because they were less certain of how this would be perceived by the parents, they had a different rule for the consumption of the sweet food compared with the more savoury items. Generally the children ate what they had made in the nursery after song time, but they were given the sweet things to take away with them to 'eat with parental permission'. They were then regularly eaten on the way down the nursery school steps in the no man's land before they were clearly under the guidance of parents. Ambivalence rules! No comments were made, and how the children reconciled the differing messages they received in these transactions is unclear.

There are implications here for a child's orientation to his doctor. These children informed me that doctors were silly because they gave sugar lumps. Children in Edinburgh tended to receive their polio immunisation on a sugar lump. Doctors were clearly not people who knew about health, although they would tackle diseases. Many doctors in Edinburgh were still 'rewarding' children with a sweet after a consultation, or using them to quieten anxious children (just as Graham (1984) describes mothers doing, when out shopping with their children, in order to maintain a degree of order – a habit frequently frowned upon but carried out with close attention to social mores). In 1974 an American study had already demonstrated that 'both younger and older children (third grade and kindergarten) were opposed to doctors giving candy. For example one child said, "Candy doesn't do much for your teeth, balloons would be all right"' (Steward & Regalbuto, 1975). This result could be dismissed on the basis that it was found with children from a sample biased towards middle and upper class Californians. I use it here to show that the place of something sweet in maintaining the affections of a child after a traumatic consultation may not be what it appears to the doctor. Doctors have begun to take note, though, and on 14 January 1984 the *British Medical Journal* noted that paediatricians in Manchester had saved £1000 by no longer buying sweets for their child patients.

Dental health initiatives in nurseries are not always welcomed by the parents. In Glasgow Macaskill & MacDonald (1982 p. 68–9) reported parents as being suspicious that more contact with dentists led to the drilling and filling of more holes than necessary.

*Formal education on health and illness: teachers and doctors*

I do not intend to present here a comprehensive review of how the Edinburgh children are taught about health and illness, or the literature on the alternative ways of presenting this information. Instead I will try and present a few of the children's observations about how the schools presented these topics and how they tried to make sense of them.

The 8-year-olds whom I met had received no formal education on health or illness matters outside the dental health weeks, which continued annually up to this age using gradually more complex strategies. They avidly attended to my group sessions, conveying a sense of much curiosity about health and illness which could usefully be tapped for education. The tecahers seemed to be aware of this and it was planned to introduce these topics in that school year. A report for the Health Education Council (Davies *et al.*, 1982) had found a similar curiosity in the 10- and 11-year-old children they interviewed. They concluded (*op. cit.*, p. 400) that it would have been natural to introduce health education in the curriculum of the last year of English primary schooling, i.e. to these 10- and 11-year-olds. At present there are no clear findings to point towards there being a 'right' age for introducing such teaching. Educational content cannot be divorced from the educational method. The communicational style which will be facilitating will alter with the age of the children.

I was surprised that one of the primary school groups, when saying goodbye to me, thanked me for teaching them so much about health and illness. In fact through my form of circular questioning, and by encouraging them to check things with each other, they had clearly digested much new information from their own perspectives without my introducing them to new information. It seems that beginning exactly where they are with their current information it is possible to create a fruitful learning environment built on their own curiosity. This viewpoint coincides with that described by Tizard & Hughes (1984 p. 264) for younger children: 'Our objection is to the notion that these goals [disembedded thinking and academic skills] are best served in ignorance of the skills and interests that children manifestly possess at home'.

The majority of the 13-year-olds received biology teaching which introduced them to some theoretical ideas and which included information
about bacteria. But the ways in which infective agents were introduced
meant that they tended to have little application to the pupils' understanding of their own illnesses. They were left to make applied sense of it from
their original lay perspective. The applied knowledge came most in home
economics, taught to both the boys and the girls, which particularly highlighted the role of food in health and disease. As they then used this
knowledge in their handling of food in the lesson, it appeared to be better
incorporated into their existing beliefs. This perspective, the importance
of the link between food and illness, coincided with the set of values found
at home (discussed further in chapter 7). I believe that because the viewpoints were shared children could integrate them more easily and they
became especially salient.

The schools do have visits from a school doctor and nurse (I am not
here referring to the welfare assistant). Their roles were poorly understood
by the pupils, in contrast to the role of the welfare assistant whose decisions
affected their regular school routine directly and more often. The doctor
and nurse were involved in measuring and quantifying various aspects of
function, including carrying out ear and eye tests, and not in making
decisions about child illness at a time of acute discomfort. They were there
to check and control, not to participate in the children's daily negotiations
involving illness. There was apparently little integration of their participation with the rest of the school microsystem, to the regret of the teachers
who wished for an expansion of the school doctor's role into formal education. Parents by contrast seem to be content in a passive uncritical way
with the way in which their children are examined by the Schools' Health
Service (Macaskill & MacDonald, 1982 p. 69). School doctors were not
interviewed as part of my enquiry.

The school medical service is also involved in initiating immunisation.
The 13-year-old girls were very aware that rubella immunisation was immi-
nent (due to occur in the weeks immediately after my contact with them).
Immunisation was seen as one of the important preventive measures, and
together with the examinations made of the children, provided the cornerstone to preventive medicine at this age. Regrettably there was no
discussion of the ways in which people talk about illness and make decisions
about illness which could well have complemented the preventive measures.
The dilemma faced by these children is whether they are being provided
with information to control them or information which is for them to use
for taking responsibility for their own health, their own bodies. The ways

in which the information is provided can facilitate the children taking responsibility for themselves and it affects the moral order associated with illness themes.

Thus the school system introduces information to the child as well as making decisions about the child's health and illness. Just as with the families these two dimensions relate to the two modes of the mathetic and pragmatic which the child has to integrate as he learns what illness means. The way in which they are currently segregated in the school makes this task more difficult.

## The framework of social explanations and rules

In this chapter I have presented various of the different possible frameworks and contexts which determine the meanings of the children's messages. I will recount the messages given and the children's understandings in the subsequent chapters. This chapter provides the structure necessary for interpreting the children's offerings, the structure which can help the decision as to what degree the accounts received from the children are warranted as well as intelligible. It helps to see how the illness and health categories deduced by Herzlich and described earlier (in chapter 3) can come about.

Some general considerations require more discussion. One characteristic of these various contexts is that they appear to be identifiable through the different strategies employed therein. Slightly different processes are occurring in different settings when an ill child is present. One result of this is that if a child 'wishes' to present a message with a consistent meaning, 'I am ill' (or rather as he experiences it more often 'I am not my usual self'), or, as is more commonly the case, to exaggerate the message in order to be certain that he is heard, he is required to be aware of these slightly different ways of reacting to him – to know what makes a difference to the others. Different dimensions of the message will be more salient to different people, as well as at different developmental phases. In this way illness behaviour would evolve, not as a conscious process, but shaped as a part of natural development from solely crying and fractious behaviour to a verbal discussion of one's discomforts. The range of illness behaviour would reflect the salience of the behaviour for the different microsystems encountered by the child in relation to how important and how emotionally charged those microsystems were to the child (Berger & Luckmann, 1966), as well as his illness experiences (and times of being half-ill/'under the weather') within each of those systems.

The illness behaviour that evolves will also have a complementary effect of modifying the decision-making processes which led to the evolution of that behaviour, provided that those who make the decisions remain with the child (a situation which will not pertain with changes of teacher). It is essential not to imply a uni-directional influence of structure on the child's behaviour, as the child's behaviour alters the structure of the family and school to cope with it. This is seen most clearly with chronically ill children, where there is a major permanent impact on the family organisation in terms of decision-making and rules concerning illness (Burton, 1975; Shapiro, 1983). In addition normal schools may not be able to adapt their organisation sufficiently and a special school placement providing an alternative structure may need to be found.

In social anthropology (Needham, 1962) and more recently in family therapy there has been debate between structural (Minuchin, 1974) and 'strategic' ways of accounting (Selvini-Palazzoli *et al.*, 1978; Haley, 1976). Debates have centred around whether the structure of a group, be it family, school or community, determines the strategies available to those within the group (which would include illness behaviour to convey 'I am ill'), or whether the strategies employed by those within the group determine the group's structure. This debate appears misplaced due to the way in which structure and strategies have been conceptualised independently of each other. I hope that my presentation so far has illustrated the way in which structure is a term which does not imply solely physical structure, but also the framework of social explanations and rules. These latter then become incorporated by individuals as their own strategies to exist in that structure during development. The way in which children develop, and words and contexts gain meaning for them, provides a model for the integration of structure and strategy as a coherent whole rather than one simply causing effects in the other dimension.

This notion is very important because it relates to the whole classical idea that children's views and strategies in the face of illness are caused in a linear sense by the things done to them. In contrast I would suggest that the mutual responsiveness of the child and his context is one of mutual adaptedness which can be described as coevolution. They are elements in a recursive system. Consequently in order to change the children's views and strategies it would be necessary also to change the structure within which they develop, the rules governing their microsystems of family and school as well as the mesosystem. If change were attempted through small steps in either the realm of structure or strategy alone it would be anticipated that the homeostatic forces in such a recursive system would work to return it to the status quo.

In order to explore this suggestion it would be necessary to do one of two things. One possibility would be to follow individual children from the time they were 3 until they were 13 years of age and note the changes that evolved in the individual and his microsystem or the child's views, and note the impact on the other elements of the child's world. One way of changing the microsystem is through altering the exosystem influences, or seeing what happens when a family culture undergoes a change of macrosystem by moving to a new place. A way of changing the child's views without altering the microsystems would be to introduce a third microsystem independent of the other two, as occurs when children join an independent group which has no contact with the rest of the family or school (fig. 4.5). As parents take responsibility for their young children this latter course is not totally possible as the third microsystem would require to be in contact with the parents, but to an extent it reflects the situation found when children are seen in individual or group therapy in child psychiatry departments. It is also found with the peer networks established especially in adolescence.

Like any other qualitative research these interpretations of the data require further testing in a second stage of the research to clarify their validity within a positivistic framework to find out the degree to which they are warranted. The longitudinal study of individual children would provide evidence on the durability of viewpoints and family structure over the years.

Although an outsider such as the researcher can interpret the framework of social explanations and rules he can adopt a metaperspective to the microsystem, remaining outside its rules and conventions but at the same time able to engage with it; this is much more difficult for those brought up within the microsystem's guidelines. Piaget (1932) identified how young

Fig. 4.5. An indpendent microsystem for the child.

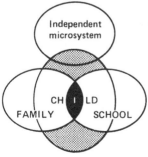

children believe that rules for children's games such as marbles are immutable, abiding by a set of absolute God-given guidelines. In the same way I would like to postulate on the basis of my observations that children see the social framework of rules regarding illness behaviour in the same manner, but that through the forms of communication established around illness themes that point of view can be exaggerated or diminished.

One result of being exposed to discussion between the parents, where mother and father may be negotiating what to do about the child's condition, is that the child is introduced to the idea that rules about illness are not absolute but negotiated on the basis of alternative understandings. The child can come to be introduced to one set of rules at home, as was the case with the two families where mothers were nurses, no discussion between school and parents, and then a different set of rules at school. Because of the rigid independence of the microsystems the child would be expected to take longer to develop a position from which he can assess the various rules as not being absolutes, as he has no model for the negotiation required. It would seem likely that if the child has a lot of trust in the parental values he could come to be dismissive of an alternative set of rules at school, or vice versa. He comes into a bind of right and wrong approaches to illness, rather than participating with others negotiating what will be most helpful for him.

The effect of presenting 'pretend' complaints is one that I elaborate later in chapter 8. One effect is that for some children their psychological discomforts can come to be recognised through observation of the functional consequences of being ill. As this area of decision-making appeared difficult for adults it can lead to the use of health professionals to identify whether the child is physically ill, distressed or a mixture of the two. I would suggest that an implication of this for health professionals is that they need to be aware of the functional consequences of illness as much as the physical nature of illness so that symptoms can be fully accounted for. The functional consequences can only be deduced through knowledge of the child's world from the child's perspective, and the frameworks of the micro- and mesosystems. In order to test the validity of deductions about function, elements of these could be altered to see whether the illness symptoms changed in response to altered consequences for those symptoms.

In addition to that implication for the management of the consultation, there are potential implications for arrangement of health service provision. The rigid boundaries between systems, such as that which occurs should a doctor wish solely to see ill children rather than respond to the parents' wish for help with their own decision-making problems, make for worse communication and a greater likelihood of a clash of perspectives. How this actually affects the child's views on illness is not yet clear, but potentially it leads to the child's confusion in integrating different perspectives and the maintenance of inappropriate, or rather unhelpful, models of illness. The same process can occur at school if there are sharp boundaries between the roles of the school doctor, welfare assistant, guidance teacher and class teacher – let alone parents. Sometimes there have been blind requests for more communication between different groups looking after children. I would hope that the request here for more communication is not limited to the conveying of information, but that the information is respected for what it means for those giving it, and that the decision-making processes are addressed. The function of the request for the discussion at this moment in the child's illness must be elucidated. This will involve exploring the potential problems in the coping strategies of the adults and their psychological discomforts. There would then be a requirement to check the impact of such changes in communication practices before deciding that they were necessarily an improvement in the service provision.

# 5

# Germs and bugs: causal agents

The previous chapter described the ecological systems within which the child learns of illness, the systems' structures of rules, the questions and explanations, and routines and rituals. In addition the range of ways of communicating about illness and their variety of effects were described. The subsequent chapters will present the children's views of illness which evolved within that framework. I will often focus on causality, as the causes of illness are seen to have a very central place in organising people's conceptual frameworks about illness. It appears to be around causality that we attribute intentions and construct the moral order pertaining at times of illness; our concepts here organise to a high degree our ways of responding and determine our expectations of appropriate behaviour from others. Nevertheless I refer to causality rather than causes. As the nature of the child's understanding of sufficient causes for illness is presented, it will be seen that straightforward ideas of cause and effect are hard to find.

The children's views reported here emphasise what they regard as facts about illness, rather than the possible functions of illness within a system. The latter were mentioned in the previous chapter and incorporated by the children in two ways: they mistakenly become part of the child's facts about illness, as well as enabling the child to be effective in altering systems through illness. With growing reflection it is seen how the effects can be turned to advantage in negotiating status on the basis of illness rationales.

In recent years there has been much criticism of what are loosely termed 'medical models' of illness, which by implication are bio-medical or structural functionalist models. These models have been said to be in the ascendant since the early success of the germ theory of disease in making intelligible the nature of disease processes and directing treatment to particular agents causing the disease rather than to the patient's state of illness (Twaddle, 1981). The children's germ theories presented here show how an apparently bio-medical model serves a multitude of other, usually hidden purposes. The earlier medical approaches to management, directed to the patient's environment in ways analogous to those found in naturalistic systems, are actually very active in the current folk applications of the germ theory. What the germ theory has come to mean for these children is apparently an elaborated mixture of the earlier naturalistic approaches and the personalistic, the latter providing the framework expected on the basis of the role of infective agents in the bio-medical model.

The three different forms of interview with the children all contributed to the data, but only views which were coherent across the differing settings of peer group, individual and family sessions are included here. There had to be a shared set of logical assumptions behind what a child said; the views could not be presented solely for an immediate effect on me or as a rationalisation (Williams, 1981). I was thus aiming for the children's mathetic rather than their pragmatic knowledge, although their efforts in the pragmatic revealed assumptions about the research situation which were in themselves interesting and affected the ways in which I interpreted the other information. The apparent surface contents of the largely functionalist messages were similar to the predominantly mathetic messages as the children drew on the range of views prevalent in their microsystems. Research is not yet at a stage where voice analysis could have improved the distinction between these different kinds of message. This distinction comes to be of greater importance when responding to the messages from the children rather than trying to establish the range of views which they have about illness.

## Germs and bugs

### The beginnings of a concept

The research method used verbal transcriptions of audiorecordings and so will tend to overemphasise the importance of the children's words for reflecting their views and knowledge. We must return at intervals to the descriptions in chapter 4 in order to look at the origins of their vocabulary, which has its roots in the non-verbal responses to each child and the words used about him.

The word *germ* is one of the first crucial words concerning illness which the nursery school child tries to master. It is introduced in many different situations, and for some children these all occurred outside the home. The word becomes endowed with much explanatory potential as it is construed as an agent with many magical powers – much as to be expected in a personalistic system but also coherent with the children's concepts of animism and their beliefs about how events are caused in the world. Their curiosity is aroused about an apparently powerful yet invisible agent. Initially the word tends to confuse the children as it is used interchangeably with the word *bug*. When they try to reduce their uncertainty about what is meant when germs are referred to they naturally make associations with the more familiar word bug, which is used synonymously with insect. As insects are visible and tangible it is not surprising that the children assume that germs are insects also.

These views are coherent with those described by Nagy (1951, 1953), even though she was partially researching in a different language in Hungary. (Regrettably I have no information on the words for germs, bugs and insects in different cultures.) For Nagy's British and American subjects insects were the most commonly referred to of her category of 'animal models' of germs (75% of all the animal models obtained were for arthropods). Her explanation was that 'animals are often carriers of germs, as children learn from posters and other forms of health propaganda. Being at the same place they will be considered to be identical, or at least similar' (Nagy, 1953). Research on linguistic ambiguity suggests that only by the time children are between 7 and 11 years old (or, using a different framework, at Piaget's stage of concrete operations) can they begin to appreciate the multiple meanings of words (Whitt, Dykstra & Taylor, 1979). These results would be consistent with that view.

Although the 13-year-olds interviewed had begun to move away from the analogy of germs to insects – a metaphor which had become real for the younger children – adults sometimes still cling to it. One 13-year-old put it like this: 'It makes bugs sound like things that fly round in the air and you can see them – and you can't.' The relics of these verbal confusions will be seen when images of germs are discussed later. It is not surprising from the way the phrase 'tummy bug' is used in everyday speech that the germs most commonly viewed as insects by a group of suburban London adults were those said to cause gastrointestinal symptoms (Helman, 1978).

These semantic confusions help explain comments such as 'Mummy's sickness was caused by a "wee" bee in her tummy'. Here there has been a personal translation of the term tummy bug by a 4-year-old. The fantasies which can be encouraged by such confusions can easily exaggerate the fears associated with illness, as well as the well-known fears of insects and especially the stinging varieties such as bees. For other young children the distinctions between the alternative meanings for bug did not appear confusing. It could be that for them the word was encountered only in the phrase tummy bug rather than being associated with insects – for example in the definition of bug as 'When a nasty germ gets into your tummy.'

When a word is introduced for the first time the possibilities for confusion are rife. But because there is much uncertainty about whether the meaning is correctly understood, the child finds it easy to give up his first understandings in the face of new information; initially a child's constructs are particularly flexible. There was only one child at nursery who appeared to be hearing about germs (from her friend in the school interview) for the first time. Her guess at the meaning relied on her current knowledge of words with similar phonetic elements and she came up with the following: 'I don't know what a germ is but I have heard of a German person.' As will be seen later (p. 116) there are possibly other factors in how she came to to mention a foreigner with the potentialities to be an illness agent. As children play around with words they indulge in a language game of a similar form to that envisaged by Wittgenstein for bringing out the connections between the speaking of language and non-linguistic activities (Kenny, 1975 p. 163; Harré, 1983 pp. 92–3). The words gain meaning and flavour from the ways in which they are used and responded to. They are shaped towards the culture's predominant use in a process of enculturation (Kvideland, 1979).

Several parents said that they had not mentioned germs to their children; yet only one child appeared to hear of germs for the first time in the interviews. This shows the importance of a child's other microsystems – the nursery and the peer group – as sources of information. Because of the ways in which germs are endowed with powerful functions, such as an ability to change the whole body and make it perform differently and uncontrollably (for example when vomiting or having diarrhoea), they become a particularly interesting topic of conversation amongst 3- to 4-year-olds. Knowledge of germs is associated with a child finding out about how his body functions and an understanding of a sense of physical self.

The child's imagination is given full rein as ideas about the nature of germs cannot be tested: they are invisible and so known only through their functions. Curiosity is aroused and germs become a topic of gossip independent of adults. Nevertheless many parents included germs and their capabilities in the reasons they gave to their children for why they should do certain things and avoid others; these were as parts of preventive strategies, rather than explanations for things that had happened. The preventive strategies are untestable for the degree to which they provide the children with mathetic information, and so these effects of germs are attributed to a mixture of the pragmatic and mathetic modes, poorly incorporated with the other concepts.

## The growth of the bug family

The primary school children aged 8 years remained fascinated by germs. Their definitions still retained close links to bugs ('Small poisonous bugs' and 'They're in the bug family or bugs are in the germ family'), but their ideas were becoming more elaborate as they tried to discriminate the separate applications of the words. One child explained 'Bugs can be inside or outside you. Germs can just be inside you', while another said 'It's a germ 'cos bugs just give you tummy aches, or most do. You've both the same thing exactly, but maybe not the same illness'. They typically saw both germs and bugs as tiny, 'dirty' and 'bad for you' ('Bugs are bad; bugs have swords that can kill you'). But realising that sizes are relative they did wonder whether they would 'ever see giant's germs?'

Some of the 13-year-olds were clearer about the distinctions between the adults' use of strategies to get them to comply in family routines (the pragmatic) and their conveying of information neutral to any pragmatic considerations (the mathetic). Information given primarily to explain could too easily be attributed to the pragmatic – an error in logical type – even though it was what others would consider accurate. The nature of metaphors is clearer to this age group so they have begun to doubt the nature of the agents described by the parents: 'Parents say bugs just to simplify it all. No such things as a bug really'. Others were trying to convince the group of their superior knowledge: 'For someone who doesn't know anything about them, a bug is exactly the same as a germ'. But the speaker could not elaborate on the differences when pressed.

The nature of the illnesses which tend to elicit the terms germs and bugs respectively have begun to lead to functionalist definitions of the two words: 'Bugs are things that travel from one person to another person and keep spreading. Like if you had a bug in the school, quite a lot of people in the school might have it'. But there were very contradictory understandings of the two terms, as became clearer in the unravelling of the statement (said as though self-explanatory) 'There's a lot of bugs going about but "I've got germs"'. There was apparently more illness status in having a germ. One could lay claim to having a germ, whereas bugs were regarded as universal and not necessarily carrying illness. Bugs are just 'around'. Germs were more contagious and so you were more smitten if you had a germ. But the world of these 13-year-olds is open to much confusion and the contrary viewpoints were also found, as in the two statements 'Bugs give you more trouble' and 'Germs may not all carry illnesses'.

These germs all had a 'bad' feel to them. It was a necessary part of the definition of a germ for the majority – 'That's why they're called germs'.

Nevertheless the children had developed ideas about complementary 'good germs', invisible agents affecting the body in magical ways contrary to the deduced modes of action of the germs and bugs described so far. The term was used in a few family interviews in the process of the parents explaining things to their children. This theme is explored further in chapter 7 in the context of the children's understanding of defence against infection. It needs to be noted, though, that the same metaphors of war and defence were used for the mode of action of any agents in the body, whether good or bad. These are encouraged by the way the medical profession talks about bodily processes, both between themselves and in consultations (Hodgkin, 1985), as well as by the similar 'challenging' metaphors adopted by scientists and taken up by society in general (Blaxter, 1983). For a metaphor to be acceptable in a wide enough part of the macrosystem it appears to need a broad base in different sectors which then each keep the metaphor going in the other sectors in a self-perpetuating fashion.

As the effects of germs and bugs were being discriminated there developed a need for a more refined vocabulary to distinguish certain conditions which were responded to differently. The 'bug family', the expression used in my samples, was getting bigger. These older children had come across viruses and fleas. Viruses tended to be referred to in the definitive as 'the virus', presumably because of the way in which adults refer to catching 'a virus' in the singular – in contrast to germs and bugs which can easily be plural. Blaxter (1983) had another explanation for the use of the definitive article for viruses, believing it to be used 'to mark [viruses] out as common, familiar almost friends . . . Diseases given more "technical" names would never be accompanied by an article'. Nevertheless Blaxter's Aberdeen mothers were sceptical about viruses: 'they've found a new word'.

Viruses were variously described by the 13-year-olds as 'a thing you catch', 'A fever' and 'It's a bug. You catch it. It spreads'. In the last example the spread was over the affected person, not especially amongst the peer group. The common exanthemata of childhood have a viral cause and are easily seen spreading over the body. Viral infections do not primarily require antibiotics, yet the nursery school literature showed that the expectation was being created for a prescription as a necessary ingredient of the treatment. The use of antibiotics (or not) was not observed to play any role for these children in discriminating germs and viruses.

Can you get certain infections more than once? This question provided a constant source of discussion amongst the children as the explanation for why it should be was surrounded in mystery. Powerful arguments were put forward for and against in the group sessions. One element of these discussions began to make itself felt in the children's ideas about viruses: a virus was seen as 'like chicken pox. Once you've had it you can't have it again'.

Some ideas about viruses seemed to a degree to be imported from the playground games of younger children, as in the statement 'You can get French and German'. The Opies (1969 p. 75) referred to French Touch as a game involving the principles of contagion which they believed obtained its name through general views in society that bad things are seen as foreign. French Touch is said to be played by 8-year-olds but it was not immediately evident in the playgrounds of the two primary schools in the sample. 'German' could have come in the same way, but is more probably linked to the semantic confusions named earlier between germs and Germans and to the existence of German measles. A belief in the origin of illness outside the self (the exogenous system described earlier) could have provided the basis for attributing the source of the 'bad' as far away as possible – a foreign place. These views can be part of the primary structure around the child from birth, as an important part of the way parents account for states of health and illness. For example, Newson & Newson (1963 p. 22) reported a view elicited about taking babies to see the health visitor at a clinic: 'Well, you see people of every nationality there. Well, it's not that I've got anything against foreigners, but all the babies have to be undressed, and I think they pick up things'.

The following rather elaborate story was typical of the way in which being foreign was implicated in illness causality in my sample:

> Well maybe if my sister's had something she passes it on to me. Because when my little sister used to go to nursery school, this wee Chinese boy, he hadn't got one of his tetanus booster jags and he had the disease and his mother didn't know about it. And he was going around the playground with it until Mrs M. she told the mother that her little boy had a disease. Isn't right. He's got purple spots or blue spots.

There are several confusions integrated into a whole through the linking theme of foreignness. Scotland might have German Measles, but Norway has the English sickness (rickets). I would expect this phenomenon to be similar in all cultures, but have no evidence on how widespread it is. I am not aware of any country choosing to name an illness with its own national identity!

Some of the colour to the children's concepts is revealed through the associations they make to the different words. They described there being more similarities between dirt and germs than between dirt and viruses. The 8-year-olds knew they could get viruses, but viruses were not used as a rationale for why a particular element in the social order should be retained. The way in which rationales for doing things are often based on a health/illness dimension which uses germs much more often than viruses is discussed in more detail in chapter 6. For example children are encouraged to wash their hands to remove germs. This seems to lead to beliefs in the ubiquitous nature of germs, rather than a distinction between germs and viruses being based on any knowledge about the requirement of viruses for living cells for their growth and multiplication. Another of the definitions of a virus could come from associations with such knowledge, as a virus was said to be 'like a germ, but it goes away'.

Assumptions about different modes of transmission for germs and viruses may have been the origin of one 13-year-old's view that viruses 'travel easier than germs. Well viruses go person–person, while germs go by the dirt'. Dirt and other people have different places in the social order (Douglas, 1966). Foreigners, though, are attributed with bringing germs and are indirectly likened to dirt for the way they can disturb the established social order.

The relation between germs and viruses remains complex. One child said 'I thought virus was lots of different kinds of germ'.

The other new members to the bug family are fleas and lice. The children were acquainted with these usually through direct experience or second-hand information from others who had had them. There is currently an epidemic of head lice in British primary schools which has necessitated regular head checks. The pupils were puzzled, though, that only nits and not lice were found. More familiarity with the reproduction of insects might have helped lessen some confusions here. Eiser *et al.* (1983) found that 70% of 6-year-olds and 100% of 11-year-olds in England could describe nits in the hair, and 65% and 85% respectively knew about treatment.

There was little knowledge of the difference between lice and fleas. Knowledge of fleas came from looking after pets. The children's images of them bolstered the insect analogies for germs which were still prevalent.

One of the 8-year-old boys had been living for several years in Bangladesh and uniquely had a belief that germs 'are like small worms that you can't see'. He was familiar with a need to avoid going round in bare feet in that country because otherwise worms might burrow into the skin. These ideas were met with much incredulity, but also rapt curiosity, when put forward to his relatively new classmates. As an aside it is curious to note a medical condition called Ekbom's syndrome, in which the patient believes he is infected with worm-like microorganisms. This syndrome is rarely reported in Britain but when found has been described as a 'monosymptomatic hypochondriacal psychosis' or a 'neurotically determined dysmorphophobia'. A developmental history of the patient's contact with cultures where models of infection involving worms is found; alternatively the images of death where worms are a potent symbol for what happens to the body after death (see for example Ariès, 1977) may help elucidate some of the reported cases (see for example McLaughlin & Sims, 1984) without recourse to diagnosis of a psychosis.

## What are germs?

The questions adults ask of children lead them to question the world about them in particular ways. I am here concerned with how a child conceptualises germs as objects – a very necessary step in view of the great emphasis laid by most parents on the 'What is that?' type question.

As we have seen the first concepts of germs were attached to the functions attributed to them. The ways in which effects were attributed to germs gave the children a model for their functioning, but they were short of answers as to what germs were. Their first ideas were built up on the analogy to bugs as mentioned above. These were the ideas of germs as insects which have definitely been present for forty years at least.

Nevertheless the children soon latched on to alternative images which were proffered. It appeared as though they were keen to drop the functionalist definitions in favour of concrete images in a process of reification. The most important image for the 3- and 4-year-olds was provided in television advertisements for a proprietary bleach cleaner called Domestos. Although some of these children had come across alternative images in children's books and some television documentaries for children, the enduring image was that germs were round, blue and between 2 and 20 centimetres in diameter. The colour blue was never used in children's descriptions of germs on Foula, the most remote inhabited island in the United Kingdom, which does not have the influence of the Domestos advertisements (Sheila Gear, personal communication).

About the time that I was interviewing the children there had been both a television documentary and recurring advertisements for Domestos. The most important point appeared to be that the advertisements came again and again and that they were linked to the daily activities which the children were aware of at home, such as the cleaning of 'toilets, sinks, wastepipes and outside drains' as the advertisements duly recited as a kind of litany at the end of each offering. These cleaning rituals were part of the way in which 'purity' was established at home; they reflected part of the moral order of the household. In this way the children seemed to latch tenaciously on to the image provided in the advertisements as the presentation was salient for them. They could not use the information provided in the introduction to the advertisement which said 'imagine these are germs'; instead they made the metaphor concrete.

The Domestos advertisements were timed to catch housewives viewing in the early evening. This happened to correspond to the peak viewing time of these children. When I arrived for a home visit one 3-year-old had just finished scribbling. She had been playing whilst her mother pottered around at home and the television was on. The Domestos advertisement had come and gone, but the effect was more lasting. The girl's scribble was of a mass of blue crayoning over the backside of a person. This, she had said to her mother, was a drawing of germs. The Domestos advertisements have employed several similar images, but the germs were always blue. In some they appeared as a kind of cloud in water, in others as though they were round globules. The setting was often the toilet with germs in the water in the toilet. The essence of the advertisements was that the germs were destroyed by Domestos and then one was 'safe'. The girl's response seemed to be coherent with the theme of these advertisements with regard to both colouring and placement. Of course the colour blue has been used in this culture for ointment bottles and things to do with medicine for hundreds of years, but the interpretation that the image comes from the advertisements is very suggestive.

It can provisionally be expected that the influence of the advertisement will be greater in those households which use Domestos. Lewis & Lewis (1974) researched the impact of television commercials on the health-related beliefs and behaviour of fifth- and sixth-grade American students (aged 10 to 13 years). Although these students are older than the nursery school age children in my sample some points are worth noting. Forty-seven per cent of the American children accepted all commercial messages touching on health-related beliefs and behaviours as 'true' all the time. This was related to parental use of the product being advertised. (Regrettably I have no information on the use of Domestos in the families I interviewed.) Seventy per cent of the television messages overall were believed, yet Lewis & Lewis reported that according to a panel of experts 70% of the messages were inaccurate, misleading or both. They concluded that given children's current beliefs about the truth of television advertisements 'television viewing as presently programmed might be labeled as hazardous to the health of future adults'. As they also noted that degree of belief in television messages decreases with age, their findings become even more convincing when considering nursery age children.

The effect of the advertisements was noted by Lewis & Lewis to be 20–30% greater on those from a lower socio-economic background. As persuasibility varies inversely with perceptions of self-worth (Donohue & Meyer, 1984), this social class effect may result from differences in self-efficacy, learned helplessness and external locus of control factors. Unless a health education programme includes steps to improve people's self-concepts any of the usual mass of information from the media will overrun the tentative hold people might have been getting on more useful health information. As will be seen later the differences in the health of the sexes is almost as great as that between the social classes. Television also has important effects on sex role development, 'higher amounts of television watching [being] clearly associated with stronger traditional sex role development' (Frueh & McGhee, 1975).

Adults may believe themselves less open to being influenced in this way. Doctors, for example, tend to assert that they are not influenced by the pharmaceutical companies' advertisement propaganda. Yet a recent survey in the United States showed they were predominantly influenced by just that rather than by scientific papers (Avorn, Chen & Hartley, 1982). Parents should be as worried as Postman (1985) about the effects that increased emphasis on images instead of words can have on their children's development. Commercials have a special place here as they ask the viewer to believe that all problems are solvable, and that they are solvable fast, through the interventions of technology, techniques and chemistry. All this must be put over in as short a time as possible. As Postman puts it vividly, television is inherently hostile to thought, logic and contemplation. The children in my sample showed, nevertheless, that the image of a germ they adopted could lead to much further thought and contemplation; but it can be difficult for others to know where the child stands with his ideas when they do not share the same image. The result can be the same as that reported by Tizard & Hughes (1984 p. 110) whereby when 'adult and child become locked on to different meanings of the same word [these] are particularly difficult for the adult to detect'. The group discussions I had in the schools where the children shared the same images were much more fruitful than when the images were not shared, as in the families.

One problem for the children associated with the image of germs adopted from the Domestos advertisements is that it is potentially confusing when germs are invoked by the parents at home as part of their rationale for why the children should do certain things. When they are asked to wash their hands 'to remove germs' when they have been to the toilet, there are clearly no 20-centimetre round germs sitting there. The confusion does not appear to create anxiety or uncertainty. This may be because the constructs are loosely held and can be discarded or taken up again depending on the needs of the moment. Nevertheless I had a sense of live science fiction when the children kept telling me that they would 'see one one day'. As there was always another day in which they might see one and confirm their hypothesis, they had presented themselves with untestable assumptions.

It is not known whether interpretations of the television advertisements for Domestos have played any role in cases of children ingesting bleach. Unfortunately the statistics do not discriminate the different brand names and the timing of these episodes have not been noted in such a way that any conjunction with the advertising campaigns would become clear. Self-poisoning with bleach could be seen as a sensible attempt at self-treatment for a tummy bug. At the time of this study bleach was recorded as the second most frequent cause of childhood poisoning (Craft *et al.*, 1984).

Amongst the nursery school children one other image for a germ was presented: 'They are like kidney beans'. For this child there appeared to be a semantic confusion with the notion of 'germination', which was illustrated in this particular nursery through the germination of kidney beans.

By the time the children are 8 years old these initial ideas have been relegated to some distant cupboards in their memories. The children of this age were fascinated by the ways in which things which were invisible could be revealed with special tools. Microscopes could reveal the world of germs. Only a handful of children had come across microscopes, but they were all aware that a special piece of equipment existed which could make visible the invisible. They viewed germs as invisible or tiny:

Boy 1: You said they were invisible.

Boy 2: Yes, but they've got to have a size.

The existence of tools to make visible the invisible had the effect of creating the idea that things could exist as objects which were invisible. Functional definitions then returned at this age as germs were defined for me by what one needed in order to see them, their size becoming their determining characteristic. This type of functionalistic definition cannot handle the concept of there being a hierarchy of sizes in the bug family. I heard that germs were bigger as well as smaller than fleas, and that viruses were about the size of lice. The differences between the various members of the bug family were created through the use of a strength category. Fleas were believed to be the strongest, but it remained unclear what 'strong' stood for as the children found it impossible to clarify its special use in this context.

The 13-year-olds were beginning to adopt the models of bacteria as presented in biology. Germs became 'one cell', 'little round things' and 'bacteria are long thin things. Viruses are dead small, thousands on a pin head'. A quarter of these children still retained definitions of germs based solely on the functions attributed to them. Two children this age thought of them as blue, but the majority allocated them no particular colour. The image of a germ could come to be quite a composite picture:

> I imagine them as sort of blood cells. I've seen blood cells under a microscope and on TV, all sorts of round blobs. I just think that they look like that except with black legs.

### How germs act

Another type of question often presented by parents is 'How?', as in 'How did that happen?' (In Edinburgh 'How?' questions are sometimes used idiosyncratically instead of 'Why?' questions, but here I will use the word how in the standard sense.) A child is encouraged on the basis of 'How?' questioning to look for and expect to find causal mechanisms along the lines of those acceptable to the parents. At the same time the causal mechanisms must make sense when taken in conjunction with the images of germs which the child has built up and the functions attributed to germs. The children in the sample were developing ideas about how their various images of germs carried out the effects attributed to them.

Many of the 3–4-year-olds were happy enough to explain the effects simply as 'It just happened'. Other children of this age elaborated constructs to explain the roles of germs in contagion. The children were aware that proximity to an ill person was associated with an increased risk of illness: 'If I have an illness and go near someone, they might catch it – especially if it's near to the bit that's sore', or 'Someone has it first, then it goes to someone else'. A puzzling addition was encountered amongst the 13-year-olds, who told me of a belief that you can catch an illness either 'from someone who's got it' or 'from someone who's had the flu'.

When considering the views of the nursery age children it must be remembered that they were not yet involved in the playground games involving contagion themes which appeared amongst the primary school children. These games, then, are not the introduction of the children to these themes but build upon and elaborate ideas which some of these children already have.

These early ideas about contagion/contamination are more advanced than those elicited by other researchers (eg. Kister & Patterson, 1980). I believe that this represents a function of the research method. In the research reported here I spent much time building up the children's trust in me in a slow and patient way prior to obtaining their views. The children were therefore probably prepared to share the views which they held more tentatively, their looser constructs. The closeness of my relationship with the children minimised the importance of immanent justice as an explanation for illness as I was an unthreatening person who was unlikely to judge them, and no actions followed from what they said to me. Kister & Patterson had found an inverse relationship between knowledge of contagion and belief in immanent justice as explaining the origin of illness. I do not believe that they have excluded the possibility that their results reflect both the quality of the relationship within which the views were elicited and their research method. It would need a different form of research design to test the hypothesis that the children's views on immanent justice reflect the quality of the research relationship. Piaget had believed this to be a possibility as he felt one could 'remove all traces of moral realism, [if one placed] oneself on the child's own level, and gave him a feeling of equality by laying stress on one's own obligations and one's own deficiencies' (Piaget, 1932 pp. 131–2). Cosminsky (1977) has suggested that research methods can affect the results in the direction indicated through her comparison of survey and case study methods in eliciting the views on illness of adults in Guatemala.

I have concluded that children 3–4 years old do have clear ideas about contagion but they find it so difficult to make sense of these that they rarely share them with others. Their problem can be appreciated when it is remembered that they are left trying to make sense of how 2–20 centimetre round blue germs (the predominant image employed by these children) could get from one person to another. Some explanations were that germs 'float . . . as a magic parcel', they were 'being given as a present – a bad present', or in one case with the germ for chicken pox there was an elaborate story of how the germ rolled down one person's leg and then across the floor before climbing up someone else's skirt or trousers. Only in this last case was a specific germ described for me by these youngest children; in other descriptions all germs were linked together as similar and able to cause any illness. The older children described different germs for different infections. There were 'mump germs, measle germs, german germs'. They did have a variety of problems with these ideas as it was believed that mumps 'could be any sort of germ. Any sort could give you a little bit of mumps, but only a special sort give you a big lot of mumps'.

In these ways, floating and rolling, the germs are seen as arriving at their new victim, but how do things proceed after that? The ways the 3–4-year-old children saw the germs getting inside people were only vaguely described, but they included up the leg (as above) and more especially through the mouth. The latter route is important because of the frequent ways in which parents make their children aware that things which are unhealthy for them can contaminate their food. The rituals about food preparation and general hygiene are embedded in the child's growing personality, their secondary structure, having had such a prominent place in their primary structure. But the concept includes more ideas than these. There is something special about the food prepared for each individual, so that if 'we eat each other's food we're passing on germs'. The hands are given a special place in the eating and handling of food, but the constraints about what you can and should do with your hands in order to remain healthy build on these early ideas and continue to emphasise the mouth as the high road to the inside of the body. Germs are said to enter the body when you suck your hands. But they were also seen as being able to enter the body directly through the hands when you 'wash the person who's been ill or their plate'.

The mouth can give much pleasure as well as being a source of vulnerability. These children's attachments to their parents were often affirmed through a goodnight kiss or a kiss at other times. But kissing could also transmit germs. They noted that 'you can't kiss your parents if they're ill'. But how do they make sense of the fact that their parents still thought it in order to kiss the children when the children were ill? How come the parents are so invincible? Maybe it is just as well that they convey this strength in this way at these times. But kissing and mouth contact means already much more than child/parent closeness and these nursery age children were aware of this. It is not just kissing but the foreignness of the other person you kiss which is associated with increasing your vulnerability to catching something. Even after a kiss on a cheek the germ is seen as travelling over the cheek on a very short route direct to the mouth. A particular moral order is established through rules about the acceptability of kissing particular people, as is a hierarchy of distance. This was reflected in the comment that it was especially dangerous to kiss 'someone else's wife or husband'. At the same time it was quite logical for the children to acknowledge that the degree of intimacy of the kiss played an important role; those kisses where 'we lick each other's tongues' were especially daring in view of the danger involved of catching and transmitting infection.

The older children had more complex ideas about how germs could act.

The 8-year-olds felt it was not possible to be ill without 'bad' germs. The 'good' germs referred to by some children (see p. 172) could be converted into bad ones through the eating of sugar, but the process of this change remained obscure. The concept remained unintelligible for me. But not all bad germs are equally potent or effective: 'Some things can't be caught as easily as others'.

This age group thought that bad germs could enter the body in the ways already described by the nursery school children. One said 'It's a sort of bug which can get into your mouth with what you eat'. Ideas of contagion remain important, as in the statement, 'My sister passed it on to me and two days later my sister had no chicken pox'. The interpretation of this natural resolution of the sister's illness is affected by the close conjunction in time with the 8-year-old becoming ill. The conjunction in time increases the child's belief that there is a connection between his sister's improvement and his deterioration. This was associated with a recurring theme that germs are passed on as an entity, and in order to get better you need to pass the germs on to others. This seemed to represent a form of 'conservation of matter' (Piaget & Inhelder, 1966 p. 47) in which germs were not seen as multiplying. The same ideas are encountered in some adults with sexually transmitted diseases who believe that the best way to be free of the infection is to pass it on to someone else.

This idea of transmission of germs as an entity could account for an observation from the nursery school age children. Some of them had recounted how important it was for the doctor to lay on his stethoscope as this was a part of the treatment during which the germs could leave the body through the stethoscope. It resonates with the importance of the 'laying on of hands'. The idea is also found in the children's games of 'Lodgers' and 'Germs' where the germs are passed on as a unit of constant size with none left behind (Opie & Opie, 1969 p. 77). One would expect to find these games or variants amongst 8-year-old children.

The 8-year-olds seemed to lay more weight on what happens when they breathe rather than when they eat. They believed that they could breathe in germs when close to an ill person: 'When they are playing, if they hold hands maybe, or one of them came very near to their face. P. might have breathed in, then breathed out again, and G. might have breathed in P.'s air then she might have caught it'. Nevertheless the previous ideas are still present, but as shown in this example more closely related to breathing: 'We were both talking together. I didn't have it but my pal had it. He coughed, and my mouth was open at the time so I caught it – caught the germ – and then if affected me'. These observations are in contrast to the earlier ones of Nagy (1953). She found very little evidence of 5–7-year-olds having any ideas about how germs entered the body, and amongst the 8–11-year-olds the predominant mode of entry was believed to be through the mouth when eating rather than breathing (79% compared with 21%). The overwhelming importance of the mouth led to her labelling the children's beliefs about illness as adhering to 'a theory of oral infection'.

The above views, which include a need to respect distance between people, can then play a part in creating problems for children depending on the level of anxiety which they have about catching illness. Other children find advantages in this rationale for controlling overintrusive parents and so negotiate for more space for themselves. One father complained that his sons would say 'Don't you breathe on me, I don't want your germs. That type of thing'.

The 13-year-olds seemed to doubt the conservation of germs yet continued to be puzzled by what happened to the germs as they got better: 'Say you've got a cold, like if you've got it from Monday to Thursday, it will still be there on the Friday, just lingering. Like there's not enough there to make you feel there's a cold. You've still got some which is taking its time to get away'. 'You never get rid of a cold – just the germs pushing their way back and forward trying to get towards you and give you another cold'. The latter suggestion resonates with the ideas of the need to establish balance in order to remain healthy that are found in those medical systems which are predominantly naturalistic in form, and also with Herzlich's (1973 pp. 58–62) description of health as a 'state of equilibrium'. The mother of the first boy quoted felt that she had helped create his viewpoint through saying to him that he needed to blow his nose in order to get rid of a cold. At the same time she observed that he regularly had a blocked up nose so he 'probably does not know whether he's ill or not because he's blocked up'.

All the mechanisms whereby germs exert their effects have been described so far in interpersonal terms. It seemed quite understandable when I was told how erecting barriers between people could then protect them from germs. These ideas first appeared with the 13-year-olds. They described the value of windows and doors being closed to protect them from the transmission of germs through the air from other people. But a lingering doubt remained about how effective these strategies could be in view of relics of earlier animistic thinking which included attributing intention to the germs. They were 'little live things which try to get into your system to breed and multiply and make you feel awful'. Different degrees of effort were attributed to the different germs. The children were hopeful that these efforts would continue to be defeated by the germs having to find their way around closed doors.

The children also expected washing to prevent the spread of germs, because the germs could no longer make their way over the body to enter through one of the orifices. Nevertheless washing was not always effective due to the efforts of the germs – the explanation deduced by one girl to explain the following story:

It was in her breath I think. Something could be wrong inside. My Mum's breath comes out and it goes onto my Daddy. My Daddy washes his face normally, but the germs still don't come off. And germs start spreading across the face and eventually they get to the mouth where it causes quite a bad cold in his throat.

One of the orifices not mentioned so far is the ears. These were mentioned on only two occasions, by 8-year-old girls who saw them as a potential source of entry for mumps. The immediate interpretation seems to be that the discomfort they experienced was in the neighbourhood of the ears, and so they explained this with a generalisation from their other ideas about how germs entered the body: through the mouth for infections affecting the tummy, through the mouth or nose for infections affecting the breathing such as colds.

Besides the normal orifices the only other way into the body was through a cut. Germs were seen as getting into the body through cuts if there was dirt present: 'If cut knee and don't wash it out, might get poisonous' and 'If you trod on something like a dirty pin and get it in your foot, well that would give you some germs'. Germs were also seen as able to enter the body through blisters, in fact any place where the skin was damaged. Some 3–4-year-olds held the idea that germs could enter directly through the skin, but there was only one reference indicating no doubt about this approach route among the 8-year-old children. Another felt the need to hypothesise that the germs would need tools in order to get through the skin – 'Maybe they go round with wee drills'. If the germs got directly into the blood stream through a cut they could then cause problems according to one 13-year-old, but otherwise they were harmless.

The understandings which the children have shown in the examples so far have not necessitated them looking at how the germs exert their effects once they have crept into the orifices or got in contact with a person. But the children did reveal more ideas about what the germs were up to. These seemed to represent a clear development from the earlier analogies of germs to insects. Insect bites could lead to one getting red spots which were seen as similar to the spots and rashes one might get with the exanthemata of childhood. With these coincidences possible origins can be seen for ideas such as 'germs bite – like these little sacks like snakes have but not poisonous', and 'you can get chicken pox by a bite'. In order to discriminate insects from germs one child used the characteristics of different bites to help: 'When you don't feel them they're infectious, but when you do feel them they aren't infectious'. With this analogy there was some difficulty knowing how the effect was brought about, and they presented the suggestions that 'germs give you viruses' through the bite and the corresponding insects give you germs. Within the group discussion some disagreement arose:

K. I was bitten by a flea in my hair. I felt well.

J. You didn't feel well.

K. I did feel well.

A bite was seen by J. and others as necessarily being associated with illness and one could not rely on subjective validation. A similar confusion seemed to be present in the statements from three 8-year-olds to the effect that 'germs sting, but aren't sore'. I never quite felt I knew what they meant by that but could not pursue the theme too long because otherwise their assumptions that we shared enough common concepts from the 'taken for granted world' would be challenged and their trust in me would be too threatened (see also Berger & Luckmann, 1966).

Germs were also said to be bionic. This word was picked up from television programmes about a Bionic Woman, a lady with incredible powers and yet normal appearance. Her ability to leap great distances provided a model for lice and germs jumping between people: 'They just jump because they are bionic'. When these ideas retain their flavour of being an analogy they can be helpful for the child in imposing some temporary order on his ideas, but as we have seen some children fail to distinguish between playful ideas and the serious. For them these ideas could eventually become unhelpful if held as part of a tight construct (Bannister & Fransella, 1980 p. 30).

A rhetorical question still remained for some of the children: 'How can they harm you if they are tiny?' Maybe this provided the strength for the bravado of the 13-year-old boys who often said they were 'not afraid of germs and bugs'. This is a domain in which one would have to look much more closely at how society construed boys' behaviour contrary to that of girls in order to find out the interpretation which was warranted. The pressures on them from adults and their peer group encourage them to take this 'tough' stand and equate size with strength.

## Germs and spirits

The following definition could well cover the children's understanding of germs:

Something whose existence and presence is postulated by its powerful effects, but about which little else is really known because it is unseen. (Miller 1980 p. 45).

This is actually the definition of a Nepalese *deuta* which Miller goes on to describe in this way: 'These powers can be and usually are called "spirits" in English but I think "invisible powers" corresponds more closely to the sense of the Nepalese term *deuta*' (*op.cit.* p. 45). Jung was interested in these phenomena and he adopted the description 'primitive energetics' for these magical powers (Storr, 1983 p. 69). These basic energetics which give life to our concepts appear to have been the same forces which Newton called upon to explain gravity, in other words they stand and have stood at the centre of our understanding of the world. Storr (1985) quotes Sullivan's report of Newton saying 'that gravity should be . . . essential to matter . . . is to me so great an absurdity . . . Gravity must be caused by an agent acting constantly according to certain laws; but whether this agent be material or immaterial, I have left to the consideration of my readers'.

When I was with the children I did not have any clear ideas about roles which their religious beliefs could have been playing in the formation of their views. If I had I might have been more open to the roles they could have attributed to God in the causes of illness. A Norwegian female priest explored children's concepts of illness and noted their comments in the contact which she had with them in hospitals in 1984–5. She obtained several views which seemed to reflect a less central role for germs and bugs and a more important role for religious powers such as represented in the power of God or Christ (Kristine Værnes Anthonisen, personal communication). The parents of these children were not noted for their religious observance, but the interpretation offered was that they had developed their views through contact 'in passing' with religion in the local community. The danger with any such results is that they are attributed to the lack of neutrality in the person who collected them. The complementary danger is that similar views could have been excluded from my awareness. I mention them here as they would be coherent with the children's frequent dependence on a variety of invisible powers for explaining the important daily changes in their lives.

Through having an image of the unseen germ, the children deduce some of its properties. These properties need to be coherent with the social system of explanations within which the children are growing up. The ways in which they then perceive themselves as affected by the germs gives them further information about the mysterious unseen germs, as well as information about themselves as people. We grow up and develop through illness. If the images provided are dissonant with the children's earlier functionalist definitions there is scope for problems, especially if there is poor discrimination between 'pretend' images and 'real' ones. In the same way there can be grounds for misunderstanding in a consultation when different images are presented without clarification of the perceived *function* of the complaint. Personal intellectual growth can come about through resolution of the various paradoxes presented by the differences in the information contained in the pragmatic and mathetic modes – the process Piaget referred to as accommodation.

# 6

# Dirt and fresh air: the exogenous system

*'So long as identity is absent, rubbish is not dangerous.'*
*(Douglas, 1966 p. 160)*

The previous chapter explored the children's views on causal agents such as germs and how they acted; this presented elements of the 'personalistic' medical system found in this population. These causal agents were regarded as representing the children's deductions of 'facts' from the various ways in which information was given to them. The systems in which the information was given were described in general terms in chapter 4, but without specific details of how illness rationales maintain boundaries between the systems and are used to facilitate particular social strategies. Here the threats to health inherent in the environment are discusssed.

How people respect the community's conventions about dirt appears to be particularly important for establishing the moral order around health in that social system. It is necessary to look more closely at what I mean by moral order, because I am here adopting an understanding of morality which differs from the stage models usually used. The concept of moral order comes from Harré (1983). (The interested reader who wishes a fuller presentation of why the stage model of development of morality is no longer adequate should refer to Harré's exposition.) The key concepts include the idea that the development of morality is best seen as socialisation towards the predominant value system of the society, in which the successive 'stages' represent approximations to the adult viewpoint without these approximations being seen as more advanced in developmental terms (see also Harré, 1979). This socialisation is viewed as the progress of an individual's moral career through which he gains honour and respect by negotiating hazards. In this context I find it useful to consider the negotiation of illness episodes as one sort of hazard, and the threats to health inherent in the environment as another. As it is the latter which I am considering in this chapter it will become clearer that the exogenous causes of illness are closely concerned with the moral order of illness/health and the ways in which people show respect for others and gain respect themselves.

At the same time it is necessary to remember that an individual can have a different moral career in each microsystem of which he is a member. Different reputations about vulnerabilities are gained depending on, for example, how school and home microsystems are negotiated. How dirt and pollution are conceptualised in a society will lead to them assuming different degrees of hazard, and so different possibilities for gaining status in one's moral career. The conceptualisations of smoking as a hazard either to be avoided or successfully negotiated characterise two opposing trends in ways to gain status amongst subgroups of adults and adolescents respectively. It is with such notions of hazards in the environment, as part of an 'exogenous' system (or 'naturalistic' medical system: see p. 47) that we will be concerned in this chapter.

Instead of viewing development as three stages (corresponding to Piaget's egocentric, concrete and formal), Harré follows the social constructivists' claims 'that there are three kinds of social order, distinguished by their conventional imperatives, to which a child (or an adult) can belong, not necessarily in the order of succession presumed by Piaget' (Harré, 1983 p. 222). What happens during development is that children become able to take more factors into account when evaluating a social order. Within these orders people can be viewed as having particular rights which change according to the sort of order established. To use a medical example the rights which parents have to question doctors about their child in a consultation are often established through a particular conceptualisation of the social order of the setting and this conceptualisation differs in different cultures. Harré (1983) then presents a proposition about what constitutes a moral order: 'In a moral order . . . the three characteristic forms of conduct – rituals, confirmations of respect and contempt and displays of proper character and moral commentary – are permitted only to those who in this or that collective, have the right to perform them' (*op. cit* p. 245). The rules of conduct for that situation govern who has this right. These rules can include superordinate rules that there are differences between how adults and children should perform. For example, has the parent but not the child the right to question the doctor in the consultation?

Both the apparent functions of adults' instructions to the children for creating a moral order to their world, and the children's views, will be presented here. These two aspects are intimately bound together. Some of these pragmatic considerations relate to decision-making about illness, but the majority represent the way in which adults socialise their children into the world of health and illness through special rituals and routines. These pragmatic modes of communicating with children about illness themes become one of the ways in which a particular social order and morality is constructed. The rules of conduct so established have both constitutive and regulative functions (Harré, 1983 p. 229). They constitute part of the primary structure (the social order) and regulate interpersonal relations within that structure at the same time.

Douglas (1966) wrote the classic description of how dirt and pollution are incorporated into the social value systems of a variety of communities. She showed how these views were reflected in and by the religious orders in these communities, which at the same time developed rules of taboo which needed to be respected in order for the community's members to remain healthy and accepted. Identity and health became associated with religion and order. Disorder and dirt appeared synonymous. The reader who wishes an overview of the adult world of 'dirt and pollution' is referred to her classic study. My interest here is the child's world and how it fits into the adult world.

The adult world is the setting within which children are endeavouring to extract 'facts' about the causality of illness. Not surprisingly their efforts in the mathetic mode become bound up with pragmatic considerations. Causes become mixed with explanations and rationalisations. The respective roles of individual and collective responsibility are fashioned through the meeting of these considerations, and illness gains its social and individual emotion-laden meanings.

The way in which the exogenous system is seen to influence health and illness is through the setting up of conjunctions between events, or states of the environment, and body states. These are key ingredients in naturalistic medical systems, and it is to this type of medical order that the social organisation of the concepts of dirt and fresh air makes its greatest contribution.

### Dirt and cleanliness

Winnicott (in Davis & Wallbridge, 1983 p. 157) said that 'the dictates of hygiene . . . get between the mother and her baby'. This reflects the way in which acceptable practices for looking after babies incorporate the standards of hygiene in the community. These standards are not built up with attention to the whole range of developmental requirements of babies and their mothers for mutual responsiveness but reflect a much more primitive value system built up over centuries in which the rights of the mother to impose things on her child (and so overrule the basic intersubjectivity) are rationalised through the dictates of hygiene.

Today in obstetric practice the same dictates of hygiene can come between the mother and her baby and lead to much friction between different schools of obstetric practice. The difference depends on what sorts of hazard obstetricians believe appropriate to allow mother and baby to negotiate, and to what degree they believe mothers can and should make informed choices. The same phenomenon seems to be reflected in the particularly high malpractice insurance needed by obstetricians in the United States, where claims are said to be mainly against those who carry out high-technology obstetrics. The *use* of high-technology procedures at birth has become linked to dictates of the ethics of hygiene as the applications of the techniques have evolved. The medical community has come to the conclusion that applied in certain ways this new technology is part of good medical practice. As the dialogue about what constitutes good practice has been carried on above the heads of the mothers and babies, this is another example of how the early contact between mother and child is affected by dictates other than their own potential desires for contact and interaction (which as described earlier lay the foundations for the development of sensitive communication). The alternative moral orders meet the affective human element, stating their cases in languages difficult for the others to understand. The ways open for negotiating their respective requirements are very rudimentary at present, but it seems an appropriate field for the assistance of child psychiatry.

One further example of the dictates of hygiene coming between mother and baby occurs in neonatal intensive care units where the usual sight is of parents approaching the incubator containing their child with hands held firmly behind their backs. They keep their distance and everything is done so as not to contaminate their baby. The staff and parents would need to discuss their ideas about the dangers of dirt in order to get over the most pressing discomforts parents can feel when they begin, at one level, to associate themselves with the potential to pollute their baby's environment to the extent that it could kill the child. The social order in the hospital is determined by the medical staff and so it is not surprising that parents can come to believe that it is the medical staff who 'cause' them to be pollutants – such is the convoluted thinking induced in such situations.

Parents introduce the adult normative standards of cleanliness to their 2-year-old children, at least in the United States (Kagan, 1982). This timing is probably dependent on the child first having a sense of self, so that the child's deviations from his sense of what is constant can be noted, disorder is distinguished from order and unclean discriminated from clean (Douglas, 1966 p. 160). In the same way, before this sense of constancy has arisen,

I would not expect the usual state of the body, health, to be discriminated from the more intermittent discomfort associated with illness. In contrast the potential daily discomforts of hunger, loneliness and cold are incorporated in normal development into the sense of a healthy self. Should the child be ill so often in the early months and years that the discomforts of illness are as frequent as these other more normal discomforts, his subsequent development of ideas about illness and its causality would be expected to deviate from the normal.

The parents of the 3–4-year-olds in my sample were introducing them to various social routines and rituals associated with different bodily functions. The children were encouraged to wash their hands before eating food. They were introduced both to the idea that this is necessary in order to prevent problems later as well as that the parents would be pleased if they complied. The emphasis here is firstly on visible 'dirt' which if not removed may enter the child. The parents make the situation as concrete as possible to fit the child's phase of development. Only a handful of the parents extended the explanation to the nature of the problem with dirt being that it contained germs, the causal agents of disease, although the link between germs and dirt in relation to cuts was already quite widespread amongst these children. The children described the importance of washing cuts in order to remove a kind of 'dirt/germ' entity, a poorly differentiated rather loose construct, a sort of noumenon.

In one family interview a mother was trying to elicit her 4-year-old son's knowledge of germs for me: 'Why are you made to wash your hands before eating?' But he remained preoccupied with a first-order explanation involving dirt, unconnected to the food which would subsequently be taken in by him – 'So my plate doesn't get dirty' – rather than the second-order element about the nature of the danger in dirt. The mother, not surprisingly, was dissatisfied with this explanation which remained at the concrete level and did not yet reflect the underlying dangers. What she believed these dangers to be remained unclear and unspecified for the boy. She had asked the question in a family interview when the theme had been germs, so I assume that dirt and germs are closely related for her, and that the danger in the dirt is in the germs and the ways in which dirt can affect health and body integrity. The routine of washing was not yet established as a ritual. Her own feelings about the danger in the dirt were not yet transmitted to the boy's total construct about the hand-washing routine, which continued to lack a charge in order to establish its effectiveness. Piaget & Inhelder (1966 p. 21) summarised the relation between these two elements in the development of behaviour in this way: 'when behaviour is studied in its cognitive aspect, we are concerned with its structures; when behaviour is considered in its affective aspect we are concerned with its energetics . . . These two aspects . . . are inseparable and complementary'.

What constitutes dirt is open to wide interpretation according to the ways of negotiation and values of the microsystems and macrosystems. Here the parents are introducing the child to personal strategies to cope with the dangers of dirt, dangers which are not and cannot initially be spelt out but only transmitted to the child through alterations in the parental responses to him. These alterations are in a way experienced, rather than observed and reflected upon, at this age. For example the dictates of hygiene are instrumental in establishing the distance between people which comes to be a part of how they live their lives.

Later at home the child lives with a particular ordering of his daily life. He experiences that everything has its proper place and time. The things which happen are responded to and ordered according to how they are classified by the adults who structure the young child's world. In this way events are linked with actions to restore order; the consequent reactions – haste and turmoil, or relaxation – which then enter into the parents' relationships with their children set the tone and colour of the event through non-verbal interaction. Housework (see Davidoff, 1976 for the social organisation of housework) appears to be very important for transferring these values to young children, who learn through the parents' explanations and through observing their behaviour about the proper place for things, the rationales for cleanliness and who is responsible for cleanliness within the order of the home. Undoubtedly the provisional hypothesis must be that the majority learn early on that it is the mother who guards the family against the dangers associated with disorder and dirt (see further below). It remains unclear what role this plays in the child's understanding of the moral order around illness and the development of the special interests of males and females in cure and care respectively.

The way in which parents organise the child so that he develops personal rituals to cope with dirt introduces the child simultaneously to the family's social routines and its sense of what constitutes dirt and is dangerous. In this way, by introducing the idea that something such as dirt can disrupt the usual family order, a shared way of organising the disorders of the daily world is established. This is coupled to a moral value system about the nature of what is dangerous. The particularly powerful effect of this form of development is that the child's understanding of dirt, danger and social order arise at the same time on the basis of particular routines and rituals begun in the home by those people to whom the child is most closely attached. The nature of the dangers is subsequently elaborated for the child using a variety of models which vary over the years but appear to reflect the different themes of development with which the child is preoccupied, and which simultaneously the parents hope the child will develop.

With the 8-year-old children germs were more commonly invoked by the parents in their discussion of the dangers of dirt. A father of an 8-year-old boy explained that 'We've had a recent splurge on germs because . . . we've noticed he's not washing his hands as much'. The children of this age more often felt that germs were necessary for all types of illness. This appears to represent an overgeneralisation of explanations initially put forward by the parents in a way which is consistent with the results reported earlier. Accidents were, however, excluded from this system of explanation by both the 3–4-year-olds and the 8-year-olds, contrary to what Kister & Patterson (1980) found with their two younger samples (mean ages 4 years 8 months and 5 years 6 months) from the United States. Accidents clearly belonged to a different category of event for these Scottish children, which I will describe as being of a different moral order.

For the 13-year-olds the situation has changed: 'I used to hear from parents about washing hands when younger. Now you are supposed to know that, or do that anyhow. Parents have stopped going on about it'. By this age there has been a shift in the degree to which the children are expected to take responsibility for their own state. Discussion about how these children come to be ill now lays more weight on personal responsibility. They were more reflective on their earlier upbringing. One added the following recollection of his younger years: 'I wouldn't eat picnics 'cos you couldn't wash your hands'. In the process he emphasised that he had moved on from a stage of socialisation in which the parents were organising him to fit in with family rituals. These budding adolescents appeared much more preoccupied with the social norms of society and their peer group, the origins of these and the ways these norms were maintained. These alternatives restored and rejuvenated their sense of personal choice and facilitated their developing sense of agency.

In the United States Campbell (1978) noted that especially boys aged 10 years to 12 years 11 months of relatively more educated mothers were encouraged to be dependable and determine what they should be doing themselves. In this connection it is interesting to note that these same mothers 'attached relatively little importance to obedience or to neatness and cleanliness'.

Although the influence of food on the child's world of illness is discussed in the following chapter, a brief digression on children's sweets and how these differ from those thought desirable by adults is appropriate. It is here that adult standards concerning food, hygiene and what they consider 'rubbish' meet the child's understanding of why these standards are being imposed and lead to apparent acts of defiance against the otherwise accepted adult standards. Children's responses at school and with their peers to sweets of particular kinds play an important part in establishing them as members of that fraternity.

The topic has been studied by James (1979) in the North-East of England. In this area the dialect word used by adults for rubbish, or useless articles, is 'kets'. (It was originally applied to 'something smelly, stinking, unhealthy or diseased'.) Kets has been appropriated by the children for their 'revered sweets'. James shows that the sweets classified by the adults as rubbishy or ketty are just those regarded as desirable by the 11–17-year-olds she interviewed. An element in identity is developed through opposition to the established adult standards. When the contrasting children's standards are employed they create a sense of power independent of the adults'.

This leads to alternative eating habits for the children such as playing with the sweets and taking them in and out of the mouth. Bubble gum, for example, is stored for later re-use. More closely related to the idea of the dangers associated with dirt is the fact that these sweets are characterised by not being wrapped. Kets are exposed to dirt, fingered at almost every opportunity by a variety of people and according to some standards of hygiene it is as though eating them 'courts disaster'. 'The normative conventions, instilled by parents during early childhood, are flagrantly disregarded' (James, 1979). Kets are typically very sweet, and so offend the standards of what is desirable to eat as established in dental health weeks and through advice from 'those who know better'. Some other qualities of kets are worth noting in relation to the discussion in chapter 7 on the place of war metaphors in the child's world of illness and the child's understanding of the functioning of the body. A battle flavour is established through the names chosen for kets – 'Fizz bombs', 'Fizzy bullets', 'Supersonic flyers', 'Robots' and 'Star ships'. These sweets are said to have explosive tastes. They often have 'inedible' colours such as fluorescent oranges or luminous blues.

Children of these ages often dare each other to eat the inedible, be that sawdust, 'fag-ends' or earthworms. If they insert the dirty object it is as though it loses the associated dangers warned against by adults. If adults force the eating of things they regard as food the children may label it as 'shit' or 'snot'. James points out that school dinners are a case in point where 'the foods which children are forced to put inside their bodies by adults are given the status of the excretions which pass out'. The power of the label and who controls it seems to preoccupy these children as they experiment with alternative orders and ways of accounting for dirt and its dangers.

In other social routines established by adults the nature of the dirt referred to is more intangible and often connected by the adults to powerful causal agents. After children have been to the toilet they are told to wash their hands. In these circumstances there is no visible dirt and the parental explanations to the 3–4-year-old children ranged from 'You've got to', to having to remove 'germs' which the children could not see. It has been suggested that this latter explanation can transmit a parental fear of germs (Becker, 1971 p. 68) which engenders anxiety in the children for whom there is otherwise no need to remove germs beside complying with the parental wishes. Nevertheless some children of this age already question their parents' explanations (which may have been linked to doleful consequences if not obeyed) because they observe, as though scientists, that 'Guinea pigs don't have to wash paws if *they* don't want to'.

Body excrement has a particularly profound impact on the meaning given to dirt. In common parlance especially obnoxious dirt can be called 'shitty'. Animal faeces are seen especially in the 8-year-old group as being particularly dirty and as a source of infection. One child said 'We've got a little boy in our street and he's always going near dog dirt and he's getting too many colds', and another 'I think if you go near it [faeces] it's got a special thing in it like a germ. And if you go near it, or do anything silly with it, the bug might just jump onto your clothes'.

There can be a more diffuse sense of uncleanliness associated with urination and defecation for some 8-year-olds. 'When you sit on the toilet you don't know where "you know what" [a bottom] has been' and 'When people go to the toilet you never know where they have been' were how two children put it. This latter child, a girl, said that the reason her mother used Domestos, a proprietary bleach cleaner, in the bath was because there was an outside chance that the bath had been used instead of the toilet. Here there is the same sort of link between body excrement, germs and Domestos as was noticed previously. The meaning to a cleaning ritual is established which integrates these otherwise disparate elements.

In addition the commonly used phrase 'dirty old man' connects dirt to sexual perversion. Without the epithet 'old' the phrase would mean something rather different, more in line with the usual use of dirt. What is important to note here is that these men are believed to be especially dangerous – dirt and danger are united in special sexual mores. Cautionary tales about dirty old men are often introduced to both girls and boys at this age. Women are not warned against for their powers of corruption in the same way.

Bathing and washing the body were seen as important for removing dirt and maintaining health for both the younger age groups: 'More likely to get germs if I don't clean myself' or 'Germs are dirty things. They give you diseases. You get them if you are dirty'. The strategy becomes refined and emphasised by the 13-year-old girls, who were quite scathing about their male peers whom they felt paid no attention to this. It was as though they were keen to draw attention to those routines which were different in degree for the two sexes so as to emphasise their own sexual difference. There was an accompanying awareness of some advantages of increasing the salience of cleanliness for rationalising, in the first instance, some of their beauty treatments. In addition they understood the boys' behaviour as being due to their laying greater emphasis on football and other sports. These were seen as healthy things to do as they involved exercise and fresh air, although they left the boys filthy and sweaty. This agrees with Davidoff's (1976) observations that it is masculine to be dirty. But the place of dirt in this order of things can only be understood in relation to the balance between the relative salience of fresh air, exercise and dirt for boys of this age from this culture.

Maccoby & Jacklin (1980) report a study from the United States which asked college students to reflect on their upbringing and compared their impressions with those of their parents. They found that 'Young men are more likely than young women to recollect that their mothers didn't allow rough games, and tried to get them to keep clean. Mothers report, on the other hand, that they hold up stricter standards to daughters than sons when it comes to avoiding rough games and keeping clean'. The mothers were seen as expressing a *value* for cleanliness that applied especially for the girls. The problem with this type of retrospective study is in knowing the validity of alternative intepretations.

The 8-year-olds had mentioned hair care as important for health when they were working out what to do in cases of nits. They had all had their hair inspected at school for the presence of nits. From early ages children can be exposed to mythical people in cautionary tales which are used to stress the importance of particular health rituals. Kvideland (1979) reports several of these from Scandinavia. One is the tale that 'if children didn't want to wash or comb out their lice, they were threatened with the louse-man; the lice will make a rope of your hair and pull you down to the lake'.

Amongst the 13-year-olds in Edinburgh it was only the girls who continued to mention hair care as an aspect of health care, being concerned that 'I don't think that we get enough of hair testing in the school'. The same links between beauty treatments and health, as mentioned above, seemed to provide the basis for the maintained status of hair care as part of health care for these older girls.

The children had been made aware from the very earliest ages of the social routines to be used when coughing and sneezing in order to prevent spreading diseases. One 13-year-old had come to some deductions because of this: 'Everyone's got one germ, because if you sneeze you're supposed to put your hand over your mouth so you don't spread your own germs. Everybody's got their own germs'. For these older children there was the awareness that when sneezing one was not necessarily ill with a cold. Yet their understanding of the social routine was such that it was predicated on a germ theory of sneezing, and hence their deductions about their own germs to which they were immune but which were potentially dangerous to others.

Douglas (1966 p. 96) has pointed out that 'danger lies in transitional states, simply because transition is neither one state nor the next, it is undefinable'. Coughs and colds, and niggling tummy aches, belong to this category of transitional state as they can be signs that something is afoot. Times of maximal uncertainty will be found when these states begin before a pattern of dealing with them is established. The anxiety can be expected to be the highest in those who have had experience that these states can lead to serious consequences. Here personal experience plays its part in raising the level of anxiety and uncertainty, and correspondingly the need for coping strategies to keep the uncertainty within bounds. Establishing clear routines to be observed when these states begin is one way of minimising uncertainty, as with routines for coughs and colds. If these routines follow the accepted mores in the community the individual knows that all that was required has been done, and so there is no need to feel a sense of personal responsibility should there be serious consequences for his own health or the health of others in the community/family. These are key ingredients in naturalistic systems. The strategies have both a personal and an interpersonal element. The ways in which people cope with the initial uncertainty, almost always present at the beginning of an altered body state, are analysed in chapter 8, where tummy aches in particular are discussed.

Earlier in this century spitting was included with coughing and sneezing as a way in which diseases were spread. Spitting had been very prevalent particularly in the working class population. It appears to have been built up on a rationale for health which included the need to get rid of one's phlegm, much as the younger children described here had a need to pass on their germs in order to get healthy themselves. Personal strategies were at the expense of the interpersonal, and especially at a time of prevalent turberculosis the health of the community suffered. At a personal level the problem was one of how to dispose of the bad without giving it to another. This previously normal social behaviour, which could be seen as a sign that people took care of their own health, has now largely ceased. I only obtained one reference to spitting, from a 4-year-old who remarked on it as a way in which infections could be transmitted. The interpersonal effect predominated over any model he might have met for spitting being a personal health strategy. The parents did not include injunctions about spitting amongst the family health guidelines. It is important to note this because the marked shift in what constitutes approved social behaviour has now reached the point where the socialisation of children into this current value system appears to occur without much direct focusing on it by parents or teachers. The model for spitting behaviour is no longer so widespread. The health ethic is no longer applied to the behaviour in such rigorous ways as previously when tuberculosis and purulent bronchitis were common. Instead spitting exists as a specific aggressive act to illustrate disdain. A behaviour which was reduced through linking it to the health/illness domain has now moved over to be an element in social posturing.

A common social approach to life is established through these personal strategies encouraged by the parents on a basis of dirt or germ rationales, these being shared to an extent with the values of the child's other microsystems. Some views on causality are established as common for a culture. Others are established as only being found in various of the building blocks to the macrosystem, the microsystems. The child's problem is knowing where he is in this building as he meets a variety of strategies and hears a variety of dialects.

The strategies are built up through emphasising the individual's own part to play in preventing things going wrong. Clearly this can only occur if an individual child retains his sense of effectiveness in altering things (Bandura, 1977), or as others put it his sense of agency, a sense which is vulnerable to lack of empathy in early development. At the same time the children recognise the situations in their environment for which these strategies are necessary and so their responses to their environment begin to alter. The environment becomes characterised by danger and order, pollution and cleanliness. The first step for this with animal excrement was mentioned above. Respect for conventions in human relations are beginning. Meanings to these conventions are formed.

'If you're walking in a street and it's very dirty, the dirt will go up your nose . . . [and cause illness]' and 'You can catch them [illnesses] at the seaside because it might be dirty water' were two statements by 8-year-olds that showed the children did not equate the dirt with germs, but were building up an approach to their environment. The seaside was seen as a risky place to be by two other children. This contrasts with the health virtues attached to seaside holidays in the early 1900s. In one case the risk seemed to exist because the girl's mother had caught food poisoning from eating a crab. This food poisoning was attributed to what the crab must have eaten, and hence the sea was dangerous.

The seaside is not the only environment to have shifted from being a healthy place to a polluted place. The same shift has occurred as regards inner cities. In 1840 the school inspectors stated how they evaluated sites for schools (Paterson, 1986): 'Spatially, one way of securing a school's exemplary status as a purveyor of a healthy and morally correct way of life, as well as ensuring its accessibility to the population, was the stipulation by the Minutes that the school had to be in a central location which was free from the dangers of moral and physical pollution'.

There were several references by the children to pollution as a cause of illness without the pollution having to work its effect through the intermediate agency of germs. Flies seemed linked to this notion as they conveyed 'pollution'. They provided a link to theories invoking germs as the agents of pollution, as flies also carried germs and were virtually indistinguishable from bugs. The exact nature of pollution could not be defined, but tended towards anything that might be undesirable – similar to the views on dirt conveyed by Douglas (1966). Attitudes to dirt reflect the society's value system, which itself reflects that of the more powerful groups within the society. At the same time children need to develop a sense of why one has respect for the predominant value system in order for it to retain its powerful organising potential. Around health themes respect for individuals and for society crystallise out together and it is possible to develop strategies which to a degree respect both the needs of the society and the individual's integrity.

At the time of this study there was much media coverage of a syndrome labelled 'Allergy to the Twentieth Century', and this was reflected in the children's views on pollution that it might be anything to do with the twentieth century. The growing interest in things immunological is related to the current growing interest in immunotheories of disease.

I would hypothesise that fear of radiation in the environment would be tapping similar sources of disquiet, especially because of its invisible, all-pervasive nature which gives it qualities similar to those of germs and pollution. Pollution never has an absolute quality, but always reflects the value system of those who define pollution as such. The ultimate disorder is seen to occur in the wake of a nuclear explosion.

Several 13-year-olds came up with the idea that 'Dirt *is* a germ'. In the evaluation of what constitutes dirt the values of the health/illness domain have predominated. And for those who make this equivalence a system of agents predominates over a system emphasising symbolic connections with things which have happened. The personalistic predominates over the naturalistic. Others said 'Dirt itself is not a germ, but things that always come with dirt are germs' and 'Cos there's all these dirt particles and they've got their own germs in them'. They were trying to make sense of the links between dirt and germs which had been so strongly emphasised since early childhood to cater for the child's question of *how* dirt affects them, and *why* they should not do certain things. Those who have come down in favour of a more characteristically personalistic system seem to have shown a relative neglect of the question 'Why did this happen now?'

### Fresh air and exercise

It has been seen so far that the children showed poor discrimination between dirt and germs. It is unclear whether the theory they were building up was of *agents*, such as germs, causing illness or of illness being caused by the *environment* i.e. having been in a dirty place. The distinction between a predominantly personalistic or naturalistic system is not clear. Germs are also used to explain what *has* happened. This contrasts with how they are used to organise forthcoming social behaviour, based on how adults structure the child's microsystems on a rationale of what dirt and germs *will* lead to. Before coming to how germs can be used to explain what has happened I will refer to another distinction between dirt and germs which introduces the idea that some factors can lead to personal vulnerability to illness and so represent a hazard.

For some 8-year-old children dirt is becoming something which does not cause problems for them, but enables germs independent of the dirt to affect them. One child from this age group said 'They [germs] can't attack you because there's no dirt around near you'. This idea enables an interpretative link to be made to the very prevalent notion of fresh air, often described as clean air, being protective. This is in contrast to the views described in chapter 2 that exogenous influences conveyed illness;

fresh air is here seen as an exogenous protective influence. The children were aware of some importance of fresh air from 3 years old and upwards. The parents regularly encouraged the children to go outside by saying that fresh air would be good for them. Several parents opened the bedroom windows at night to let the fresh air in, although for others it was to make the room smell nicer. The salient quality of fresh air then seemed to be that it was outside and usually cooler. Florence Nightingale's working hypothesis was that 'fully one-half of all the disease we suffer from is occasioned by people sleeping with their windows shut' (Nightingale, 1860 p. 12). Nevertheless Helman (1978) reports some adults from near London now saying that 'children get sick if you leave the bedroom window open at night'.

Cool air was often seen as fresher than warm air. Yet this resulted in a potential danger which Florence Nightingale (1860), amongst others, worked hard to avoid. As she stated (*op. cit.* p. 73) 'I need hardly repeat the warning against any confusion of ideas between cold and fresh air. You may chill a patient fatally without giving him fresh air at all'. Her first canon of nursing (*op. cit.* p. 8) was: 'TO KEEP THE AIR HE BREATHES AS PURE AS THE EXTERNAL AIR WITHOUT CHILLING HIM' (capitals in the original).

Maybe there is a persistent underlying folk belief which emphasises being cool for getting a good night's sleep. This would be coherent with sleep research which has shown that poor sleepers are hotter by night and by day (Oswald, 1986). I am not aware of any systematic attempt to induce more satisfying sleep by lowering the ambient temperature at night and noting any shifts in body temperature and sleep states. Later in this chapter as well as in the next the vulnerabilities one is exposed to when asleep will be discussed, as well as sleep's protective and restorative qualities. The rituals established around this time of greatest vulnerability assume special protective powers.

Some of the children saw it as possible to become ill if one 'doesn't get much fresh air, and you're all just in a stuffy room', especially a room filled with cigarette smoke. The children from 8 years old made definite links between smoking and cancer. The characteristics of a stuffy room are covered in the following quote: 'If you don't have proper air, have very old air . . . you can breathe in the old air . . . it kind of makes you suffocate because you don't have the good fresh air. It would feel funny in you'. One mother of a 13-year-old boy explained how they linked germs and smoking: 'I suppose germs on buses. We have talked recently about travel on buses. There's likely to be more germs floating about upstairs in a bus than there are downstairs, with all the smoking going on upstairs. We encourage James to go downstairs on a bus'. This mother was aware of the growing importance of the peer group's influence on children of this age as reflected in her statement that 'I suspect he goes upstairs 'cos that's where his friends go'. The parental influence on determining their 13-year-olds' value system concerning health and illness matters was already beginning to wane as the children gained more socially important respect from their peers.

The concept of fresh air has been central to rationalisations of a large part of the organisation of housework, and the values attached to the different parts of it. The organisation has changed over the decades in line with shifts in culture and class values, yet the concept of fresh air has changed also to maintain its place as the main organising concept, particularly for the middle classes (Davidoff, 1976). (Due to the nature of my sample I was unable to test hypotheses about any class linkage of the concept of fresh air.) A recent review of the role of women in maintaining the health of the family (Graham, 1984) suggests that because mothers usually have a central role in allocating and justifying the distribution of household resources it tends to be their value system as regards health which predominates in the family (see also Mayall, 1986).

The concept of fresh air has an ancient basis, dating back at least to the miasmic theory of contagion described by Sydenham in 1676. Acute illnesses were said to be due to invasion of a person's body by atmospheric miasmata which were Sydenham's disease entities (Taylor, 1979 p. 7). The same words were actually used in two families of 13-year-olds, much to my surprise. A 15-year-old sister said, 'It's the bad night air. It's the miasma from the back garden'. Whereupon her father corrected her a little, 'Miasma from the canal'. Subsequently the father seemed to stress the properties of damp air coming from the canal. The ill health associated with dampness was a general theme. As one 13-year-old put it, 'Damp places – that causes some illnesses like a cold or something. Really damp places make you really ill'. A damp climate is said to lead to similar problems. The same concept of fresh air mediates between the establishment of the moral order in the house and protection against the threatening influences in the environment.

Yet paradoxically, at the same time, being outside carries its dangers. The children were aware of the need to wrap up carefully to protect themselves when going outside. The semantic confusion in the English language between 'being cold' and 'having a cold' may exaggerate this effect in this sample. Different languages express this in different ways. In Norwegian, for example, when one *has* a cold one *is* 'forkjølet' (made cold) and so the problem for the child's ability to discriminate being cold and having a cold is even more taxing. The connections between cold and rhinitis become deeply engrained. An 8-year-old described colds coming because of 'Not putting your coat on on a cold day. And sometimes it just goes away if you put your coat on'. For others of this age group, though, there had been the same change as observed earlier in the relation between dirt and germs, where the dirt was seen as potentiating the danger of the germs. One 8-year-old girl said 'You feel cold outside and the coldness makes your body feel cold, and then maybe something in the air is bad and it comes down and gives you a cold or something'. A mother of a 13-year-old described limiting the importance of these sorts of instructions to preventing colds, as though this was the only danger one was exposed to if one became cold outside. These routines were well maintained in the families of these 13-year-olds.

All families referred to going out in 'proper clothes' for the conditions, but what these clothes should be differed markedly and appeared to reflect different cultural values about the dangers inherent in the environment. In some families woolly hats were seen as very important for preventing colds and earache; partially it seemed through a local protective effect as they were worn pulled over the ears. The practice was not associated with histories of earache in these families, but they looked to their strategy as having been successful in enabling them to avoid ear problems and therefore it being necessary to continue wearing woolly hats. Anxieties about illness made it apparently unethical to try a 'controlled experiment', although adolescents subsequently tended to find this out when testing the values of their parents' routines. Putting on warm clothes to go outside was particularly important if you had been ill as illness was seen as increasing one's vulnerability to catching a further cold, yet paradoxically 'being outside' was also 'a good place to be' after one had been ill. The children had to make sense of these apparent paradoxes on their own.

The likelihood of catching a cold was seen as the chief danger of being outside. The 8-year-olds were aware that this might be just a Scottish problem: 'You'd get heat spots instead of a cold if you lived in Iran'. There was some advantage in one's local fresh air compared with foreign air, which could be a source of germs. One child said that germs came from Greece. Another thought they came from Italy because of hearing 'a story about the canals smelling in Venice 'cos all the toilets go into it'. This is a further aspect to the conceptualisation of the threats seen to be posed by things foreign. Different countries seem to emphasise the positive value of their own fresh air to different degrees, and so indirectly increase the contrast with the dangers of foreign air; for instance fresh air (often combined with exercise) appears to have a very central place in Norwegian health strategies. Possibly if the fresh air were not awarded such positive connotations in Norway the apparent dangers of cold would lead to very unbalanced health strategies in winter.

Heat and cold are central concepts in several different health cultures. Folk models of health and illness try to make sense of environmental factors, bodily sensations and, in some cultures, the measured bodily temperature. As many elements as possible are involved in constructing a coherent account of why they are in the state they are, in the environment they are, knowing of the dangers they are aware of. For an exposition of an English folk model which integrates folk concepts of heat and cold in connection with adults' theories of illness see Helman (1978).

Wrapping up adequately was not just to keep warm, as illness could arise because 'You could be outside with no coat on; 'cos our street's quite dirty and you could catch a bug out there'. On exploring this idea further it became clear that the coat represented a form of bug-proofing. As described above, cold comes to be seen by some of the children as a vulnerability factor rather than a causal factor and it is possible that describing coats as bug-proofing is a metaphorical way of presenting this idea.

There is a large difference between a foreign country and 'foreign' parts of one's own country. Just as Herzlich found that those in her urban sample regarded the countryside as a healthy place to be, so also did these 13-year-old town dwellers: 'In the country it's fresher than in the middle of town because of exhausts and things'. As was seen in the school inspectors' report from 1840 quoted above this view is relatively recent. I can provide no comments on the views of children who have to live in the country. Those adults constrained to live in the country in Herzlich's sample saw it as an unhealthy place to live. In contrast to adults the degree to which children's way of life is urban or rural is always chosen and created for them by their parents or alternative primary care-givers. Their sense of helplessness in the face of their environment arises within their smaller microsystems rather than the macrosystems stressed by Herzlich (see chapter 2).

When the children are sent out to get fresh air, often independent of the parents, it appears as though it may be a parental strategy to get a bit of peace and quiet or space for themselves. Several of the older children seemed to interpret it as a regulative rule on this basis, used for pragmatic reasons rather than being presented as information about what is good for them. As such it would be expected to lead to much more discussion and potential for renegotiation, rarely being taken at face value.

Some families make a point of getting out together for 'a spot of fresh air'. In this situation the rules about fresh air stand less chance of being interpreted as regulative and one would expect the place of fresh air in the family's value system about health to be regarded as one of the constitutive elements – the mathetic would predominate over the pragmatic. When the family gets out together it is often to *do* things. Exercise in the fresh air is additionally seen as 'good for you'. In other families exercise was emphasised as an activity for children which need not bother adults. Here particularly one would expect the children to interpret the rules around sending them out for fresh air as belonging to the regulative category.

Children of all ages in the sample regularly associated fresh air and exercise as combined reasons for doing things. The forms of exercise which were mentioned as healthy included swimming, football, judo and jogging. The exercise approach to health was particularly prominent amongst all the 8-year-olds and the 13-year-old boys. There may be hidden dangers in stressing the benefits of fresh air. It may be that excessive emphasis on being outside, when the child is not with a responsible adult, is one of the causes of childhood accidents. A health strategy thus comes to be potentially dangerous, but because of the health premises to the rationale which lie deeply embedded in the moral order it can be expected to be resistant to change.

Too much exercise was seen by my respondents as harmful but mainly through leading to injury rather than illness. The establishment of the child's exercise norm could lead to much negotiation within a family, with discussion of both the advantages and disadvantages of exercise, rather than there just being a general instruction 'Exercise is good for you'. Through this discussion the nuances of the construct 'Exercise is good for you' are elaborated and a set of values put forward by the adults which represent the combined viewpoints of those involved.

One other special sort of 'strain' was mentioned: that which results when 'I've watched TV without my glasses on'. Even then the parents had been making the point at a time of encouraging the boy to get outside for some fresh air and exercise rather than sitting watching television. Depending on whether the child already has a view of this strategy as regulative or constitutive he will be likely to start arguing about it, provided he perceives the social order of the setting as giving him that right, i.e. the regulative strategies being regarded as open for debate.

## Personal responsibility in a 'hostile' world

Throughout their development children's relation to the environment is reflected in, and comes to reflect, their developing sense of locus of control. The form to this will be related to their rights in particular settings characterised by the differing moral orders of the microsystems. The views they develop of being 'at the mercy' of dirt and pollution in the environment, or of being able to take care of their vulnerabilities, are reflected in their attitudes to their own responsibilities in settings with differing characteristics. These attitudes are here hypothesised to have developed in relation to the factors presented so far in this chapter.

I will now proceed to look at how further questioning introduces the child to points of view about germs and environmental factors which do not mean that a germ theory excuses the child his personal responsibility for his state (see earlier discussion) but lead to an exploration of the complicated relationship between causal agents, such as germs, and personal responsibility. Where the responsibility is allocated will not necessarily correspond to who takes it, responsibility sometimes appearing to be a rubber ball bouncing carelessly amongst the people concerned. It is useful, though, to explore the child's sense of personal responsibility for his state in more detail.

At the same time as germs are being used in the establishment of appropriate social behaviour and order they are presented to the child as an explanation for things which have already happened. Vomiting is a common condition of early childhood requiring explanation. The children are commonly curious to find out why it happened, why their body suddenly seemed to be out of control. The parental explanations for the vomiting which I encountered seemed to take two forms: either food met a germ or bug in the tummy, or something had happened to the food before the child ate it. It is in furthering these explanations, together with explanations concerning tummy ache and diarrhoea, that the roles of dirt in physically affecting the body come subsequently to be elaborated. Nevertheless some of the children seemed to have been trying to understand how their bodies came to perform in the way they did – an enquiry about themselves as vomiters rather than the food or stomach in particular and the role of contamination.

Some 3–4-year-old children were content with the parents' first-order explanation mentioned above, whereas others reiterated the question to ask how the germ got into the tummy, or how the food was affected. Whether this particular form of extended questioning is modelled on their own experiences of being questioned by others, or reflects curiosity (or both) is not known. They shifted from why to how questions. Only with this second-order questioning comes the possible introduction of an explanation involving the child as agent in causing the introduction of the germ or contamination of the food.

The 3–4-year-olds in my sample felt they had no part to play in being responsible for their illness, with no hint of it being a form of immanent justice; in other words they gave the same sort of response as was observed by Brodie (1974) in healthy children. They appeared to be greater believers in neutral chance following the neutral questioning I adopted than social and developmental psychologists following the stage model would have us believe. They did not see chance as an 'obstacle to deductibility' (Piaget & Inhelder, 1966 p. 113). I believe this to be a result of my experimental method, which avoided either forcing the children to take a moral stance in relation to their illness or making a guess at what sort of expectations I had. The method used will always be reflected in the information obtained. The import of these observations is that given the chance children will believe in chance. If the ethos is that chance plays a limited role in causing things to happen, the children's views are likely to reflect that ethos. Additionally it may well be that alternative factors, such as separation from parents, affect how children interpret their condition when they are hospitalised, such that immanent justice ideas arise on that basis rather than because of their understanding about illness (Perrin & Gerrity, 1981).

The relationship between concepts of justice and illness causality is complex. One 3-year-old girl was aware of two sorts of doctors: those you go to when you are good and those you go to when you are bad. The latter sort of doctor was typified by 'Dr Guthrie'. This doctor gave his name to two List D schools for delinquent children, one for boys and the other for girls, in Edinburgh.

The 8-year-old children were much more aware of a part they might have played in causing their own illness. They frequently echoed the responses I obtained independently from the parents, who would say that the illness happened because the child failed to follow a social rule. They became ill because they were 'going out in the garden with bare feet', 'eating a sweet off the ground. It would have bugs in it', 'rushing around too much', or 'eating food too quickly – especially chocolate'. The parental response to the older child who is ill often involves some irritation as they believe that their careful social instructions have not been followed. Parents believed that the 8-year-old children were old enough to be taking more responsibility for their own state through observing the socially approved rituals. The statement 'My mother gets very cross when I get sore ears, because she thinks I haven't used my hanky enough' was given with the explanation that 'germs will go through a little tube to your ears and make your ears red and sore. If you sniff it gets worse'. Here it can be seen that the tone to the parent–child relationship affects the emotions which accompany *post hoc* explanations. Illness beliefs and ways in which social order is maintained can come to be tinged with the same emotions.

The same phenomenon could affect illnesses which appear to arise at school, with parents expressing irritation at the teachers for not encouraging the child to wear their gloves and scarves or follow some other home-based social rule. In this way additional properties of the mesosystem (the relation between the microsystems of home and school) affect the child's concepts. The child caught between the two can be the vehicle for the adults' discontents in a functional way so that the child's mathetic view of illness becomes distorted. Nevertheless parents are aware that they are really concerned about something other than factors which increase the child's vulnerability to illness when 'carrying on' about some of these strategies. I believe that they are referring to the importance of following the appropriate set of rules for the moral order. In relation to other microsystems, such as school, they are aware of the importance of establishing the 'right' moral order. One of the mothers said that she herself 'knows dressing up is a fallacy' but that she still gets quite 'worked up about it'. The emotional colours to the social rules of the parents' own childhoods appear to be very enduring. Through the emotional tone of the relevant moral order the colours are produced for their own children's illness and health behaviours.

In accounting for some further actions of the children which could have appeared to result in 'illness' the children nevertheless absolved themselves of responsibility. The majority of accidents were attributed to chance and were not seen by the children as causing illness. There was no use made of germs to explain accidents as a form of contagion. This is contrary to the results of other researchers (Kister & Patterson, 1980), and I believe reflects the social orders of the different research situations.

Occasionally children were introduced to other ideas about accidents. One mother put it that accidents can make 'people ill, perhaps in your mind'. On exploring this idea she seemed to be thinking of the result being increased anxiety regarding a repeat accident.

Two 8-year-old children described getting mumps secondary to falls in which they knocked their heads. One girl, who said 'I fell and hurt that side [of the face] and it grew and grew to mumps', clearly attributed the cause of her resulting lump to the fall and saw the lump as the precursor to her mumps. At the same time she told me, 'The doctor said because when I fell I probably got something infectious', which I interpret as her way of integrating a germ theory of illness to her conceptualisation of the cause lying in the physical origin of her lump. The other child said, 'Think I must have fallen out of bed and landed on something. Germs could be on smelly socks', which suggests a similar line of thinking.

These explanations for illness that *has* occurred are then resurrected in argument and negotiation when parents are trying to persuade their children to do things. This can take the form of almost threatening them that they are likely to become ill if they do not do a particular thing. It is not surprising, then, that children search over events which preceded their illness, as in naturalistic systems, to decide where the cause of their problem lay.

Piaget (1932) sees this form of response as a prerequisite for the child's development of 'moral realism':

> The rules imposed by the adult, whether verbally (not to steal, not to handle breakable objects carelessly etc.) or materially (anger, punishments), constitute categorical obligations for the child, before his mind has properly assimilated them, and no matter whether he puts them into practice or not. They thus acquire the value of ritual necessities, and forbidden things take on the significance of taboos. Moral realism would thus seem to be the fruit of constraint and of the primitive forms of unilateral respect. (*op. cit.* p. 129)

Using Harré's terminology I would say that it resulted from a particular kind of social order, characterised by a hierarchical relationship, such as is normally found between children and their parents, in which the rules of respect are such that only certain individuals in the microsystem have rights to respect.

At the same time as children are being exposed to the adults' views of dirt and danger, parts of the naturalistic system, similar emphasis is being given to germs as a kind of agent similar to those found in personalistic systems. Elements of both types of system appear to be introduced to all age groups bound together in a complex way. The children are trying to make sense of the rules and regulations, and to distinguish the pragmatic from the mathetic. The overall impression seems to be that chance events were the cause of 'our' problems, but that others become ill because they failed to carry out some protective strategy. Whether this is because of the forms of questioning and modelling the children have been exposed to or not remains unproven.

## Sleep and helplessness

*'Sleep tight. Mind the bugs don't bite'.*

So far I have explained the adults' systems of explanation and the resulting ways in which children then become socialised within an illness rationale. In order for this to be effective the children have been awake and active participants. Many 3–4-year-old children saw themselves as waking up ill in the morning. This is not surprising because if one's state is changing slowly it is difficult to notice the difference unless there has been 'time out'. Consequently the immediately preceding events were a mystery to them and their personal theories of causality tended to neglect their own potential role in causing illness.

Parents of children this age read them many fairy stories of events happening in the night (see for example Bettelheim, 1976), usually immediately prior to the child's bed-time. In addition Father Christmas is said to visit during the night (for further discussion of the way in which children make sense of Father Christmas see Tizard & Hughes, 1984 pp. 114ff), as do tooth fairies. I was not surprised, therefore, to hear from one child that illness comes down the chimney at night. Parents are also known to tuck their children up in bed at night and recite the superficially silly rhyme 'Sleep tight. Mind the bugs don't bite.' Is bed-time a time of danger? The predominant view amongst these 3–4-year-olds was that illness just happened, although night-time and sleep remained a mysterious time.

Another possibility for what can happen at night-time was noted in connection with measles. Maybe the child had not noticed the first red spot before he went to sleep; perhaps there had always been one little spot of rash: 'Measles comes from weeny spots which get bigger; the rest of the measles pushed it onto the tummy'. This spread then occurs when the children are not watching, primarily when they are asleep. For chicken-pox there was an alternative explanation for the spread of the rash reflected in a slightly uncertain belief that 'The itch makes it spread', which on exploration seemed linked to ideas of scratching itches and so making more red spots.

Night-time was seen by these young children as a time when they were very vulnerable to getting illness as illnesses 'come' when their eyes are closed. In addition it was a time when they felt relatively separated from their parents, which was in itself seen as increasing their vulnerability to illness: 'Germs are not there all the time, they come when mummies go away'. In similar circumstances one 4-year-old felt as though he hardly existed during the time he was asleep when the illness arrived. He did not know where his illness had come from – 'don't know how it happened as I wasn't there'. Bed-time rituals have an important role to play in helping children cope with these vulnerabilities through establishing order (Wolin & Bennett 1984). This is especially important prior to the child entering the, to him, anomalous state of sleep during which he is neither here nor absent.

These ideas of night-time being the vulnerable time are still present for the 13-year-old children: 'germs come at night'. However there was an evolution of this viewpoint as germs were more often said to come 'when you're feeling tired'. Here the state of sleep as being the vulnerable state has given way to the state of pre-sleep, sleepiness, as though the state which preceded sleep caused the problems which you woke up with in the morning (in the way that important socially approved preceding events could in naturalistic systems). The parents of 13-year-olds were having a greater struggle to set bed-time limits for their children, so they had also begun to develop their rationalisations about tiredness and its links to states of ill-health. They began to refer to the importance of getting a good night's sleep. There appears to be a coevolution of parents' and child's ways of accounting associated with joint negotiation of a phase of their social life together, but they are developing their ways of accounting from different perspectives. The role of sleep in building up the body's resistance is discussed further in the next chapter. The advantages of sleep, when taken together with the child's vulnerabilities whilst asleep, introduce children to another paradoxical state having similar qualities to those of fresh air, in that it is potentially both 'good' and 'bad' for them at the same time.

In other cultures night-time is the time when witches are about and one has to take precautions to ward off that danger. Whether bedroom windows are closed to keep out miasma, 'sins', witches or germs, I suggest that the underlying fears are similar regardless of what explanatory structure is built up to account for them. As was seen with germs, a definition for a *deuta* lies very close to that for a germ. When we act to keep things out we run the risk of excluding that which can give health, such as fresh air. I believe that further research on locus of control factors and how these develop and relate to people's approaches to dangers in the environment will be helpful here. They may also be found to relate to sleep patterns, as an initial result suggests short sleepers have a higher internal locus of control (Kumar & Vaidya, 1986).

## Giving the problem an airing: a summary

In this chapter I have presented a range of the environmental factors which were associated in the children's minds with causing illness. It was as though dirt was seen as a potential source of germs, or potentiator of germs; faeces were the most potent form of dirt in this connection. The social rules that help children find their way through this potentially threatening environment are then established through the parental and school strategies towards cleanliness. The basis of particular moral orders is established.

Fresh air was described as a social construct representing a healthy environmental influence. It was closely linked to taking exercise. As with dirt, fresh air was defined idiosyncratically within families, usually functionally. These pragmatic considerations then coloured the children's constructs about exogenous factors causing or preventing illness, and the degree of their personal responsibilities in causing illness. In this way a certain moral realism is established around 'appropriate' behaviour; this stage has been described in other settings as starting at about 6–7 years old (Newson & Newson, 1976 p. 190), which is in line with the observations here. By appropriate is meant approximating more to the predominant adult set of values. A balance between 'good' and 'bad' aspects in the environment facilitates the child's sense of choice and effectiveness in his relations with that environment.

When children are asleep their personal responsibility is suspended. Sleep can then be seen as dangerous if one has few personal strategies one feels competent to use for warding off illness. Alternatively it can be seen as a relief if one's personal responsibilities, or the requests made of one to exercise them, have become burdensome. It is not yet clear whether there are links between views on illness as liberator or destroyer and the above feelings about the dangers of sleep. These may turn out to be related to locus of control factors and particular styles of upbringing.

# 7

# My castle and the good germs: the endogenous system and its boundary

In the descriptions so far I have looked at some of the microsystems within which the child develops his views on the causality of illness, the role of causal agents and how they might act within that system. I have presented how rules and a moral order are established which govern the child's relationship with his environment with regard to both health and illness. In this chapter I describe the individual's view of his contribution – the endogenous influences – which enable him to cope with the causal agents. This gives more insights into how children view the agents as acting and their bodies' resources for combating these. I suggest that the ways in which the children are socialised, with particular values becoming salient for them, foster to varying degrees their self-efficacy in maintaining their personal health. Lifestyles become established and to varying degrees under personal control.

### The castle walls

Many of the younger children's comments suggested that they regarded their skin as an important boundary, protecting them from intruding environmental factors such as dirt and pollution as well as germs. The weak points are at the body's orifices such as the mouth and ears. Genitalia were not included by them in these discussions. The views persisted with the 13-year-olds, who thought for example that '[you get ill when you are] . . . sleeping with your throat uncovered when it's cold'. The same views are to be found amongst adults in England (Helman, 1978).

The skin is also weakened if it should be broken in a cut. An 8-year-old girl said about a cut: 'If you don't clean it there are germs in it. Then once it starts to get worse, when it starts peeling off, you get a big bump of poison in it. That's what I saw. That's what Lorna got 'cos she didn't clean her knee and all the dirt didn't come out'. Here the understanding and the emotional response to the importance of washing the cut is linked to the world of dirt and the moral associations made in that domain.

These children had not experienced surgery. Blaxter (1983) reported the belief amongst a group of Scottish women that trauma and surgery 'might leave weaknesses or permanent gaps in defences against the environment', much as though one is left with permanently weakened skin.

Some of the youngest children had felt that germs could enter directly through the skin, for example through the hands which washed an ill person's plate, whereas others thought the germs would have to travel over the skin from the hands up the arm to an orifice. Skins differ though. There is some evidence to suggest that both boys and girls between the ages of 5 and 7 years, in the United States at least, view women as having weaker skin (Ullian, 1984). The social construction of sexual stereotypes has led to the 'fragility' of the female being reflected in her capacity for reduced resistance relative to males, and this is present in the views of young children. The boundary wall of the skin could be built up externally with additional clothing in the views of 8-year-olds. It is easy to hypothesise that the different ways boys and girls dress will be seen as reflecting the greater 'need' the girls have for protection on the basis of the girls' skins being seen as weaker. The degree to which this interpretation is warranted remains unclear.

The children had also developed ideas about what was happening within them to build up their defences. These ideas took form for the 8-year-olds in the concrete metaphor of a castle with walls and busy defenders, a metaphor which becomes reified rather than just poetic, and hence becomes the child's reality. This view was put forward by one of the 8-year-old boys in the following manner: 'It's like a castle, right. Germs knock down a wee bit of the wall. Red blood cell scampers upstairs to the white blood cell and they come down and patch it up'. Some others in the group who had not used the idea before, avidly recounted it later in a subsequent research session saying that they now thought it was true. It appeared as though they found the concept helpful for their current problems in making sense of what was going on. The organising potential of the idea gave it credence. A way of expressing the importance of metaphors such as these is provided by Leech (1981 p. 38): 'through its power of realigning conceptual boundaries, metaphor can achieve a communicative effect which in a sense is "beyond language"'.

Although most children used the idea of the castle as though the walls were their total surface area, another 8-year-old had the idea that maybe castles were erected in the stomach out of potatoes. Food was seen as having a concrete action in building up the defences inside one of the entrance ports, rather than this effect being mediated via several intermediate steps following food absorption.

Davies *et al.* (1982 p. 388) found similar views among 10-year-olds in England who envisaged germs being fought with white blood cells, antibodies or good germs. They said that 'The analogy of "armies in conflict" was a particularly strong one'. The metaphor had been put in its place by my 13-year-olds. They described their recollections of castles when reflecting on views which they had held previously: 'Red cells and that are fighting off the germs – a castle and all the germs – I thought that the germs actually were little green men, eyes and nose and little hands, and used to go with little pitchfork things trying to get into the castle'. The castle idea generally seems to have been a loosely held construct which was held over a period of between 3 and 4 years.

The metaphor of 'battle and warfare' has also been observed in Aberdeen women (Blaxter & Paterson, 1982*a*) and Welsh women (Pill & Stott, 1985). The profession of medicine seems to be full of a 'warlike' approach to patients and their diseases as reflected in the turns of phrase used (Hodgkin, 1985) – 'battling' against overwhelming infections, or engaged in the war against cancer, etc. The castle metaphor seems to reflect all levels of society's thoughts about disease processes and the body's resistance. It permeates all discussion whether it is between children or adults. It would be expected that the prevalence of war-related metaphors would fit in with the children's capacity to relate illness causality to questions of immanent justice and punishment for misdeeds.

In earlier times the metaphors employed were more to do with the nature of 'balance', but these now seem to have been largely superseded and I found no references to them among the children. Sontag (1979 pp. 64–5) suggests that the change got under way in the 1880s with the identification of bacteria as agents. Others have suggested that the culture of modern science is responsible as it has adopted a predominantly masculine value system. A return to metaphors of balance, cooperation and interaction could be useful clinically, especially as these would reflect some of the key elements in an intersubjective psychology. But a return seems unlikely in view of the ways in which the war-related metaphors are so embedded in our culture. Balance metaphors, though, could help people get away from viewing their bodies as objects containing diseases, for 'What we will find in ourselves will be a function of the metaphors available' (Harré, 1983 p. 283).

## Food

The role of food in maintaining the boundary walls involves more than just erecting potato castles in the stomach. Food was important to the

3–4-year-old children, who had frequently been presented with the parental injunction to eat something because 'It will do you good'. This seemed to reflect parental anxiety about whether they were giving their children enough of the right types of food, with their concerns being transmitted to the child's value system. An alternative interpretation would be that it was a control strategy legitimated on health reasons. At that age the children appeared to be particularly aware of the virtue and value of eating those foods which they were encouraged to eat at home, were mentioned in the Dental Health Week and were approved of in the nursery. Home-made food was seen by several families as more healthy than bought food.

Although the parents referred to 'a balanced diet' in many family interviews, this concept was rather nebulous and enabled the children and parents to include most things of which they were rather fond. A balanced diet had to include lots of fish and chips for some, fruit for others, whereas diversity was important for still others. It was only in connection with diet that metaphors of balance appeared in the family interviews. Eiser *et al.* (1983) have reported that English children of 6–11 years assign a central role to diet in maintaining good health.

The 8-year-old children viewed the feeding issue as so important that they described the principal job of a nurse being to 'shove' food into people because it was one of the ways of making 'Big healthy people, and if you don't get food you die'. The German proverb 'A good cook is the best doctor' can either be interpreted along the same lines or suggest that it is important to make the food as tempting as possible for those who are ill, and who maybe have a poor appetite. If the food-stuffing view prevailed this would be a recipe for large scale obesity, but this was not the case partially because of the widespread view that being fat increased the likelihood of a person becoming ill. The actual foods eaten are seen as important, 'wrong' foods being associated with ill-health, but I remain uncertain why 'If you eat too much sugar you get worms', as one 8-year-old told me. The characteristic of 'bad' foods is that they contain a lot of sugar (6–11 year olds: Eiser *et al.*, 1983). The problem for advertisers of fizzy drinks is how to present products which are sweet and liked, and yet establish a more socially responsible image. The motto appears to be 'Talk dry, taste sweet'.

Food was quite a frequent battleground with the parents. Health rationales predominated as a negotiating tool in these confrontations between parents and children. For example, the parents often used a stock phrase for milk and meat that 'It will make you big and strong'. The 13-year-old children would on occasion disregard their parents' advice on health matters to do with food, even if they agreed with it, 'In order to get our own way'. In this situation the content of the message was agreed upon but pragmatic issues predominated and so the mathetic element was apparently disregarded.

The same problems arise with presenting information to the public. The method of presentation and its timing are crucial for impact and effectiveness. It must be presented in a way which makes it clear that it is not being presented to score points over others, but solely to give information to enable people to make their own choices. Advertisers go to great lengths to establish the right climate of acceptance for their products (see for example the presentation of sugars and fats as scientifically approved 'non-fattening' agents in an analysis of media functioning: *British Medical Journal*, 7 June 1986 pp. 1520–1). The audience will always be wondering about covert messages as they have been used to manipulation from childhood onwards as regards what constitutes a healthy diet. This makes the current situation where there is lots of conflicting advice very confusing. One would hope that official reports could steer clear of these dangers but, for example, when the Committee on Medical Aspects of Food Policy (COMA) reported in 1984 the above 'nettles' were left ungrasped (see Winkler, 1985), so that the issue of how the agreed information on dietary factors in cardiovascular disease could be used to shape a new policy regardless of political motives (the pragmatic implication) remained.

The 13-year-old children were obtaining further information on food in their home economics lessons, independent of the pragmatic elements of home instruction but instead incorporating the rules and regulations of the classroom. They were very aware that not all food was good for them, but this was especially thought to be the case if it was not prepared correctly. From the way things had been highlighted for them in their lessons I was reminded that food must not be left uncovered, must be fresh and properly defrosted. Freezers were seen as potential sources of ill-health if food was not used by its expiry date or properly defrosted. I was left wondering how this affected the negotiating balance at home in the confrontations over food.

A common strategy on finding someone is ill, especially a child with a tummy upset, is to reappraise what has been eaten recently. This strategy is the same as in naturalistic systems. The cause is not necessarily attributed to some 'agent' in the food, but it can be the food itself or some problem in its preparation. The preparation of food involves obeying a lot of different guidelines, the transgression of which is seen as predisposing the eater of the food to potential harm. The role of germs, the agents of a 'Western' personalistic system, are incorporated into the rationales for the different rituals of preparation, but in the end the problem is felt to be with the food and not the germs referred to in the rationales. Allergies to food seem to be gradually taking a larger place here as potential causes for unexplained illness (see below).

One 13-year-old girl who uniquely in the sample had American connections and belonged to an out-of-the-ordinary religious sect, put forward the view that water was also very important for health, on the basis that if one washes one's outside to remain healthy so one must drink plenty of water to rinse out the inside. This view was repeated by her mother in the family interview. This view was found in earlier times. The inside of the body had to be cleansed or purged just as the outside. Culpeper had described these cleansing and purging roles of medicines in his *Complete Herbal* in the seventeenth century (Culpeper, 1850 edn, in *British Medical Journal*, 2 April 1983, p. 1105).

### Vitamins

The 3–4-year-old children were aware of 'vitamins' as a special element in the food. Vitamins were allocated an important place by parents and nursery staff but not as an active agent with animistic qualities as had occurred with germs. As the invisibility and intangibility of germs elicited the children's curiosity, so too did the nature of vitamins. This nature remained a mystery, but vitamins were clearly important for modifying social behaviour through being used to justify social value systems.

They remained important as the children got older and were referred to in biology and home economics lessons. Davies *et al.* (1982 p. 398) found war metaphors prevalent here for 10-year-olds, who saw vitamin C as important for strengthening antibodies before they go off to fight 'the other army'. I heard of no concrete images of vitamins (in contrast to the situation with germs), the emphasis remaining all the time on the functions of vitamins for growth, strength and warding off infection. Two quotes from 13-year-olds were: 'Said to give you energy, especially vitamin C' and 'Vitamins are things which keep you from getting diseases, or keep your energy up'. On enquiry these qualities seemed to reflect ideas of building stronger walls against infection as well as of being a kind of anti-germ. In other words vitamins provide both resistance ('It helps you build up a barrier against the germs') and a cure for illness ('Very good at times, because they help make you better when you're ill').

Although the 13-year-olds were hearing much more about the nature and use of vitamins, they had ceased taking them at home. Three-quarters of the 13-year-olds used to take them at home when younger but only one did currently. One said 'Taking vitamins is babyish', and another 'You don't really need it now'. Whether this reflected the belief that the castle walls were established by now, or that mind should begin to triumph over matter remained unknown to me. It may be that the pattern of giving vitamins as additives in the diet fostered one view that vitamins were not found in food but only as powders which were added to fruit juices. The 'megavitamin movement', perhaps relatively localised to the United States and Australia, did not seem to have influenced these children.

## Medicines and poisons

Pills were distinguished by the children from medicines, which was a term reserved for syrups. Pills were seen as being required to treat the more difficult illnesses. Hence being given pills was a sign of the seriousness of your illness. In 1982 in Edinburgh the principal pharmacist in the region was warning that chronically sick children who were taking medicines sweetened with sucrose had much more dental decay than other children and she encouraged the greater use of tablets. Whether this led to a change in prescribing habits and how the children reacted is unknown, but they could have viewed their condition as deteriorating.

Medicines were not viewed as special sorts of vitamins or food but instead more like one of the agents in a personalistic system: 'It's got something in it that just kills them [the germs]'. On elaborating the premises behind the statement that 'You get rid of them with medicine. But not just the medicine, because sometimes it's just like strawberry water and it hardly does it', it became apparent that medicine was seen as a facilitator of the body's own defences. It may be a special sort of poison, 'Poison which kills germs but not us'. Poisons were seen as good things in some cases: the children had been given the information that plants developed poisons as self-defence and logically assumed that people needed their own protective poisons also.

In spite of the way in which medicines were portrayed in several of the nursery school story books as being necessary for recovery from a variety of viral infections, 10-year-olds in England have been found seldom to expect medicines to cure them of a cold (Davies *et al.*, 1982 p. 389). Of those that did hold that belief, four out of the five thought that the medicines would 'kill the germs'.

The 8- and 13-year-old children were also aware of poisoning as in 'food poisoning'. In these circumstances poisoning had a slightly different range of meanings: 'Something that won't agree with your body', 'Eating wrong sort of crab', 'If you eat something that's eaten something else that your stomach doesn't like, you're ill'. (All these quotes were from 8-year-olds.) The same phenomena are seen as happening with some medicines, and the 13-year-olds knew of idiosyncratic and allergic responses to medicine. In these cases they tended to describe the medicine as one that 'doesn't agree with them'.

*Allergies*

The importance of dislike for things leading to illness seems linked to two other concepts. The first was referred to earlier and is that illness or health reasons are used to persuade children to eat or drink things that they do not like. It is hardly surprising, therefore, that children use the same value system of 'dislike' or even 'disagreement' in relation to illness. The second concept refers to the growing awareness of allergy. Allergies appeared to be very important in the playground and at mealtimes at school, but to a much lesser extent at home. The 8-year-old children rarely distinguished between not liking and being allergic. If they wished to avoid sprouts at school dinner they believed they were more likely to succeed if they said that they were allergic to sprouts rather than that they disliked them. The belief seemed to become consolidated as part of an identity as an allergic person rather than as someone who has dislikes. Similar observations have been reported for adults who have excused their food avoidance as 'allergy' (Pearson, 1986). A 13-year-old gave the following example of the uses of allergy: 'My cousin can walk past dogs, but big ones he's scared of and he says he's allergic to them. But nothing happens, all he is is scared of dogs'. This illustrates an awareness of the rules of this particular 'negotiating game'.

Parents also use allergies to maintain limits on their children: 'My mum told me I was allergic, but I don't know what it is. She said that you can't go near that. So that's why I always tell my mum where I'm going as she will know whether it's safe there. She still hasn't told me what it is yet. She says "I'll tell you when you're older"'.

Allergies were seen as particularly threatening to the boundary walls as they were associated with changes in those walls – skin rashes and runny noses – and hence the child was made more vulnerable to illness. In addition the children were aware that the effects of allergies could be local at the exact point of contact, such as an allergy to sticking plasters. Skin conditions which were seen as remaining on the boundary wall were felt to be particularly hard to get rid of using the strategy whereby the causal agents such as germs were handed on. It was as though the illness was not really part of them so could not be dealt with in the usual ways, remaining on the surface rather than being incorporated as part of them to give them an identity as an ill person with all the associated advantages and disadvantages that accrue in the family.

When the 13-year-olds pursued their ideas about allergies, endogenous factors in causing illness became emphasised for them. They believed that people 'can be born with it. In some cases they can catch it. Also it's something to do with the nerves or something like that'. 'You've inherited it'. Another stressed the mental contribution: 'I think a lot of it's in the mind probably'. It was also said that people with allergies 'have a bad resistance against something'. These ideas give food for thought when taken together with recent psychiatric research on patients 'with supposed food allergies' (Rix, Pearson & Bentley, 1984) which have stressed the psychiatric morbidity in that population.

The immunotheory of disease appears to be going through a critical phase of its development at the moment where disinformation about allergy can distort its applications. Potentially the theory can leave children either feeling that they are responsible for their immunological state or not depending on how adults account for children's states. The key ingredients for the 13-year-olds seemed to be environmental dangers and reduced resistance due to poor mind over matter strategies. Although some have seen immunotheories as reducing personal responsibility my observations of these 13-year-olds suggest that the role of personal responsibility is currently in the balance. But the tendency is to allocate responsibility to the allergic individual. A provisional impression in Norway is that the situation is different and emphasis is laid on environmental factors. Children there hear that carpets are unhealthy for the ways in which they can make it more difficult for people with allergies.

I believe it is important to note that these observations refer to other people's allergies. These older children are now coming across illnesses which they have not experienced in themselves. In this situation it is potentially easier to impute a role for the individual in the origin of his allergy where that individual is not yourself. Although they are saying that the cause of allergies may be endogenous in these cases, it is endogenous in a person apart from them. It is nevertheless as though they are saying that the cause arises outside their own self, only in the affected individual. This contrasts with the one child who had asthma who saw no role for his own inheritance or mental state in causing his condition in spite of being well aware of the allergic nature of his particular asthma (see also Blaxter (1983) for similar observations in Scottish women). These older children appear to be adopting their parents' pattern of imputing the cause of illness in others to actions or inheritance of those others, in those cases where the disease is one from which they are not personally suffering. Similar conclusions have been reached elsewhere; for example, 'people do not ascribe their own sickness to moral transgressions, but they use these concepts in describing each other' (Cosminsky, 1977).

The children also mentioned another basis for allergy as a response to overloading the body with something: 'You're resistant to everything, but if you have too much of it it [the resistance] breaks down'. 'When I was a baby I had too much of it and I got allergic to it'. The body's reaction to the overload is what gives rise to the symptoms: 'Your body's trying to get rid of the penicillin so it's breaking down to lots of spots'. The rash is seen as a message to the body, 'It tells you that it can't take it – a rash or something, or sore stomach'. What cannot be taken is then deduced through recollecting preceding events as in a naturalistic system.

I was concerned to hear of a door-to-door salesman whose tactics emphasised another dimension of the social construction of illness and health behaviour. He appeared to play on the family's fears of the unknown.

> Lot's of people who've got asthma, their mothers and their fathers have to hoover the bed before they go in to get rid of them (bed bugs) [sic] 'cos they irritate them. They're minute things. You can't see them. Jane's got this, like a hoover. A man came to the door selling it. £200. He tested it. Ran this hoover thing over the sheets in the bedroom, tipped what looked like nothing into this little jar. Tipped it under the microscope. And the man looked at it, and showed all those little things moving about.

Similar fears of the unknown are played upon in England at the moment by people selling check-ups for microwave ovens so that the owners can be reassured the ovens really are safe for health with no microwaves escaping.

### Immunity

Awareness of another method of strengthening the boundary walls comes with the recognition that some infections can only affect you once. Although the 3–4-year-olds had been receiving immunisations they had not mastered the idea of immunity in relation to some of the infectious illnesses they had had and did not use the concept.

In contrast the 8-year-olds were fascinated with this idea – 'I want to get mumps to get it over with' – at the same time avidly searching to see whether there were exceptions in true scientific fashion: 'But I know someone who had chicken-pox twice'. Immunity, as well as being something specific, was also seen in general terms as increasing gradually throughout childhood: 'Probably as you become older you become more immune to colds'. This may be one of the origins of Herzlich's category, 'Reserve of Health', which she saw as being built up throughout childhood and providing the basic resource for the 'career of illness as an occupation' (Herzlich, 1973; see also chapter 3).

These 8-year-old children were aware of the effects of their immunisations: 'I won't catch it as I've had the injection, and I've had the lumps before'. The 13-year-old girls were especially aware of their forthcoming rubella immunisation and the way that this could even protect a foetus. The ideas of the 8-year-old girls were a little less sophisticated: 'If you have measles [sic] and you're just about to have a baby, the baby's brain could be damaged. The tube that's collecting the food from the mummy to the baby – probably dented or damaged'. The 13-year-olds' explanations were more informed: 'Sometimes if you catch something like another thing, you don't get it again because your body can fight it off easier'. ''Cos the blood cells and thing in your body, they know what it's like 'cos they've managed to . . .' (tailing off into uncertainty as the subsequent words were mumbled). The 13-year-olds reported a potential danger in being in contact with people who are immune to some diseases as 'Some people carry germs 'cos they're immune to them, 'cos they've had them before'.

*Exercise*

Strength and fitness from exercise were also seen as leading to a resource for the child which could be linked to ideas of strengthening the defences and a 'Reserve of Health' as this 13-year-old believed: 'Some people are fitter and they can fight off diseases if they get more exercise and fresh air'. Exercise and fresh air were often linked together as was seen in chapter 6, and I will not go further into the children's views on exercise here. Exercise is seen as very very important ; 75% of 11-year-olds in Eiser *et al.*'s (1983) sample from England 'Saw health primarily in terms of exercise and being energetic', compared with 40% who thought eating good food was the most important factor. Perhaps the latter belief is currently reflected in the growing popularity of Health Studios, which is now a synonym for a health-conscious gymnasium where exercise is the order of the day.

*Closeness*

The boundary wall is most under threat at night-time. The same belief is found amongst adults from a variety of cultures (see for example Douglas,

1966). I have already described how 3–4-year-old children see themselves
as most likely to get ill then, and that this effect is exaggerated if parents,
especially mothers, are away. The most dramatic extreme of this position
came from one 3-year-old who said 'If you're ill and nobody comes you
die'. This should help to reduce surprise at the findings of Mattsson &
Weisberg (1970) in the United States that some ill children under the age
of 4 years had 'short-lived return of earlier fears of animals, monsters and
the dark'. They report that these fears apparently disappeared as soon as
the children's health began to improve. There was a marked increase in
the use of comforters at night-time, as well as during the day. Being afraid
of going to bed could well continue after the illness, even for older children,
as reported by Shrand (1965) for an English sample (8/33 1–4-year-olds,
1/20 4–6 year-olds, 3/36 6–12-year-olds).

   This is a child's way of emphasising the importance of social networks,
which are being much researched for their consequences for adults' health.
The important elements in what goes to make up a protective social network
for adults are being teased apart. Several different parameters appear to
be important (McKinlay, 1981). Some of these are similar to factors perceived as important by the correspondents in Herzlich's study. For example
people who were used to a rural life but had to move to the city experienced
an increased incidence of coronary heart disease and were at greater risk
from lung cancer (when the level of cigarette consumption was allowed
for) than were those who had lived in cities all their lives. Herzlich referred
to this as part of her 'way of life' factor. There are problems associated
with residential mobility when this leads to a marked discontinuity between
how people lived as children and how they live now. Ways of life, social
networks and forms of attachment are closely interlinked but tend to be
conceptualised from predominantly social or psychological standpoints
rather than being integrated comprehensively. Social networks are protective both for adults (Hammer, 1983) and for children (Haggerty, 1980).

   The next stage is to find out how these effects occur. It has been suggested
that they mediate the form of 'help-seeking behaviour' which is adopted
after symptoms have been discussed with one's near social contacts. It
appears to be especially important how close the ties are within the social
network. For example, 'weak tie networks, with their diversity of contacts,
may provide information which is confusing or conflicting. In such a
situation, individuals may seek professional help earlier than they would
if their networks were of the strong tie form' (Reeder, Marcus & Seeman
in McKinlay, 1981).

   Social isolation as a category does not identify the coherence of viewpoints within the limited social system, but it has been used as a category in follow-up research. For example, social isolation was found to be of life and death importance for those who had suffered a myocardial infarct as it predicted 3-year survival (Ruberman *et al.*, 1984). In addition it is necessary to note as an aside that the least educated men were the most isolated. This underlines another dimension to the relationship between health and education already pointed to by Pill & Stott (1985) (see chapter 3). I underline these points here to make the reader aware of possible links between early socialisation, both at home and at school (see Tizard & Hughes (1984) for an elaboration of these processes) and later consequences in coping with physical illness through a beneficial lifestyle. Haggerty's (1980) review of the roles played by social supports for children concluded that a good social network mitigated against illness. Maybe one appropriate interpretation of the clingy behaviour of children during illness which arises and is identified so early in development (Shrand, 1965) is that it represents a biological predisposition elicited by states of illness and reflects the important place of attachment in all future health behaviour (see also Bowlby, 1969). After attachments have been under moderate stress those involved often report and react as though the attachment is stronger afterwards. I believe Shrand (1965) is describing this phenomenon when he says that 'many [children] came to "love mother more"' after minor illness treated at home. This occurred for children in all his age groups, i.e. from 1 to 12 years old.

To return to the children, it is not surprising, therefore, to hear the complementary view from the parents that the best form of help for the ill child is 'cuddles' and closeness to parents. The children particularly appreciated having temporary beds made up for them in the living room so that they maintained their closeness to the rest of the family. Otherwise they particularly liked people with them in their bedroom. Very few children apart from the 13-year-olds liked to be alone when ill, in contrast to the situation in the United States where children over the age of 3 years tended to withdraw (Mattsson & Weisberg, 1970). The 13-year-old children were withdrawing in a much more active and self-secure fashion than the younger children were reported as doing. These younger American children were described as having 'experienced an "emotional separation" from their mothers during this state of relative withdrawal'. The separateness of the older children was associated with their more often keeping secrets about their health from their parents, which they said was partly to protect their parents from worrying about them.

Closeness could also paradoxically be dangerous because if you were ill you might pass on an infection. It seemed as though this dilemma was resolved through a belief that one's own family was 'permissible' and likely to be immune to catching something from the child. A group boundary was then erected between the ill child/family and the child's peers, who were often particularly missed during illness. This quarantine-type boundary then became a constraint if relations with others were missed, or a useful defence if things were going badly with one's peers. It was as though the child temporarily required the boundary walls of the other family members, especially the mother in this group.

When the child is made to feel better with this closeness, it is as though he were made better. Feeling better for the older children could involve personal effort and this led to the following quote: 'Sometimes if you don't feel well, the more you think you are ill the worse you'd get in certain cases. It can be the mind that . . . If you think you're not ill you can stay on and not be ill sometimes'. This 13-year-old boy thought that the latter strategy would only apply with potentially mild illnesses. The general idea is widespread, though, and reflects the battles and warfare metaphor reported earlier (Blaxter & Paterson, 1982a; Pill & Stott, 1985) where the right mental attitude is required to fight off illness. Pill & Stott (1985) reported that the right mental attitude was significantly more often seen as required amongst those for whom the concept of a healthy lifestyle did not appear to be particularly important.

Paradoxes abound for the younger children with the conflicting demands on them. One paradox relates to the idea of sleep being dangerous for them (see chapter 6), whereas at the same time they are being told that sleep is good for them. It may be that this advice helps neutralise the fears of night-time. Another possibility is that it could make the children doubt the advice of their parents if their own fears were more salient for them and there were problems in trusting their parents' words. As the constructs are generally loosely held these contradictions often cause little concern. This is the sort of situation in which Piaget envisaged children accommodating to new constructs, as children would be unable to assimilate the ideas to existing constructs because of their contradictory nature. In other words these apparent contradictions force the children to question their logical assumptions and are a necessary part of development. The 13-year-olds had moved on to seeing sleepiness as the dangerous state rather than sleep itself, as another way of handling this paradox; for example it 'depends if you're very drowsy or sleepy. Your body can't fight them off so easily'.

## Warmth

Sleep and cuddles are also times of snugness. The time when being ill in bed was often made more comfortable with a hot water bottle and a hot drink. The value of warmth for protection was also emphasised when one had to wear lots of clothes before going out on a cold day. As the mother of an 8-year-old boy put it concerning the value of keeping warm, '[it's necessary to be] well clothed, especially the feet I think. It's one of the main parts. The heat goes, the cold comes in. And the same with your head. The heat goes out of your body'. Warmth was also seen as an important ingredient of a cure: 'You get warmer, and all the warmth goes up to your nose and stops you sneezing'. Even the medicines for a cold might act that way; one 8-year-old said 'It's not really the medicine, the medicine keeps you warm'.

The role of warmth in the treatment of colds and chills for adults has been explored in a suburban London community. The views obtained were very similar to those I obtained with these children. There was one contrast in that specifically the older adults saw it as dangerous to leave a child's bedroom window open at night, because it let the cold in (Helman, 1978), a view which was not reflected in the families in my Edinburgh sample.

With warmth, just as with food, medicines and exercise, too much of it was seen as bad for you whereas usually it was healthy. A reasonable balance is required. But this concept was more a reflection of the collective views of the groups of 8- and 13-year-olds rather than of the individuals. The beliefs in the dangers of heat, such as a 13-year-old's comment that 'heat causes germs to breed', balanced the advantages described above when the collective situation was analysed. Hot air was additionally one of the attributes of stale air, 'the unhealthy kind'.

Although I have constructed a picture here of how warmth, food and exercise build up the 'castle walls', an alternative approach has been to regard attitudes to clothing, diet and exercise as reflecting lifestyle. The importance of these factors for maintaining health has been incorporated into as Salience of Lifestyle Index (SLI) (Pill & Stott, 1985). The socially constructed concept of resistance to infection based on the development of health routines is only one aspect of the development of a lifestyle which increases people's awareness of what they can do for themselves to maintain health. It is incorporated as part of their 'effectance motive'. Pill & Stott's study of women showed that those who had the highest scores on the SLI were significantly more likely to feel that illness could be prevented, and to have a 'more positive concept of resistance'. Resistance for the others, 'the fatalists', was based on an 'immutable genetic factor'. Not all who recognised the relevance of lifestyle choices for illness prevention retained a sense of their own effectiveness to alter outcome. The effectance motive seemed to be highest in those with higher educational backgrounds and to a lesser extent those with greater religious commitment.

## Good germs

Although vitamins had been described by the children in functionalist terms much as though they were good germs, when the 8-year-olds talked of good germs they referred to white blood cells. The white blood cells were seen as fighting the 'bad germs'. 'There are invisible bad germs and they just go out and fight the good germs'. 'The white cells are sort of germs – sort of like a war'. 'They [germs] get inside your lungs. The white corpuscles, they are trying to fight them, the germs in your body, 'cos everybody's got germs in their body'. Only one 4-year-old had alluded to anything similar when he had said 'the white things come and rescue them', but it was impossible to elucidate his underlying premises and even what was being rescued.

The rescue operation is not an inevitable process: 'Sometimes there are good germs which fight the other germs but not often', an 8-year-old said. If you have been lucky, though, the 'good germs enable you to get well without going to the doctor'. There was a decrease in the use of the term 'good germ' with the 13-year-olds. Helman (1978) found no references to good germs in his adult English sample.

This sort of moralistic and semantically confusing language about germs can add to the children's confusion and draws them to make analogies with other properties of germs in order to describe them. An 8-year-old girl said 'white blood cells are clean, but some times mummy and daddy say they're dirty, so I am not sure'. In addition the moral order appears to reflect one's own standing in this internal battle. If 'a bit of the bad germs attacked a good bit, that means you are getting less goodness in your body, and the badness is coming up and up'.

There was a feeling that white blood cells could be transmitted from child to child in the following way: 'white blood cells may go from me to you. I may have two less and you two more'. This movement had the same quality as found with germs, which seemed to go from one person to the next with conservation of matter.

These white blood cells were seen by some as bigger than the invading germs. They acted in various ways, according to the following 8-year-olds:

'They are a bit in the body like string. They trap the germs [like a modified spider's web]. Captured. Then throw it out when you go to the toilet'. 'Sometimes they go up to your mouth to stop the bad germs from getting in, by throwing them out in attack'. They are seen as working in tandem with the red blood cells as already mentioned. Additionally 'white blood cells keep out germs. Red blood cells go round the body cleaning it, giving it energy'. A boy in the group took up the above 8-year-old girl's comments, asking 'Using a broom?' her reply was 'It's not like that. No broom. Has to go back to the heart, say every hour, to get to breathe. Blood gives them energy'.

These processes within the body tended to be only vaguely referred to by the 8-year-old children, who were often puzzled by how things go to other parts of the body, be it spots spreading or medicines affecting distal pains. Some 3–4-year-old children had had an idea that medicines were most powerful near where you took them. They entertained the idea that for headaches the 'power' of an aspirin went directly through the roof of the mouth to the ache; but then again this is exactly the same idea as propounded by Culpeper in the seventeenth century for how potions for relief of headache worked.

One other historical note will be included here to set the castle metaphor in an even older context. Jung refers to 'the thousand-year-old Chinese text on the yellow castle, the germ of the immortal body' (Storr, 1983 p. 235).

### The illness routine

These strategies that have been described for bolstering health were frequently found together in a family's routine responses to illness. Usually a child was tucked up either in bed, or on a made-up bed. They may well have been kept warm with a hot water bottle. Family members remained close and tried to cheer up the child. Special foods were given to build up the child's strength and make the child feel good. Good luck charms were not referred to by these children or their families.

Some families appeared bound by fixed routines which then became constraining and frustrating to all involved in them. These families appeared to fear the consequences of modifying their routines, resolving any uncertainty they experienced by slavishly following guidelines. For others, though, an essential ingredient to the routine was restoring maximal choice to the child within certain broad limits. In these families, contrary to their normal way of relating, the child could choose whatever foods he wanted or television programme to watch. Obviously this strategy would not work for those who imposed bed rest on their ill child in order to make certain that he really was ill. Through emphasising the child's ability to choose it seems that his sense of helplessness in the face of his illness is minimised and he is least likely to perceive his illness as 'destructive'. If at the same time the limits to the child's choices are maintained within bounds illness does not become totally 'liberating'. Too much choice leads to sensations which can be rather scary for a young child.

Family rituals rooted in childhood are an important stabilizing influence through times of uncertainty (Wolin & Bennett, 1984; see also Douglas, 1966, for the place of rituals in giving form to disorder for adults). The rituals give social relations visible expression (Douglas, 1966 p. 128), which is especially important when illness threatens the security of normal attachments. At the same time there is the possibility of the child learning the socially approved ill/sick role in which he plays an active role at getting better, a movement towards illness as an 'occupation' (see chapter 3) in which effectiveness in one's 'way of life' is maintained even in illness. Constructive lifestyle decisions can be taken.

Shapiro's (1983) review notes that 'mother's reaction to the illness is the most important etiological factor in any subsequent behavioral disturbances in the child'. If the illness routines diminish parental confusion about what to do and facilitate 'a feeling of mastery and accomplishment' then they will be beneficial for the adjustment of the child.

# 8

# 'Pretend illness': an analysis of how communication patterns can foster particular forms of complaining

*'It is in what people pretend that true morality may be discovered.'*
Bishop Butler quoted in Gillon (1985).

In order to show how physical complaints are established as part of the child's world of illness I will now proceed to link the observations I made in my study with research carried out into abdominal pain in childhood and somatisation disorder in adults. This will point to ways in which children develop special dialects for complaining, an understanding of which opens up a variety of new treatment approaches.

It has been seen that when children are growing up they have a wide range of views on illness and how it is caused. Their views change over the years in a sequence described as though conforming to the stages outlined by Piaget (Neuhauser *et al.*, 1978; Carandang *et al.*, 1979; Whitt *et al.*, 1979), the stages being the same in hospitalised children (Simeonsson, Buckley & Monson, 1979). Piaget's approach had predominantly been an ego-psychology which did not stress the ecology of the developmental process. As we have seen it has been necessary to place more emphasis on the form of the relationships with the child, how questions are presented to the child (Donaldson, 1978; Samuel & Bryant, 1984) and how the child presents his questions (Tizard & Hughes, 1984). The questions asked must make sense to the child with his experience of the world and especially his relationships (Hobson, 1980, 1982). It is these aspects which must be looked at both in consultations and when parents try to understand their children's offerings.

The communication processes going on between children and adults colour the content and provide the child's illness language with a grammar. As has already been seen the content of children's views is not directly related to those of their parents (Mechanic, 1964; Campbell, 1975; Blaxter & Paterson, 1982*a,b*). From the communications analysis presented here it will be seen how some of the colour to the child's world of illness is produced, and how particular family-based languages for sharing discomforts are developed. As with learning other languages, when a language not in one's repertoire is encountered it can appear very foreign, even if it is just a specialised dialect. The languages which are developed for sharing discomforts in childhood are very durable. Zeitlin's (1986, p. 108) analysis of adult patients at a psychiatric hospital who had also been patients there as children showed that there was a continuity of symptoms irrespective of the psychiatric diagnosis. Symptoms reflect both signals for a person's discomforts and the nature of those discomforts.

I will now analyse the ways in which adults who care for a sick child make decisions about that child and how the child subsequently can come to present the adults with different forms of illness behaviour. This appears to be based on the child's experiences, the illness language he is introduced to and on his assumptions about what the sick role constitutes for those adults.

The ecological perspective lays stress on how the child has learnt and continues to learn to communicate through a dialectic between illness behaviour and sick role, or in other words establishes a balance between the demands placed on him by his state and society's interpretation of his disease and the required sick role. The detailed nature of the relationship between them and the longer-term consequences remain conjecture. The pressures on the child from the powerful others in his microsystems to take a sick role modify the illness behaviour he presents in a way which is still ill defined. This transactional model nevertheless clearly gives possibilities for deceit and play with the learnt signalling system, and it is these factors and the rules which families seem to develop to cope with them which will be discussed here. This will lead to insights into the morality of illness and how it is created. It will suggest why some people preponderantly use a body language based on what has occurred in a somatoform relationship (see below). Additionally it will suggest important communication skills to be taken account of in future research.

My study did not include a description of parents' responses to crying infants or the ways in which the care-givers discriminated the different forms of crying. It is probable that this early stage, when it is already possible to allocate the sick role to an infant in accounting for his distress, will turn out to be critical for the infant's subsequent development of illness behaviour. Infants' cries differ at birth depending on their maturity and other factors, making it more difficult for the parents of premature infants to respond helpfully. Already at very early ages some parents are preferentially attributing physical rather than psychological reasons for their infant's distress. This early development of a particular form of interactional 'dance' around the infant's discomfort must be taken into account when interpreting the results of the adoption studies I refer to in the section on somatoform disorder and somatoform relationships. The attribution of physical causality is sometimes aided by the questions which specialists in physical medicine are likely to ask and statements they selectively respond to (helped of course by the fact that these parents have already chosen a physical specialist as the one most likely to be able to solve their problems).

The parents of the 3–4-year-olds reacted in contrasting ways to their children's complaining, from the extremes of saying that children of that age always told the truth to resenting that they could never believe a word they said. For the parents who never believed a word that their children said the children's behaviour was not yet labelled as 'pretend' as they laid no particular emphasis on what the children said, effectively ignoring their verbal presentations of their discomforts. As described earlier, parents of 3–4-year-old children decided whether the children were ill largely through noting any alterations in behaviour (see also Spencer, 1984), particularly their normal daily routines such as getting up (which would occur more slowly), whether their appetite was worse, or whether they were reluctant to go to nursery. In addition parents noted their child's mood and appearance. Only hesitantly were the children beginning to use words, such as 'sore', to share their discomforts. This hesitancy appeared to make it easier for some parents to ignore their child's verbal complaints if they thought they were 'a load of rubbish' – and indirectly add to their child's hesitancy in the process. The whole decision-making process was more difficult where family routines were poorly established. Generally parents were responding to what they observed, and many simultaneously labelled their children's behaviour with words.

In contrast to the lack of importance for the parents, the consequences of illness to the 4-year-old child can have been very different. He experiences the effect of illness on his relations with others, such as not being able to play with friends. Although the parents can say that it does not matter very much whether he goes to nursery school that day, and err on the side of keeping him at home, for the child the decision can appear much more momentous as important relations are temporarily threatened for some uncertain and unclearly labelled reason. He must develop his own way of accounting for these variations in his routines.

Between the ages of 4 and 8 years children's 'pretend' illness becomes much more important for the parents to unravel. The consequences of getting their assessment of the child's behaviour 'wrong' have altered due to the importance of school. Society is reacting more to how parents bring up their children as the children increasingly come out of the family. 'Pretend' illness is important to varying degrees depending on the value system of the individual family and their local culture. I will analyse the parents' evaluation of pretence in their 8-year-old children in more depth as it reveals important influences on the development of illness behaviour.

What I present represents an account of the communicative competences which can lie behind the observations I have reported. This represents a hypothesis the validity of which needs testing. I did not attempt to alter the family structure in order to test it out and so elaborate its connections with the particular views and illness behaviour of the children. This micro-sociological analysis of the structure and its moral system is deductive and difficult to corroborate. The family rules are implicit and multidimensional (Ford, 1983).

## Play and pretend

The central dilemma for parents is knowing what weight to attach to their child's complaining. This involves identifying and differentiating between those occasions when the children are playing, pretending or misleading. It has become important for the parents to make these distinctions with their 8-year-olds. Illness-type behaviour with accompanying verbal complaints of discomfort did not get clearly labelled 'pretend' prior to the children in my sample being 8 years old, although the children had been doing similar things earlier.

I need to return briefly to the experiences of the 3–4-year-old children in order to put the above development in context. The 3–4-year-olds were learning important aspects of caring for sick people, not only through how their discomforts were responded to, but also in their play, both with their peers and when experimenting on their own, making sense of what had happened to them. They learnt that things are acceptable in play which are not otherwise acceptable. What occurs in play comes to belong to a different moral order in which things are not labelled as more or less right in the same way as can occur otherwise. In the play of 3–4-year-olds the salience of different health and illness beliefs is not revealed in the same way as it appears to be for older children and adults who, within a different moral order, must take notice of their own states and act accordingly. With growing responsibility for taking action to respond to their own discomforts rather than waiting for others to respond to them, their health beliefs begin to occupy a different place in their value system (see Gochman

(1971a), and Dielman *et al.*, (1980) for Rosenstock's Health Belief Model as applied to children: Rosenstock, 1966).

Between the ages of 4 and 8 years the place of play in the child's world is distinguished. Children are much clearer about 'as if' introductions, so that for example the advertisements for Domestos bleach referred to previously are now regarded as representational and not revealing mathetic information. Play has become tinged with a variety of emotional connotations. The children have also begun to manipulate situations to relabel them as playful in order to avoid the consequences due if the behaviour had been evaluated according to different moral categories. They have been learning how to handle play in negotiation, and how to handle those markers which can be exaggerated to lead people to respond to one as though one is playing. They have begun, in other words, to use some of the metalevel signals of play (Bateson, 1955) and turn them to their advantage through a reflective process. Although I am here using the example of play to illustrate contrasts between moral orders, different forms of moral order exist in different settings and these could have provided the basis for alternative analyses.

This development has occurred at the same time as it has become more important for the parents to make correct responses to their children's messages. The children have entered the school microsystem which has a different set of values about attendance and expectations of appropriate behaviour compared with the nursery school. The parents have been made aware of this in differing ways depending on their relationships with the school (the functioning of the mesosystem). It is in this way that the respective moralities of the teachers and parents meet and colour the consequences for the parents of getting their decision-making right at home, and similarly for the teachers at school. Society's values transmitted through the school meet the family's values. Manning *et al.* (1978) have already shown that the ways in which a child's emotional and aggressive behaviour is interpreted at school and at home can lead to serious misunderstandings if either does not know enough about how the child functions in the other place (see chapter 2).

Eight-year-olds reveal what is most important for their illness behaviour through what they believe will have the greatest impact on their parents or teachers. They discussed this in terms of how they believed it important to pretend illness. Here they explained their interpretation of adults' value systems as seen from their position. They included an understanding of the ways in which the adults' interpretations of their complaints leads to the possibilities of deceit, as shown by their adept use of 'untestable' complaints such as asking permission to leave the classroom to go to the toilet. I included a number of open-ended questions about pretend illness which revealed this perspective (see appendix 2). Table 8.1 shows a selection of the responses I obtained from both the 8- and 13-year-olds, which can be seen to reflect the parental decision-making strategies used with the younger children. Nevertheless it is noteworthy that not all investigators have managed to get children of this age to talk about their favoured ways of pretending illness, and the majority at first deny that they could pretend (see for example Prout, 1986). It is appropriate to relate this to the key points in the method I adopted.

Generally these 8-year-old children could adopt roles both at home and at school in a way which made the discrimination between play and non-play situations much more difficult for those around them. The fact that the children had shifted role did not mean that the others around them had observed this shift. This 'half play' situation enabled experimentation with alternative realities in a way which was qualitatively different from that used by the younger children. 'Pretend' became pretend due to the greater reflective capacity of the children, and the responses they elicited. When

Table 8.1. *'I pretend to be ill by . . . '*

The table shows quotations from both 8- and 13-year-olds of both sexes (M and F). There was no difference in the tenor of the responses from the two age groups

| | |
|---|---|
| **Change in pattern:** | 'to not do what you normally do' (M13) |
| Getting up | 'sleeping in' (M8) |
| Eating | 'by not eating your food' (M13) |
| Appearance | 'putting on a sad face and turning white. I don't know how but I am able to do this well' (M13) |
| | 'put talcum powder on your face to look pale and put an act on' (F13) |
| | 'put fire on in the room, put your face to it and then turn it off' (M13) |
| Contact/mood | 'to mope about the house until somebody asks you if you are really unwell' (F13) |
| | 'asking to go home' (M8) |
| | 'being quiet' (M13) |
| **Complaints:** | 'to have something your parents can't really tell' (F13) |
| Tummyache | 'saying I have a sore tummy' (F8) |
| Headaches | 'with a headache, because no one can tell you have one or not' (F13) |
| Being sick | 'licking soap to try and be sick' (M8) |
| | 'coffing down the loo and saying I've been sick' (F13) |
| | 'sticking fingers down your frot' (F8) |

the possibilities for 'half-play' are taken in conjunction with the children's greater verbal skills, family and school interactions become much more puzzling to unravel.

The majority of the parents were aware of their child's greater ability to act and had 'consequently' evolved a wider range of decision-making strategies. An alternative way of accounting for this development would be that the parents had expectations that children of this age would be likely to use the functional advantages to be found in illness and so felt it necessary to refine their techniques. They wanted to prevent their children developing a sense of 'illness as a liberator' (see chapter 3). Suspicion on the part of those parents who had always believed their children were experts in 'kiddology', played a role in some families in making the children aware of the dramaturgical possibilities. By suggesting the two alternative interpretations beside each other I hope to draw attention to the possibility that the behaviour and the responses evolve together on the basis of expectations and developmental processes. These altered parental strategies were generally similar to those employed by the welfare assistants at school. When the situations regarding individual pupils were looked at there was nevertheless scope for dissonance in the way these two systems functioned and attributed salience to different aspects of illness behaviour.

### 'I have a tummy ache'

With these background comments on the nature of pretence and the acting skills of 8-year-old children in mind, I will now take as an example for analysis the child who says 'I have a tummy ache'. I will limit myself to a composite verbal example in order to illustrate the important variations in the ways parents and teachers respond. Through their responses they structure that child's world and influence his competences to communicate about his internal state. There are various signals which the parents and teachers need to interpret in order to account for the child's state when he gives the message. Is the message intelligible and warranted in this setting?

The coherence of the total picture is often used to evaluate each of the constituents to the message: the content, form and the metalevel signals. I will begin, though, with the effects of the setting on the meaning of what occurs. If the setting is evaluated first, the moral order of the setting gives the clue to the intepretative set to be used in that microsystem. One of the possibilities is that the message 'I have a tummy ache' is seen to come over within a play frame; in other words the adults have interpreted

the metalevel signals in a way which alters the 'seriousness' of the complaint. Generally parents and children, and teachers and children, will
have evolved clear metalevel play signals which include voice quality
changes and body posturing. The signals need not always be so clear due
to a variety of misunderstandings which will be more frequent between
children and adults who have found it difficult to differentiate and subsequently discriminate between the moral order of play and other orders
of daily life.

Within the moral order of play there appear to exist 'rules' which define
limits to what is acceptable content in the play frame. Is it possible to play
with illness themes, such as tummy ache? The theme of the play can be
taboo for one of the interactants; it is not warranted for them within that
moral order. This can be because it raises their anxiety too high. If that
participant is an adult who is responsible for keeping the play 'safe', it
becomes necessary for him to take the interaction out of 'play'. The message
itself is intelligible, but the context invalidates it – or the salience of the
message is such that within a family's value system it overrules their
interpretation of the metalevel signals. These latter families will have premises of the form:

We never play with situations which are serious.
'Tummy ache' is always a serious illness complaint.
Therefore any messages about tummy ache must be
interpreted within non-play frames.

Learning about play appears to involve learning the metalevel signalling
of the family and school systems, and also which topics can be invested
with what emotional qualities for the play to continue. Whilst these learning
processes continue, misunderstandings will be a necessary ingredient of
the mutual accommodation of the child to the others around him. The
misunderstandings are likely to be more frequent when the expectations
of the microsystems are different. The emotional investment in the different
topics is additionally likely to fluctuate depending on the emotional state
of the care-giver, potentially adding to the child's confusions if his capacity
to discriminate these states is diminished. The handling of the misunderstandings will be important for the direction of the child's developing
illness behaviour.

Some parents do not attach importance to discriminating rigidly between
the frames of play and non-play. There is the possibility for messages to
be taken half seriously and half playfully where there is no clear ascription
of one form of moral order or the other to the situation. This appears to
arise in two ways. It both represents a choice on the part of some adults

to introduce the child to this sort of order, and it results from the experience of poor differentiation between these two contrasting frames. If the explanation lies in the second possibility the discrimination of the two forms can only get worse in a self-perpetuating way. The children would necessarily be helpless to sharpen their discriminations between the different moral orders in a process analogous to learned helplessness (Abramson *et al.*, 1978). This development would depend on there being no alternative experiences for the children in their other microsystems which were reparative. Provided the mesosystems functioned facilitatively, these alternative experiences could be assimilated into the child's framework, the developing secondary structure in contrast to the primary ecological structure (Harré, 1983).

If the possibility of play has been excluded the parents appear to respond in alternative ways. They appear first to check the validity of the message content against their various family rules for labelling it as a sign of physical illness. In other words, is the child's signal a genuine message about his natural state? These were principally the same rules as listed earlier for the 3–4-year-olds. Nevertheless parents had become aware of the importance of their 8-year-old children's abilities to play roles and pretend. They were daily faced with their children's clear abilities to exaggerate their discomforts as they used their complaints for renegotiating their status.

The 8-year-olds had found that colds are a very valuable negotiating tool, in contrast to the 3–4-year-olds who had not viewed them as illness. The parents had modified their basic decision-making strategies. If they had been in doubt about whether a nursery school age child was ill or not, they looked for signs that the child's illness behaviour was coherent across several situations. The child had to be reluctant both to get up and to eat. If the child was reluctant to get up they would often press him to have something to eat in order to see whether he was also reluctant to take food. In order to refine their technique and remain, as it were, one step ahead of their children, the parents of the 8-year-olds were taking much more notice of the child's degree of reluctance. In order to discriminate between signals which could either represent the child's learnt illness behaviour or the child's natural state the parents quantified the signs as well as noting the qualities and pattern of the illness behaviour as done previously. It appears likely that cultures differ here in how early quantification of the signs is emphasised (see chapter 4).

After the above evaluation procedure the child's behaviour was then interpreted by the parents as being either appropriate for the state of physical illness or not. If the verdict was 'not ill' and the parental discussion could be terminated with an edict of judicial bearing, the parents then had to reassess the situation. The quality to the verdict must provisionally be related to parental expectations about how others might or should respond to their decision-making. Those who receive their decision rarely tolerate either a 'bit ill', 'under the weather' or 'don't yet know' diagnosis. Children who are brought up without being exposed to adult debate about their condition, for example the children of the two nurses in my sample, come to miss out on an understanding of the nuances of the grey half–illness states and how they are discriminated from other body states.

Parents have two main responses. The first type has the following form:

The behaviour was not warranted as that of illness.

We cannot believe the form to our child's verbal message 'I have a discomfort'.

As he was not playing, he must be 'having us on'.

The child's complaining could then get the label 'naughty' behaviour. In this situation the parents have ascribed mischievous intent to the child's message by using their own frame of reference and available skills, although their conclusion does not necessarily fit with the child's intention. The child is already familiar with a different range of microsystems where his message 'I have a tummy ache' can have a variety of functions of which the family is not aware. In most families the adults' definition of the underlying intention holds sway in accounting for the child's subsequent behaviour. This then necessarily affects the effective vocabulary available to the child for sharing his discomforts with them, but it will not mean that his efforts at sharing his discomfort in this way will diminish if he gets helpful responses elsewhere.

With the second type of parental response more weight is attached to the form of the child's statement 'I have a tummy ache'. They pay more attention to the process of complaining than to the detailed content of the message. In order to evaluate the complaint they adopted a further strategy. Already they have noted any alteration in the pattern to the child's daily routines; they now note whether there is a pattern to the complaining. Noting a pattern to the complaining addresses primarily the question 'Why complain now?' It is this same question which Balint (1964) emphasised when discussing with general practitioners how they could further assess the nature of their patients' discomforts.

These parents talked of their children having 'Monday morning feelings', the stresses of particular school days, and the problems which occur when grandma comes to visit. It was through noticing the correspondence between recurring events and forms of complaining that the origins of psychological discomforts were deduced and labelled by the parents. In this way the child's 'illness' vocabulary was broadened to include forms of discomfort besides the purely physical. This process was dependent on the parents' vocabularies of noteworthy events, relevant points of view, and their likely associated emotional consequences.

I have been looking at the situation for 8-year-old children. The research of Davison, Faull & Nicol (1986) suggests that there is significant remission of the recurring abdominal pain in 6–7-year-olds, whereas those who have looked at older children with abdominal pain have found that once the complaint is better established, and this includes amongst 8-year-olds, it seldom remits. The remissions were attributed by Davison *et al.* (1986) to the children adjusting to what had otherwise been a stressful start at school. This would mean different frequencies of abdominal pain in different cultures which start school at different ages. If the parents and others could identify the stress and the way the children present their discomfort, then it seems provisionally as though somatic complaints of tummy ache could be reduced.

It is not sufficient to extract temporal patterns as otherwise no potential environmental influences are recorded and the cause of everything is attributed to processes within the child. If one only observes that the prevalence of abdominal pain in 6–7-year-olds is 25% (Faull & Nicoll, 1986) whereas later it is 10% (Apley, 1975 p. 101), without at the same time noting the effects of and associations with starting school and school difficulties, one loses any possibility of improving the children's discomfort through simple social measures.

It is this temporal patterning which some physicians tend to record when diagnosing infantile colic. A recent example which illustrates this was that 'Crying was diagnosed as infantile colic if it lasted more than three hours a day and occurred for more than three days a week' (Hwang & Danielsson, 1985). Interestingly the same physicians found that psychological support offered similar relief in many instances to that provided by a drug, dicyclomine. But their way of identifying pattern did not give them the necessary points of view from which they could evaluate the nature and effectiveness of the psychological support, or relabel the child's complaint.

A major difficulty for some parents is to wait long enough for events to recur and so allow correspondences to be established. The uncertainty associated with not knowing the origin of the child's discomfort during the first episode must be coped with. It is not immediately necessary to provide definitive labels for the child's discomfort, but the child can be securely held (I use the term here in the same way as Winnicott: Davis & Wallbridge, 1983 p. 106–9). In other words the child is responded to with recognition that something 'is up' but the superficial details of the verbal message 'I have a tummy ache' are not responded to, and no equivalently detailed verbal label is provided by the adults. The form of the message is given precedence over the content.

If these parents have the ability to discriminate between non-verbal cues to states of stress from those for illness and other body states it makes their decision-making easier. The form to the complaining, with the accompanying non-verbal cues, can suggest anxiety, but some parents do not feel warranted in making this interpretation until they have noted the pattern. They adopt a 'wait and see' policy (see also Spencer, 1984). The message is intelligible, but the pattern says whether it is warranted to account for it as a sign of anxiety. It is the pattern which gives clues to 'causes' of the discomfort (or more correctly correlations with the discomfort), such that taken together, the pattern and the non-verbal behaviour establish a cause and effect model and the parental interpretation is confirmed. If the parents had not waited until a pattern had been established they would have found it necessary to impose assumptions from their own experiences on the first episode of complaining. This could have resulted in the child's behaviour getting a label based on the parents' experiences rather than reflecting his own, although the parents could have got it right.

Similarly paediatric surgeons (e.g. Jones, 1969) have described the advantages of waiting to take action with children with abdominal pain of uncertain origin where it appears similar to that of appendicitis (at that time 40% of hospital admissions in children for suspected surgical emergency turned out not to require surgery). Through waiting, patterns are revealed which elucidate the problem.

If children who were clearly employing a play frame are excluded, which other children could be said to be pretending illness? The word pretend can conjure up the world of Punch and Judy or alternatively pejorative overtones of forgery and fraud. In the first, potentially playful intention is imputed to the pretender; in the second, there is said to be mischievous intent. The first could perhaps be ascribed light-heartedly by those parents who are poor at discerning play roles and situations, who believe that their child is probably pretending. They are open to different interpretations of the child's behaviour with associated alternative implied intentions on the part of the child. The pejorative 'pretend' label appears to be found amongst those who relabel their child's verbal message as pretend because for them the content of the message is analysed in conjunction with the non-verbal signals for illness which are most salient for them. The form of the child's message signifying the sharing of a discomfort is not acknowledged. They are also poor discriminators of the child's other internal states besides illness, such as those associated with psychological forms of discomfort (see Papousek & Papousek (1983) for the development of parental competences in relation to recognition of infant states).

The first group of parents are hypothesised as having diminished competences in discriminating the metalevel signals for the different moral orders, such as those of play, or attributing little salience to them. Alternatively the children given less clear signals about whether they are playing. Intuitively these two reasons are likely to be associated.

In the second situation I hypothesise that the parents do not attribute salience to the form of the child's verbal message, 'I have a discomfort' – which can alternatively be interpreted as 'I am complaining' – instead concentrating on the apparent falsity of the overt content of the message. Their trust in verbal communication is diminished. I believe that this could have occurred for the parents through a process analogous to learned helplessness, where the verbal messages were not effective or used primarily for their dramaturgical potentialities and in this way came to lack salience and be seen as less real.

Whether the children came to adopt the same value system as their parents would depend on the functioning of their other microsystems and mesosystems. In isolated and disengaged families, which tend to function more like relatively closed systems, communicative competences of the children would appear to have the greatest chance of developing in the same form as those of the parents. Although the family language is likely to predominate it can be anticipated that the children will bring into the family some of the illness vocabulary they meet in their other microsystems. Within the family that vocabulary will remain relatively foreign, hence the relative incomprehensibility of 'I have a tummy ache' to other family members if the language is not the family's. The child has to use a method of sharing a discomfort which is not generally acknowledged.

The decision-making rules the parents then adopt when deciding on their own or their child's condition in the future would determine how effective complaining could occur. One possibility would be through *being* 'appropriately' physically ill, without being able to discuss the nuances of one's state with others. Alternatively patterns to verbal complaining could be identified, psychological complaints acknowledged, and associations between external events and psychological states established for the child. In the extreme case where there is lack of discrimination of non-verbal cues to psychological states of discomfort, such as anxiety, the child will be introduced to a family set of rules which not only says that one is only ill when illness behaviour is appropriate according to the parents' criteria and that verbal complaints are incidental to this overordinate rule, but that psychological discomforts will be denied, no words found for them, and no psychologically difficult situations acknowledged. One particular problem for the child comes from the moralistic overtones used to label the verbal complaints as 'fraudulent', which can make verbal exploration of this whole area for the child emotionally fraught. I believe that here lie some of the roots of a variety of disorders grouped together as somatoform disorders (see below), especially that subvariant of somatisation disorder identified by Bohman, Cloninger and colleagues as 'high frequency somatisers', rather than the alternative 'diversiform' variety (Cloninger *et al.*, 1984).

I do not wish to imply that a somatoform communication pattern where the verbal complaint must be accompanied by 'appropriate' physical drama in order to be effective is pathological. The development of this specific form of language can give rise to a pattern of complaint presentation which is liable to be interpreted as a disorder if it becomes fixed in the child's personal repertoire (the secondary structure) so that it is used in all contexts regardless of whether he is presenting discomfort to family members or not. It would probably be more correct to identify the special language as a local dialect, a sign of a somatoform relationship in this age group (8-year-olds at home with their parents). In such a relationship physical complaints and complaining have more effect than shared distress.

### Somatoform disorders and somatoform relationships

Although somatoform relationships cannot be equated with somatoform disorders, a digression here on somatoform disorders will highlight some of the processes which appear to be happening when a language, developed in one context and effective to a degree in that context, is used regardless of context. This can easily happen as the elements in different languages are similar, although the modes of interpretation vary. It is largely a change in the grammar. In order to recognise the novelty of the particular somatoform language with its own culturally dependent vocabulary and syntax, a degree of reflectiveness of all participants is required. There also needs to be an awareness that some people have potentially more than one language at their disposal, for example the somatoform and the psychological, whereas others only have rudimentary elements of one or other of these. I am not concerned here with whether it is right or wrong to consider a different language or lack of a particular language as pathological, but rather with the implications of this communication perspective for a re-appraisal of somatoform disorders and ways of helping people develop a shared vocabulary so that complaints can be heard.

According to the classificatory system of *DSMIII* (American Psychiatric Association, 1980) somatoform disorders are a rather loose collection of four disorders. The first subcategory is labelled somatisation disorder, the others being conversion disorder, psychogenic pain disorder and atypical somatisation disorder. Some of the diagnostic features of somatisation disorder are as follows:

> The essential features are recurrent and multiple somatic com-
> plaints of several years' duration for which medical attention
> has been sought but which are apparently not due to any phys-
> ical disorder. The disorder begins before the age of 30 and has
> a chronic but fluctuating course. (*op. cit.* p. 241)

Although symptoms are said usually to begin in the teen years a recent paper (Livingston & Martin-Cannici, 1985) draws attention to a few prepubertal children (aged 6–12 years) who present multiple somatic complaints consistent with somatisation disorder.

I will now look at some of the comments about these child patients, to see the similarities to those reported on in the adult literature and how these fit in with the analysis I present here. One of the earliest ideas about somatisation was that it arose as a defence in some children who were particularly stressed. This explanation would not be coherent with the analysis presented here. In Livingston & Martin-Cannici's child psychiatric sample the somatising children were not subjected to more psychosocial stressors than the other children, but it was as though they reacted to stress in a different way. For example the 'somatic complaints . . . usually appeared after he was stressed by environmental or social demands', whereas the children diagnosed as having 'anxiety and depressive disorders had significantly fewer somatic complaints', although a similar number of psychosocial stressors.

The same observations were reported earlier for abdominal pain in children (Apley, 1975). Hodges *et al.* (1985) showed that depression was not more common in children with abdominal pain (age range 6–16 years) than in healthy children, although it was in their mothers. For some of the children their experience of stress is transmitted to others in a language which leads to a psychological label for their discomfort; in similar circumstances other children's messages superficially suggest somatic discomforts. Nevertheless adolescents complaining of abdominal pain, but in whom no organic cause is found, have experienced more life events inter-preted as stressful than others attending with clear physical problems. These adolescents are not significantly different from other psychiatric patients (Black, 1985); it is rather their language for sharing their discom-forts which differentiates them.

The speech of those with somatoform disorders has been examined in adults and some support is obtained for the above analysis. The content analyses showed a low use of words from emotion categories, but the usual frequency of those from a distress category. The subjects used more negative statements, and rarely described themselves in relation to others. The conclusion was that the language of these patients showed them to have a confused, negative self-identity (Oxman *et al.*, 1985).

This is to be expected on the basis of the analysis I have presented of the alternative ways in which parents can facilitate children presenting their discomforts. We have already noted that the child's sense of locus of control is dependent on the pattern of parenting and that those children with a predominantly internal locus of control have a greater pscyhological vocabulary and a greater awareness of differentiated internal states com-pared with a predominantly external locus of control (Neuhauser *et al.*, 1978). I believe that if the locus of control status of these somatising children were investigated they would prove to have a predominantly exter-nal locus of control. Associated with this we could, on theoretical grounds, expect a greater degree of 'learned helplessness' and reduced sense of self-efficacy in that group, which would be consistent with the conclusion of Oxman *et al.* (1984).

It has been shown that it is an easy misinterpretation to make to say that children have been 'naughty', instead of acknowledging their psychological discomfort. It is necessary to look further at the observation that antisocial behaviour is a frequent occurrence in the families of those with somatisation disorders (American Psychiatric Association, 1980). The antisocial behaviour is found especially amongst the male members, whereas the somatisation disorder is found especially amongst the female members of the family. As noted earlier boys' and girls' conditions tend to be construed differently. The role of this effect in producing the above difference in the sexes could depend on a communication model such as I have proposed in this analysis.

Bohman *et al.* (1984), on the basis of an adoption study of females, suggest that both genetic and environmental factors are important in the aetiology of somatisation disorder, and analyse in detail the relationship to different forms of antisocial behaviour. Although the common title of their series of papers refers to somatoform disorders the content is limited to somatisation disorder. The incidence of somatisation disorder in adopted females in Sweden is greater than expected, so this group lent itself to the study of this theme (Sigvardsson *et al*. 1984). On the basis of both clinical and genetical analyses they propose a subdivision of somatisation disorder into two types: high frequency and diversiform (Cloninger *et al*., 1984). The genetic component in the relationship between antisocial disorder and somatisation disorder they summarise in the following way:

> Somatizers were distinguished from nonsomatizers by the com-bination of criminality, alcohol abuse, and low occupational status in their biological parents. The high frequency somatizers were distinguished from other somatizers by having biological fathers with onset of violent nonproperty crimes as teenagers and many temperance board registrations, but no treatment for alcohol abuse. The diversiform somatizers were distin-guished from other somatizers by having biological fathers with a history of either property crimes or alcoholism treatment.
> (Bohman *et al*. 1984)

It is not just these factors about the biological fathers' various forms of antisocial behaviour, here interpreted as genetic, but also environmental factors which are important in the aetiology, although the latter were interpreted as accounting for only half the variability that could be accounted for by the biological background. The environmental factors Bohman *et al*. distinguish as differentiating those women with the different forms of somatisation disorder from those without are 'occupational status and age at placement'. No further details are provided about the form of the age at placement variable, but they explain that 'unskilled occupational status of the adoptive father is associated with an increased risk of both petty criminality in men and diversiform somatisation in women. Alcohol abuse in the adoptive father is also associated with an increased risk of diversiform somatisation'. As mentioned earlier the age at adoption variable will need further investigation for its potential effect on early distress behaviour, as will the adoptive parents' expectations of their new child's personality based on the information provided to them, before the genetic interpretation is fully warranted.

I will not enter here into the debate about inheritability of criminality, but wish to stress that a mixture of factors link up behaviour of various kinds labelled as antisocial with somatisation disorder. Somatisation disor-der is most frequently diagnosed in females and antisocial behaviour in the males, but there are often associated symptoms of antisocial behaviour in the females. The conditon has a particularly important place in the genesis of both medical and social problems. Women with somatisation disorder report more social and medical problems in both their spouses and children (Hartvig & Sterner, 1985). The children of these families seem a particularly vulnerable group. These women tend to choose and be chosen as marriage partners by antisocial men (seven times as often as comparable depressed women), their children are twice as likely to have severe conduct disorders, and they are three times as likely to be reported for child abuse or have their children removed from home. These effects are independent of socioeconomic status (Zoccolillo & Cloninger, 1985). We are dealing with conditions which are very important socially, having a major impact on the fabric of society. I believe they are complex 'disorders' of communication linked to aberrant socio-cognitive development.

A recent editorial in the *British Medical Journal* (Jenkins & Clare, 1985) emphasised that the excess of psychiatric disorder in women should not be seen as implying constitutional weakness but pointing mainly towards environmental factors (Jenkins & Clare, 1985). The expression of the women's vulnerability, which they appear to have inherited according to the alternative intepretation of Bohman *et al.* (1984), seems to be determined by factors in the environment, such as responses in school and other microsystems, which construe girls' difficulties differently from those of boys. Brown, Craig & Harris (1985) regard depression in women as reflecting the way in which they have learnt to express their distress; this includes those with depression severe enough to warrant hospital treatment as well as those identified in the community. The 'tough man' syndrome can also come to be fostered through social interpretation, with the effect that these men isolate themselves at times of difficulty, whereas women tend to turn to others including professionals (Horwitz, 1977).

It seems to be that a similar communications analysis of antisocial behaviour is needed in order to reframe the 'disorder' into intersubjective terms, allowing the two conditions to be compared on a similar basis. From the analysis presented in this chapter it can be seen that it is a very small step from labelling a signal as one of distress to one of 'naughty' behaviour – a sort of junior version of antisocial behaviour. It is in order to make this distinction that parents employ their decision-making rules, trying to discriminate states of illness and distress from attempts at deception. The attribution of intention by the parents can then lead to the behaviour being labelled mischievous, although the child's state is not necessarily congruent with that intention. In this situation a clash of perspectives within a family can only be expected to escalate, as each side presses on with their message ever more stridently in order to achieve effectivity – until they give up, or, rarely, learn each other's language. The same sort of relationship has been described as developing in theory with people with somatisation disorder.

In order to facilitate discussion of some of the problems involved in trying to help adults with somatisation disorder, the term alexithymia was borrowed from the literature on psychosomatic illness to describe a difficulty in 'capacity to verbalize affect' (Taylor, 1984). It is this difficulty which I hypothesise could have its basis in the particular response to 'pretend illness' identified above. Support for this argument comes from some of the additional difficulties presented by patients with alexithymia. For example Taylor's (1984) review mentions 'the frequent presence of alexithymic characteristics in patients with somatoform disorders', their 'difficulty discriminating between emotional states and bodily sensations', 'impaired capacity for play' and 'impaired capacity for empathy'. I suggest that these are exactly the characteristics we would expect to find following the poor interactional 'dance' which develops in families where parental communication competences are reduced in the manner described above.

It seems inappropriate to describe those who have alexithymia as having a disorder, as though they were ill. It seems more helpful to talk of a different emphasis in their language, a specialised dialect. Taylor points out that alexithymia is not an all or none state, and that research suggests it is a '"situation-dependent state" concept rather than an "organismic subject-dependent trait"'. The difficulty is more pronounced in interactions with others than when subjects talk alone about their state. In the latter situation the restrictions on their limited emotional vocabulary are at their least. The language they use to describe their discomfort is the real language for them to use; it is up to the 'foreigners' to learn the language so that therapy can take new directions as required. The difficulty faced by a therapist can be to know whether the language portrays a problem which requires action to be put right, or a difficulty which the patient must live with. We live in a culture in which physical complaints more frequently imply the need for action to deal with the problem, whereas psychological discomforts more often need to be lived with. The language in use in somatoform relationships may, contrary to expectation, more often mean a discomfort must be lived with, through use of particular strategies, rather than the problem being physical in nature and requiring intervention.

The communication skills which someone lacks when in interaction with another in what I have termed a somatoform relationship are conceptualised as alexithymia. Another conceptualisation of the relationship stresses that messages are conveyed in a dialect dependent on the expression of physical discomforts.

When these people come asking for help, classical therapeutic methods have been largely unsuccessful (Taylor, 1984). Some recent developments in helping them alter the reduced psychological emphasis in their communication suggest that the communication pattern I have identified here is on the right track. I mentioned the way in which some parents successfully negotiated the 'pretend' phase by noting pattern and form to the complaining, rather than being caught up in the superficial message of the complaint. This approach forms the basis for one therapeutic approach reported in Taylor's review in which the focus of therapy is shifted 'from the content to the form of the patient's communications . . . and the patients are then . . . taught to recognize their emotions as signals to themselves'.

An alternative would be to use biofeedback techniques to give people visible feedback about their changes in emotions as reflected in pulse, blood-pressure and skin conductivity etc.

Other approaches get even closer to the pretend elements I have identified. For example, Madanes (1980) actively encourages pretend in the therapeutic session or as homework so that the family structure is reorganised as they 'pretend' new ways of relating. The complaining is approached indirectly through the world of play rather than being seen as outright fraud. Symptomatic behaviour is relabelled as a specific communication so that a new vocabulary is introduced to all those who need it, this then allows the family to renegotiate the situations where the old behaviour had arisen. Tizard & Hughes (1984 p. 57) have mentioned in passing that the most effective way for parents to modify their children's 'cheating' behaviour is to adopt a good-humoured relaxed approach rather than a moralistic one. This approach would seem coherent with that described above.

A third approach is under development by Greene & Sattin (1985). For their patients they used pairs of therapists, one labelled 'the symptom therapist' and the other 'the primary therapist'. The symptom therapist only allowed the patient to talk about his physical discomforts, and if this tailed off before the end of a standard 15 minute session the therapist enquired further of physical discomforts. The primary therapist allowed the patient to talk about anything else except his physical discomforts, the session being terminated if they were mentioned. If the patient successfully negotiated the session without introducing his physical discomforts he was allowed 5 minutes extra to talk solely about them. The patients in this approach are not told to change but they do, and they each 'rapidly developed a sense of humor about the expression of [their] physical discomfort', ceased being so isolated and joined in the ward. Their 'discomforts' are placed in different moral orders in this clearly structured but superficially paradoxical approach. The different languages are respected and when the patients live with their discomforts in new ways they are of reduced importance, especially in their effect on interpersonal relations.

Seltzer (1985a,b) has described both the families and therapeutic techniques she successfully used with children with conversion disorders (a somatoform disorder characterised by the presence of specific motor or sensory disorders where no organic problems can be found) and it is remarkable how close are some of the important factors she points out to those I have identified here. These families are socially isolated and are preoccupied with moral issues of right and wrong. In order to reduce their 'psychological mutism' she 'forces family members into fantasizing and imagining' through getting the family members to pretend alternative situations. In this way their tight constructs are loosened. As she puts it so clearly, 'the therapist functions similarly to the linguistic anthropologists discovering the grammatical rules for language spoken by peoples lacking literate traditions'.

I have described these approaches in some detail as their effectiveness distinguishes them from the more classical approaches and at the same time there is no apparent dissonance between the communicative skills For further discussion of treatment of somatising children see Shapiro & Rosenfeld (1987). In this indirect way I believe that the analysis suggests intelligible ways of accounting for the development of somatisation disorder; it will take alternative research efforts to discover to what degree the concept of a somatoform relationship is warranted.

### Naturalistic systems, psychological causes and the role of doctors

In some societies 'naturalistic' systems of illness causality predominate (Foster, 1976; see chapter 3). These are characterised by the view that illnesses are 'caused' by the events which have preceded them rather than by disease agents or by a change in the body 'balance'. Certain events are recognised as 'giving rise to' particular forms of illness. The salience of the different events varies in different cultures, but what is noteworthy is that diagnosis is dependent on establishing a culturally approved pattern in the preceding events which is then linked to the state of the individual. This connection has the same form as that between stressful events and anxiety in our society. We have evolved distinct languages for psychological problems and physical problems, although this distinction is not so clear in predominantly naturalistic medical systems. Events are associated with psychological problems rather than physical problems. 'Psychologese', to coin a word, is largely a western phenomenon, and it has been suggested that it most probably developed after the industrial revolution.

When patients from a Western culture come for a consultation with physical complaints they generally come with expectations appropriate to their predominantly personalistic system. They expect others to make the diagnosis, although keeping to themselves the relics of their childhood 'naturalistic' system and their own provisional diagnoses and beliefs about causes. Superficially they believe it is more appropriate to present their symptoms to professionals than to discuss them with their social contacts. The nature of somatoform symptoms often makes it more difficult for the often meagre support network (here distinguished from social network) to function. They do not expect the establishment of any connection between their complaints and preceding events to be relevant. Patients with somatisation disorder appear to work actively against that possibility. In contrast patients with somatic complaints from more 'naturalistically' oriented cultures are expecting connections to exist between their condition and preceding events, but they are chiefly waiting for the healer to intitiate treatment, not for a diagnosis to be made.

In Western culture these somatising patients come for treatment without expecting to take an active role in their own treatment. Their model of treatment tends to be that which fits into a personalistic system, whereas the nature of their underlying difficulties suggests that other expectations would be more facilitative for their treatment. We see similar problems with other disorders characterised by behaviours often labelled as having a primary physical basis, such as anorexia nervosa and hyperkinesis. With regard to what has been said above about somatoform disorders it is interesting to note that alcoholism, antisocial personality and hysteria are also unusually prevalent amongst the adult relatives of hyperkinetic children seen at psychiatric clinics (Cantwell, 1972). The actual expectations on coming to a consultation will, of course, be moulded by the patient's previous experience and that of the people who are important in his life.

The doctor's difficulty in these consultations appears to involve reframing the patient's expectations in a way which can lead to recognition of other factors which play a part in his condition. In this way the patient can begin to experience possibilities of control over those external factors which are playing on his vulnerabilities. He can develop a sense of competence to alter his own condition and an ability to protect those aspects of himself identified as vulnerable (the body states associated with the events).

The process increases the individual's sense of an internal locus of control and his self-efficacy, his sense of agency.

How can one avoid that pattern developing in children who are potentially at risk, those who have developed effectance through a somatoform relationship? Using the above analysis a general practitioner, for example, needs to help parents note pattern. In order to do this there needs to be enough order to the child's day, and the parents must be helped to identify significant deviations from these patterns. They can be helped to record a diary of appropriate events suggested by the history so that they can identify any pattern in the complaining. A suitable development of the health diary would be useful here (Freer, 1980). I suggest that it can be impossible, or at least unhelpful, for a doctor to draw any conclusions about the nature of the discomfort before the data on pattern exists; indeed, it is constructive for him to be initially uncertain. He also needs to have a large vocabulary of potentially relevant points of view. In this way the doctor's role can become political; there is no escape from this. I believe that child psychiatrists have important roles to play in bringing to people's notice relevant points of view.

Expectant waiting can be very difficult for doctors, as parents are often demanding a clear answer as soon as possible. The physical conditions which the doctor needs to exclude from the diagnosis add to his wish to end uncertainty about the diagnosis as soon as possible.

Parents are said to invoke doctors as authority figures to judge questions of malingering in their children. Only occasionally is a consultation with a doctor used as a threat by capitalising on a child's dislike of doctors. Otherwise it 'is not so much an idle threat as a deliberate check by the mother on whether the child feels that he has symptoms acceptable to an expert eye' (Newson & Newson, 1976 p. 388). When a child is brought to a doctor in these circumstances the doctor rarely concentrates on how the parents discussed and evaluated the child's condition. He rarely helps them elaborate their strategies and in this way keeps a metaposition in relation to the family and avoids a judicial position in the future. If the doctor erroneously limits himself to the assumption that all at home have been in agreement that the child has a problem in need of treatment, the consultation becomes charged with covert moralistic evaluations of which parent made the 'right' or 'wrong' decision.

The consultation can indirectly come to be a judicial situation around the child, charged with tension – a very different sort of moral order to that which facilitates communication as in the 'ideal speech act' (see McCarthy, 1973). The doctor is inadvertently put in a position by the family whereby support for the child becomes more difficult. Through concentrating on pattern and parental decision-making strategies he can avoid such a position. His evaluation can usefully remain unresolved until he has this information, unless there are clear indications for immediate action. By looking at the parental decision-making he is carrying out a particularly constructive sort of health education which can restore to the parents a sense of effectiveness and minimise the family's helplessness.

Additionally a doctor needs to aid the family's ability to reflect on their 'pain' language. Children more often report the same sort of pain as do others in their families, even when there is no clear organic basis for the pain. This has been reported for abdominal pain (Apley, 1975 p. 102), dental pain (Craig, 1978), lower back pain (Gentry, Shows & Thomas, 1974) and headaches (Turkat, Kuczmierczyk & Adams, 1984). Children need to develop a language for sharing their discomforts and they build on what is available. Adults with chronic pain disorder have more often been hospitalised as children (Pilowsky *et al.*, 1982) and the hypothesis must be tested that they learnt their pain language in that setting. Many children admitted to hospital with abdominal pain have associated family problems and recover in 24–48 hours (Jones, 1969; Drake, 1980). But we must ask what the longer term consequences of this admission strategy can be for their developing language of discomfort; how this affects the family members' sense of ability to nurse their child subsequently and his security of attachment to them.

In a consultation it is helpful to build on the family's language, but at the same time make the children aware of *their* language. When they say that they have a tummy ache, they have a tummy ache and not depression, regardless of how many other signs of depression an observer trained in the value system of that culture could find. The treatment of that tummy ache, though, may well involve treatments which others would regard as being for depression. Only by being aware of the limits of our language can we extend our dialect. The same sort of process needs to occur when the languages of school and home meet so that the bilingual child does not get confusingly caught between them. The functioning of the mesosystem needs to be facilitated.

## The advantages of pretending illness

I personally believe that it is essential for children to be able to pretend illness occasionally, or exaggerate, without becoming locked into one form of family style or another. This will occur naturally if the parents can tolerate that first episode of uncertainty about 'what is up'. Through their experience of parents, teachers and welfare assistants, who are always refining their techniques for discriminating physical and psychological discomforts, the children come to learn the construction of the locally approved illness behaviour. As the decision-making strategies are developed, so the children's knowledge of the minutiae of their culture's value system about illness is elaborated for them. They learn not to complain too much or too little in order to be effective. They experience the salience of different symptom constellations, and how these can come to have the same or alternative meanings at home and at school. Through being successful pretenders from time to time they learn the value system of their culture as well as continuing their individuation. This connects with the position described by Winnicott in which if the mother 'knows too well what the infant needs, this is magic and forms no basis for an object relationship' (Davis & Wallbridge, 1983 p. 66). The caveat to my approval of pretence resides in the need for successful pretence to occur only from time to time, as good enough holding can only be secure if parental interpretations of what is going on are accurate most of the time.

## Summary

In order to develop the fullest possible language for conveying all sorts of discomforts we need to be as facilitative as possible in helping children convey their various aches and pains. We need to be aware of the possibility of deceit, but through noting pattern to the form of children's complaints we can identify those situations they struggle with, and introduce them to a differentiated vocabulary of psychological discomforts to put beside the physical. Children come across a variety of different languages for complaining, but they appear to be able to integrate these only if the mesosystems function facilitatively. This will mean the family functioning as though it were a relatively open system. It is through an understanding of the different worlds of childhood that adults important to the child stand the best chance of attributing the correct intention to the child's behaviour.

Through 'hearing' the child, and 'holding' the child through periods of uncertainty the child can be expected to approach Herzlich's (1973) illness categorisation of 'Illness as an occupation'. Here he retains a sense of his own effectiveness even in illness. A balance between his illness behaviour and society's sickness role is accomplished. If it had been that his illness behaviour overrode the predominant sickness language we would have expected illness to be a liberator, or a destroyer if social pressures predominated.

In this analysis I have explored some of the potential origins of somatoform complaining in the decision-making rules applied to the illness behaviour of 8-year-old children. The ways in which these rules lead to the allocation of the sick role to the child were described. This distinction between illness behaviour (their own) and the sick role (attributed by the parents, the powerful others in this case) was lost on the children, who came to develop a language of illness behaviour based on the ways in which they have been handled when ill. They learnt to account for their states in ways which were intelligible to their care-givers and warranted by the structure to their care-givers' daily lives. In this way the child's reality in illness highlighted the communication processes occurring between people.

The communicative competences required for interpreting the content of these interactions and decision-making were analysed. Diminished use of these competences in particular areas were interpreted as giving rise to a somatoform relationship. These were particularly the skills required to discriminate the different moral orders of the prevailing systems in which the children are presenting their discomforts, together with the skills to distinguish the non-verbal signals for psychological states of discomfort, often used as one of the markers to the prevailing moral order. It was necessary to couple with these competences an ability to notice pattern in the presentation of the discomfort. Pattern is only established after more than one presentation of the discomfort and so it was necessary for the parent to be with the child through the first episode without definitively labelling it (the holding state). It is during this first presentation of the discomfort, before the child has learnt to signal it in a way which makes a difference to his care-giver appropriate to his state, that there is the greatest chance of the parent imposing his own meaning on the child's behaviour without knowing whether it is correct. It is here that the past exerts one of its powerful effects in this hermeneutic model of the development of illness behaviour.

# 9

## The consultation: a form of dialogue

*'Do not mistake a child for his symptom'* (Erikson, 1965 p. 59)


I started my search with some questions which I felt an observational study could answer. Observations are interpreted from our own peculiar perspectives. Inevitably the questions and suggested answers raised by my review of the child's world of illness will be coloured by my practice as a child psychiatrist. I hope that my analysis of the origins of physical and psychological labels for discomfort which I presented in the preceding chapter will enable the reader to integrate physical and psychological elements in the consultation.

What do these observations of the child's world of illness mean for consultations of all different kinds, be it a child with a parent or parents with a doctor about their child? What is their usefulness and validity in that context? My aim here is to propose some implications for professional consultations based on what I have reported, with limited reference to the relatively meagre literature on consultations with children. Unfortunately there is not yet enough research to comment on validity. The general tenor of research in this field has been to explore the processes going on in a medical consultation around the child, with the assumption that the children are passive attendants. My view is that the consultation setting is like the primary structure which I discussed in chapter 4 – a microsystem with its own properties. It will affect the further development of children's views in particular ways analogous to those described earlier.

The literature on interview techniques and consultation processes with adults has multiplied rapidly recently, in line with the belief that there is room for improvement in this area. Regrettably general experience is that giving information about something, such as what can facilitate a medical consultation, does not mean that established practices are likely to change. Further research is needed to look at how such information can be incorporated in a way which makes it meaningful and usable. It may be that this can be achieved when the information comes from work colleagues – general practitioners' behaviour changes most when they work together with other professionals (Horder, Bosanquet & Stocking, 1986).

My suggestions are made in the spirit of a clinician translating research findings into a practical context. It has not always been possible to check the degree to which my interpretations of the children's views were warranted. I have not tried to obtain figures for how often particular views are found, taking the view that what was most beneficial, given the current state of our knowledge, was first to establish the breadth to the children's knowledge. My assumption was that on establishing contact in a consultation it was more important to know the range of the possible than what was probable, so that individuality was respected. Subsequent research will need to look further at the probabilities of obtaining the different views from different groups in different settings so that some of the initial uncertainty about what to expect in a consultation can be reduced. But enthusiasm for this type of research must be tempered with knowledge that the price of reducing uncertainty can be a loss of individuality.

My method, founded on an intersubjective model of developmental psychology, suggests ways of establishing and nurturing dialogue with children which enable one to find out how their world of illness is constructed. The children's reported sense of guilt in causing their condition seemed to depend on the form of dialogue established. We can either play on children's beliefs in immanent justice and so increase their sense of guilt that they caused their condition, or we can avoid it, through the form of enquiry used. We can play on parents' sense of guilt about not preventing their children's illness, or avoid doing so through both the form and content of our questioning.

The form and the content of an interview are crucial when it comes to interpreting the messages we get from children – just as they are of critical importance for the children. But it was seen in chapter 2 and subsequently that the two parts to a message are really not so distinct. One only has to see how patterns of complaining evolve dependent both on the form and content of the discomforts presented, as in the preceding chapter, to be reminded of the relative impossibility of producing an intelligible coherent account which can convey all the potential interactions.

The development of illness behaviour is dependent on naturally occurring events which have evolved into a signalling system that is more or less effective depending on what the signals mean for those who receive them and how they are responded to. The consultation must address itself to both elements: the naturally occurring states and the ways in which the changes these lead to in the care-givers alter the child's vocabulary and grammar for presenting his discomforts. At the same time those who provide consultations must be aware that they are playing their part in creating a child's illness vocabulary for the future. This awareness can be the foundation for the health education element in the normal consultation.

## Consulting

The consultation is the culmination of a complicated process of provisional assessment (Locker, 1981; Twaddle, 1981). All participants have their personal histories of what these preliminaries have led to. Together these will affect the expectation people bring with them and the ease with which they will approach sharing their discomforts with others in a consultation.

Some of the factors which affect the frequency with which children consult or are brought to a consultation are known. In relation to the child's world of illness the former may at first glance appear the more interesting here, although as will be seen below the two are intimately related. Already I have referred to the Californian project where children at school could take the initiative to consult the school nurse (Lewis *et al.*, 1977). In that project 15% of the children made 50% of the visits. The high-frequency users had the same profile as found amongst the adult consulters in the local community. They tended to be female, come from more affluent families, and were often the youngest or an only child. In relation to the theme of internal versus external locus of control it was noted that the high-frequency users had no particular locus of control orientation, according to the researchers' criteria of measurement.

The consultations were not by children who had more medical problems as defined by the professional staff; it was the children who had more often been taken to a paediatrician who more often used the services at the school. The pattern of use of care by the mother was significantly associated with her pattern of use of paediatric care for her children. Campbell (1978) noted an additional variable due to an interaction between the factors of sex of the child, maternal educational level, and paternal socioeconomic status (co-varying with maternal educational level but being a less strong determinant); those mothers of higher educational level successfully encouraged a more stoic approach to illness in their boys. This effect began early in their lives, but in this study the maternal influence did not extend to the children's inclination to report illness. Mechanic (1962) had reported that for adults in the United States their 'inclination to seek medical advice was significantly related to [their] religion, social class position, dependency on others, and the magnitude of stress reported'. Jews and Episcopalians were twice as often inclined to consult as Catholics. Interpersonal difficulties increase the chance that someone will consult.

Social class effects have been interpreted in a variety of ways. Blaxter & Paterson (1982b) suggested an interpretation of their observations that mothers from social classes IV–V took their children to the doctor less often as being that these mothers perceived illness less readily. When Campion & Gabriel (1984) in another Scottish sample, but one in which there was less marked deprivation, looked at consultation patterns of mothers with their children they found in contrast an appreciably higher rate of consultation associated with lower socioeconomic status.

Blaxter (1984) has analysed British adult consultation behaviour for social class effects to try to elucidate the differing influences. Generally the increased use of services by lower social class (IV–V) adults was for 'life threatening, urgent, chronic, or incapacitating conditions, thus matching the presumed difference in need'. The social class difference for trivial conditions is less than for serious conditions. The most marked differences between the sexes for 'illness' consultations concern the youngest category she analysed (15–24 years), where the numbers of consultations a year for males were between 1.1 (social classes I–II ) and 1.5 (IV–V) while for females they were between 3.4 and 3.6. Over time the differences between the sexes diminished so that for men between 44 and 65 years consultation rates were between 2.0 and 3.4, while for the women they were between 2.6 and 3.3 In fact the consultation rate for young women was even higher than this because they often took their children to consultations. This in turn would have a pronounced effect on the developing consultation behaviour of their children, especially the girls.

It will be necessary for several possible interpretations of the data to be examined before these sex differences can be understood. It is possible that women complain about their condition to professionals as a part of their illness behaviour more easily than men, without there necessarily being any correspondence between their threshold for complaining and their physical state: Their own complaining can be related to a poorly expressed need to present someone else's complaints, for example their child's (a hypothesis I will return to later) or even to present the complaints of their husband (Graham, 1984). It could be, however, that men have a poorly developed ability for, or a high threshold to, complaining about their state to professionals, relative to the ability of the women, especially in the 15–24 age group. Expectations can play a determining role; Gochman (1970) pointed out that boys expect to remain healthy more than girls. These hypotheses could be evaluated in relation to the respective mortality rates. The male/female mortality ratio was 1.87:1 for the 15–64-year age group in 1971 (Townsend & Davidson, 1982 p. 57).

Campion & Gabriel (1984) emphasise one further aspect to consultation behaviour which elaborates on their observation reported above, and I quote them in full:

> Our finding that a 'doctor defined' significant diagnosis is more highly associated with consulting rates than any social or economic measure is important, if only to set in context the reported associations between such measures and use. Though it may be obvious that children with 'significant diagnoses' will have seen their doctor, we have shown that these children and their siblings attend more often with other, less important, complaints. The perceived threat of any symptom is heightened by the previous experience of a significant disease.

Shapiro's (1983) review on family reactions and coping strategies recorded that the pressure of a chronic illness in the family was associated with increased clinic attendance in other family members.

The set of expectations held prior to the consultation is important. Spencer (1984) reported that mothers took their children to the doctor not because they thought their symptoms were serious but beause the symptoms caused anxiety and might become serious. It will be seen below that this can pose problems because of the development of the role of the receptionist. She increasingly acts as a gate to the consultation with a doctor, so that it can become more difficult to use the doctor in this way. The dangers are that reputations will guide the receptionist's responses to the request for a consultation, rather than there being an unprejudiced enquiry in which the nature of the current uncertainties is unravelled. Bloor & Horobin (1975) reported how a group of Scottish doctors believed that patients should use their own judgement as to when it was appropriate to seek medical advice. This contrasts with these parents' wishes on behalf of their children, and can put the receptionist in an invidious position between two contrasting sets of expectations.

Experience plays a complex role here, as Pattison *et al.* (1982) have described for mothers consulting with their babies. If mothers have had previous experience of looking after babies they consult more often with their own first baby, especially if there are a lot of major symptoms at the same time. But with subsequent babies of their own they are 'expected' to be more knowledgeable and consult less. Campion & Gabriel (1985) reported mothers consulting more with their first children, and also that mothers with fewer children consult more often. It is unknown whether first children come to develop alternative illness behaviours on the basis of these consultation patterns but they are described as being more sensitive to pain (Chen & Cobb, 1960). What are accepted as normal childhood ailments will alter depending on the frequency with which the conditions are encountered. In larger families there will be a greater chance that conditions crop up time and again and become accepted as normal, and hence not requiring specific consultations. Garralda & Bailey (1986*c*) did find that in a comparison of 7–12-year-old children attending general practitioners in Manchester, England, with and without psychological disturbance (but where the presentation was of a somatic problem), the child's position in the family had a significant effect. Only 12% of the children with psychological problems were first-born, compared with 43% of those without psychological problems. The incidence was similar for only children (8% vs. 11%), whereas for youngest children the figures were respectively 52% and 33%.

I will now present elements of the consultation referring to key concepts which I have used in my presentation so far.

### The setting

When the consultation gets under way the moral order of the setting will establish the rights which the participants have and how they obtain respect for themselves and their symptoms, as well as the rights to assert their respective expertise. Current research suggests more questions than answers. I will include many of the questions as they point to the research 'menu' for the future. How the moral order is established and recognised and what the effects of the moral order are on the children, their views, and subsequent illness behaviour and consultation patterns urgently needs investigation. It will be more difficult to explore connections to morbidity and mortality.

The effects of design features in health service buildings on children's consultations have been seriously neglected as a research topic (for example the effects of whether furnishing is child centred or adult centred), and yet it is in childhood that patterns of health-related behaviour are established. We do not know the effect on the consultation of having rooms with demonstrable sound-proofing, so that the out-patient hubbub is immediately dulled or eliminated on entering the consultation room. Confidentiality – a central part of the moral order of a consultation – is clearly a myth when the whole ward or waiting room hears every precious word the child dares to share.

It is unknown what 'confidentiality' in a medical consultation means for children. They do not have the same rights to confidentiality as adults. The research reported here supports the idea that young children are more capable of sharing their own discomforts with others than is generally assumed, as well as their own views on the nature and origins of these discomforts. In the future it will be necessary to refine our knowledge of what confidentiality means for establishing a helpful moral order in the consultation with children, and to what extent the information which they give should be regarded as confidential in relation to their parents. The ethical issues here are important to explore for their effect on the consultation process and what they can do for establishing the children's sense of responsibility for their own condition. The research so far does not point to clear age-linked factors that enable children to be more or less responsible for their condition at predetermined ages.

The shop window for a hospital is its out-patient department, and for the general practitioner his receptionist and waiting room. They set the scene. Usually in the United Kingdom contact with the receptionist is necessary before entering into the consultation with the 'expert'. It is particularly at this stage that symptoms have to be presented for quick scrutiny, without there being the chance for the child to be heard. The emotional atmosphere can change swiftly in this para-consultation, which has a critical place in validating a consultation. It was particularly the acceptability of symptoms which has been described as central to many parents' consultations (Newson & Newson, 1976 p. 388). This particular role of symptom validation is now often not accomplished in the consultation but delegated, so that the consultant's expectatory set is that protopatients will present as patients. He will not be called upon to discuss the grey half-ill states. Initiation into the professionally confirmed patient role has proceeded apace prior to the consultation rather than in it. It becomes less relevant for the consultant to take up decision-making.

It is not known whether parents find presenting their uncertainties to a receptionist preferable to presenting them to a doctor. This could be the case if we extend the observation that they prefer discussing their complaints with community nurses than with doctors (Chapman, 1986). The question here is the effect which this type of setting has on the presentation of children's discomforts to a consultant, as there has been delegation of the critical role of establishing the initial moral climate. The effects of these procedures on children's developing illness behaviour have not yet been researched.

The speech of mothers to their young children varies with the social context (Dunn, Wooding & Hermann, 1977). The moral order of a clinic will be different from that of a ward in a hospital, a consultation with a homeopath or the sitting room at home. These different settings with their moral orders could be particularly important for ways in which social class effects are mediated. The communicative competences of childen from different classes are affected differently when they enter school. There is a greater difference between home and school for a working class child than there is for a middle class child (Tizard & Hughes, 1984).

When pursuing a communication model of illness behaviour it is necessary to find out more about these effects. The differences between the health of the social classes as reported in the Black report are enormous (Townsend & Davidson, 1982). But what the report did not analyse in the same detail were the origins of the similar differences between the sexes (ratio of death rates for 15–64-year-olds for social class V compared with I was 2.5 and for males compared with females was 1.9 in 1971: Townsend & Davidson, 1982, p. 57). The observations which I have reported suggest many further questions to be asked in order to explore these sex and class differences, such as 'How do the different sexes get respect for different forms of complaining in different types of moral order?'. How do our responses help children differentiate their varying internal states, and develop a language for sharing them? Garralda & Bailey (1986*b*) found that in England parents were more aware of girls' than boys' psychological difficulties, when these were part of the presentation of overtly somatic problems to a general practitioner.

In a consultation it is necessary to be aware that prior to that consultation girls' and boys' discomforts may well have been responded to in contrasting ways. Boys and girls will share the results of the consultation with their peers in differing ways due to their different ways of maintaining face with them. Analysis of these issues can account for the observation that boys say they expect to remain healthy more than do their female peers (Gochman, 1970), in spite of the long-term outlook for them being much more gloomy.

The analysis in the preceding chapter suggests some of the influences and can account for some of the differences between the sexes. Our knowledge of the setting and how it influences children's developing language is currently rudimentary.

The moral order of a setting is interpreted from clear messages one receives about what must be done in order to be approved of. At the same time there are relevant hidden bits of information. Only by making 'mistakes' will it be possible to learn what the hidden rules of the settings are (see chapter 2). In addition children will necessarily take their untested previous experiences and myths about the settings into their subsequent encounters. Those who are in a position to ask questions will stand the greatest chance of avoiding being bound by past responses. It therefore seems appropriate for the Health Education Council in Britain to have produced their leaflet on 'A guide to asking questions of your doctor', echoing the Chinese proverb 'He who asks a question feels a fool for five minutes; he who doesn't ask remains a fool for ever'.

In the communication analysis presented in the previous chapter we saw how different languages used in different settings could give rise to subsequent problems if there was not shared knowledge about how the child functioned in the different settings of home and school. A consultation must be carried out with an awareness of these factors, at the same time as the consultation itself is treated as though it was one of these special settings with its own rules. I have not looked specifically at how children construe hospitals as a special type of setting with its own moral order. But it was noted earlier that perhaps the language of pain was refined in that setting through the respect that sort of discomfort was afforded (see chapter 8).

The local hospital rules about who can visit and when, will also say something to the child about the hospital staff's understanding and respect for his experiences. The child's definition of illness reflected the importance of maintaining his relationships: the fewer visitors one receives the more seriously ill one could believe oneself to be. The long- and short-term effects of barrier nursing and isolation on children, increasingly used with developments in medical techniques, are just emerging as topics of research. Can telephones help here? Are telephones available on the wards for adolescents to make confidential calls so that their contacts can be maintained?

In 1959 Marlens (in Peters, 1978) described how hospitalised children had a much greater sense that their illness was a punishment and that they were rejected because of it. This effect of 'illness' was attributed to the process of hospitalisation rather than to the illness *per se*. These views could not be altered by the explanations which were used. Whether hospitalisation still has the same effect after the increased contact with family members which is now allowed has not been adequately checked. Haggerty (1980) has noted that 'in the developing world family support is accomplished more naturally in hospitals since there are few professionals available'. Nevertheless we must not lose sight of the fact that in the United Kingdom only half of 50 hospitals surveyed by the Consumer Association in 1980 had 24-hour visiting on children's wards. I remain uncertain why adults should continue to be treated so differently from children. As a child might say: 'Do hospitals know how important my sister is to me, and my best friend at school, or do they think that I should be content with having mum popping in every day on her way to see gran whom I know cannot get by without mum's help?'

Macaskill & MacDonald (1982 p. 72) reported that parents described a greater sense of professional distance between patients and hospital staff than between patients and general practitioners. Research has not always specified the hospital staff involved; but the reported views do reflect the hospital setting. As noted above, patients in Britain prefer to talk to community nurses rather than doctors about certain matters (Chapman, 1986). The role of uniforms in creating different types of moral order in the settings has not been explored, yet uniforms are key ingredients for a child's interpretation of a setting and what rights he has in it. Some doctors have stopped wearing white coats; some community nurses are seen more as part of the daily round whereas the often more elaborate uniforms of the hospital nurses can set them apart. More information is needed here.

What are the anxieties which particular settings engender and why? Are these anxieties to be acknowledged or denied? Will support be available? It is unethical to enquire of anxieties in children if the children are not to be supported, as it is the response to the anxiety which shows whether the child is understood and respected. Is it more helpful if the consultant does the support himself or facilitates the parents in providing it? But then again 'Am I free to tell everyone about what is really worrying me?' 'Will they tell if I let on that our neighbour's been scaring me silly?' What are the child's views about confidentiality and how does a child deduce from the setting the sort of confidentiality that applies there? 'Is my point of view relevant in this setting?' 'Am I allowed a point of view here?' What happens to a child's sense of agency in a state of illness if the answer to these questions is 'No'?

Some of the above factors have been addressed in the Minneapolis Children's Hospital's 'human ecology programme' (Wallinga, 1982). As the setting is under the administration of non-clinical staff these are included in the programme, as are all other staff groups, so that a coherent child-orientated programme is fostered at all levels in the hospital. In this way a consistent message is conveyed about the child's place in the scheme of things with respect for his special and vulnerable position, as well as his ways of talking about himself. An orientating course on communicating with children is an important part of the introduction to the programme for all new appointees.

Although the above programme shows what can be done at the local level, there is no reason why similar but larger-scale programmes should not orientate higher levels of government to children's communication patterns and their needs in medical settings so that similar initiatives can be fostered. Instead of having a health Ombudsman who concentrates on what has gone wrong, the emphasis could be more in line with the role taken by the Norwegian 'Barneombud' (Children's Ombudsman) whose role is making certain that the administration is cognisant of the needs of children, and who takes initiatives to comment on government legislation for its anticipated effects on children.

### The stance

Although a set of expectations is established by the surroundings and what they mean for us, the people encountered there can convey alternatives through their stance. (I will here limit myself to the initial stance, rather than including the continuous modulation of the stance that occurs throughout the consultation.) The stance has been hinted at before the consultation begins through the form and timing to the preparatory contact. If an appointment is set for a short time after the referral there is generally an increased chance that the consultation will proceed (for example in child psychiatry see Mearns & Kay, 1985). Although several factors affect the decision of whom to call to an early appointment, it could be that parents and children regard an early appointment as respect for the seriousness of their request for help. It is not known what effect appointment systems, which can be associated with delay in being seen, have had on the illness behaviour which children develop. Some people recover naturally in the waiting period, some give up complaining, whereas I expect that others come to develop even more pronounced symptoms in order for their request for help to be effective.

The stance of the consultant cannot really be divorced from his relationship to what he has in the room. Is it predominantly child orientated? Are there toy telephones, glove puppets, drawing paper etc. which facilitate child communication? Or is it an adult world which children enter at their peril? In 1956 Gips (in Eiser, 1984) reported that medical personnel tended to be seen as punitive and non-empathic. Children (especially aged 7–10 years) have believed that staff empathy is dependent on their expressing pain (Brewster, 1982). It is not revealed in Pilowsky *et al.*'s (1982) report on adults with chronic pain disorder at what age they had been hospitalised as children (see Chapter 8), but the hypothesis must be tested that as children they had developed the view that staff empathy was dependent on their expressing pain. If that turns out to be true it may be a case of moral order effects in the primary structure of the hospital being incorporated into the child's secondary structure, which the child has continued with into adulthood.

Generally the consultation dialogue begins with an expressive interchange, and the practical requirements follow on (Harré, 1979 pp. 4–5). This expressive phase, where the 'How are you?' is still a greeting, before it switches to being a request for factual information, sets the tone. Subsequent social progression is usually through discussion about how the patient's normal roles are affected, which is also a helpful stance to adopt in the consultation. This is commensurate with the proposition I presented about children's understanding of illness, and is very useful as a starter to exploring what the illness means for the patient, and as an introduction to his way of life.

The patient's rights are established, and differing types of respect hinted at in these preparatory exchanges. His feeling states are responded to prior to the illness state being further explored. It is here that anxieties on coming to a consultation must be addressed. The expressive phase is the sounding-out phase. Apley (1980) had a guiding maxim which was that 'a surprising number of improvements in communication can be made when the doctor reminds himself that all the time that he is appraising the child and parents, so they in turn, are appraising him'. In this way one avoids fostering childhood egocentrism.

In a concise review of the consultation literature concerning child psychiatry Hill (1985) describes those factors in the consultant which facilitate self-disclosure in the patient. These include accurate empathy involving the communication of understanding, non-possessive warmth (the creation of an accepting, safe, trusting atmosphere within which the therapist conveys his respect for the patient and withholds negative value judgements), and genuineness or consistent sincerity in overt responses to the patient.

Initial, as well as underlying, anxieties are of crucial importance to the whole of the consultation. Stress increases utilisation of services for children's ailments (Mechanic, 1964; Roghmann & Haggerty, 1973; Tuch, 1975; Garralda & Bailey, 1986b). In the presence of stress there is also an increased vulnerability to infection (Meyer & Haggerty, 1963; for further discussion of changes in the immune system in relation to stress see the review of Stein, Keller & Schleifer, 1985, and Jemmott *et al.*, 1983). At present the concept of stress is rather abstract and not conceptualised in a way which individualises it for application to the circumstances of individual children, but current 'life events' research is beginning to make advances. One of the complications of interpretation, for example, is that parental investment in the child's performance is related to the child's vulnerability to infection (Kasl, Evans & Neiderman, 1979). Doing nothing can be particularly stressful for some individuals (Frankenhaeuser *et al.* (1978) in Jemmott *et al.*, 1983).

Complementary studies on how stress in the consultant affects his stance, especially as regards his ability to establish a position from which he can identify stress in the patient and support the child and his parents, have not been developed. Yet these factors could turn out to have importance for the forms of illness behaviour in the child which are effective in a consultation and on the child's long-term illness behaviour. Is a stressed consultant predisposed to use biological models to the exclusion of psycho-social models of illness or vice versa?

What is the acceptable content to the dialogue and how is this conveyed in stance? In my research method for gathering information I stressed the neutrality required and ways of establishing it. It is my impression that professionals do not usually find it easy to say that they do not know something, yet it can be just such an openness which facilitates neutrality. Through their analysis of the discourse children deduce whether the adult is dealing mainly in the pragmatic or the mathetic mode. As noted earlier the younger children keep these modes rather discrete, whereas for adults the functions are more mixed. 'It is the intention behind the question, not the words with which it is expressed that is crucial' (Tizard & Hughes, 1984 p. 107). The consultation will be unhelpfully sidetracked if the child's deductions suggest that questions are being asked on some pragmatic basis, rather than their being for elicitation of factual information.

The difficulty comes here of conveying in the non-verbal stance, and the initial expressive phase of contact, what is acceptable in verbal as well as non-verbal modes so that therapy can proceed effectively. Doctors, being of higher socioeconomic status, are more likely to foster a stoical response to illness (Zborowski, 1969, in Campbell, 1978). They must beware of imposing their life-style values in their stance, not all of which arise because of expertise in the field of illness and health.

Specific training programmes (for example that at Yale: Granger *et al.*, 1986) do affect how paediatricians communicate with children and result in alternative illness behaviour in the parents and children who consult them. Ingredients of helpful programmes include interview teaching (see for example Maguire, Fairbairn, & Fletcher, 1986; Wilkinson, 1983 for British approaches), developmental assessment and family dynamics, which amongst other things address those influences I highlighted in chapters 4 and 8. Collaboration is fostered, with respect for the contributions all concerned can make, if training has been undertaken jointly with other professionals. The result is that paediatricians use more time to gather information than give it, they use more open-ended questions, use more time to listen, and establish more of a dialogue. This has been shown to give more satisfaction to the mothers and is associated with fewer developmental disorders, such as enuresis, in the children (Granger *et al.*, 1986). One of the ways in which these paediatricians' stance is reflected is through their keeping more toys in their consulting rooms.

*The interview*

I have already referred to some aspects of the interview when looking at the establishment of a helpful stance for a consultation. I will now discuss the process of interviewing in more detail. The research results which I have presented point to the abilities of children to be involved much more actively than has usually been the case, provided that those consulted have the ability to appreciate the child's world and his communicative style and skills.

For the interview to proceed smoothly the child needs to be able to distinguish what is said for pragmatic purposes (in some ways similar to discriminating the expressive elements in the interview) from the mathetic. On a basis of trust he establishes whether the questions are genuine or attempts at control and checking. For a question to be 'felicitous' the following conditions must apply:

1. There is a piece of information of which the questioner is ignorant.
2. The questioner wants to know it.
3. The questioner believes that the person questioned knows the answer.
4. The questioner is in a position to elicit the answer from the person questioned (Leech, 1981 p. 322).

The developmental literature to which I have referred has pointed out the role of asking questions for the way in which this potentially puts the questioner at a powerful advantage and in a position which makes the establishment of a dialogue more difficult. Wood (1982) summarised this research for the part questions played in affecting the interview with a child. Questions tend to suppress children. The person who asks them is making demands of the other. The pacing of these demands in a question and answer format may well overestimate what a child can manage; children need longer to think and talk, and more time for introspection. Continual questioning inhibits those questioned from seeking information themselves, and the questioned children ask fewer questions of others. The latter effect is especially pronounced in working class girls in the school setting (Tizard & Hughes, 1984); but effects in the consultation setting have not yet been examined. The ways in which questions are asked will mean that patients are enabled to establish, to varying degrees, their own sense of personal importance and ability to participate effectively. The

forms of questioning together with the relevant points of view they introduce can create a framework for health promotion and illness prevention
at the same time as the consultation proceeds.

Wood (1982) continues with some tips about how to establish an interview. These are coherent with the research method I used, which successfully led to the children revealing a lot of their world of health and illness.
Questions ideally lead out from the child's last statement. The questions
should be interspersed with acknowledging moves, 'uhm' and 'yes', and
statements about the topic or expression of views about it which elaborate
the discourse along relevant lines. Pictures, toys and stories can act as
props. Asking for the children's current wishes opens up the dialogue.
One way of avoiding questions being too restraining is to use a multiple
choice format.

The questions which are asked establish critical points of view from
which events and body states are evaluated. Questions asked about how
social contacts have responded to the present complaint emphasise their
relevance and can either develop the support possibilities available or
minimise them. I noted some of these effects in chapter 8. Through the
questions asked a history of the complaint is both taken and created at
the same time. Tizard & Hughes (1984 p. 47) reported how the forms of
questions which mothers asked of their children forced the children to
construct logically consistent accounts. In an analogous way the questions
asked in a consultation force the construction of a logically coherent account
of the illness episode, which for children will be based on their underlying
premises about the nature of illness and their bodies. It is the nature of
these premises which I have presented. They cannot always be put into
words by the child but one becomes aware of them through a sense of an
ongoing pantomime. They can be shared collectively without being personally verbalised.

The information which the consultant obtains about the complaint will
enable him to place the complaint within the context of the family decision-
making guidelines, and come to an understanding of what is important to
the child in his different microsystems with his particular life style. This
will mean being able to answer clearly what is being complained of, by
whom, and why it is a matter for concern. He will have found out the
nature of the pattern to the complaining, and which points of view have
been used to understand that pattern. The jigsaw will fit together with
the knowledge gained about the family and school illness languages. This
will enable respect to be paid to the child's way of defining illness when
one knows what is important in his relationships and so take care of the

points raised earlier (chapter 4) about how children, adolescents (Millstein *et al.*, 1981) and adults (Apple, 1960) define their own illness. The role of illness as part of the child's strategy for maintaining face (Goffman, 1955), and negotiating his status and respect with his peers, will place the child's views of illness into the categories of illness as an occupation, liberator or destroyer (see chapter 3). It will facilitate discrimination between signs of illness and symptoms.

Throughout my presentation I have drawn attention to the importance of maintaining a child's sense of effectiveness, his sense of agency. This can be facilitated in the interview through the ways in which the child is given choice, even if it is just choice over the timing of when a particular part of an investigation will be carried out. The parents' sense of being effective in helping their child recover can also be facilitated, through both the forms of questions asked (which can emphasise the importance of their points of view and the support which they can give their child, so that their care is acknowledged as an important ingredient in the cure) and the explanations and advice given (see below). Choice must reside in the primary care group, so that instead of working towards compliance from the child, treatment becomes a cooperative venture. The child's sense of ability to control threatening situations is fostered and he develops an internal locus of control with the consequences this will have for his developing a psychological language to place beside his language for physical complaints.

Real choice is based on relevant information. The concept of informed consent is important in consultations between adults. It is only really consent if there is a genuine possibility to refuse that consent. Its role in childhood illness, where parents give consent on behalf of the child, is unknown. At what age or state of maturity should a child be able to refuse a consultation or specific parts of it? What effects will this have on children's health and illness behaviour? This is a rather grey area where it has been suggested that informed consent is a lawyers' myth (Hamilton, 1983), because even in adults it has been shown that their knowledge of body parts is so erroneous that they give uninformed consent. The critical element is the establishment of trust. I believe it essential that doctors establish trust directly with their child subjects, rather than solely with their parents – although the latter strategy will potentially facilitate the establishment of trust with the child. The doctor must carry out the interview, investigations and treatment in ways which deserve and retain that trust. This will include supporting someone through their initial anxieties, and enabling others such as the parents to do this.

When establishing trust we expect to develop cooperation. Yet in medicine the available metaphors predominantly suggest competition and warfare (see chapter 7). The two are combined when one encourages a child to work with the doctor to beat his illness, an attitude which is said to facilitate treatment, minimise conflicts with the doctor and lead to better results. Although I have suggested the advisability of laying more weight on metaphors of cooperation and balance, doctors are dependent on using the metaphors which make sense to the children, and this may often mean using those which the family members reveal in the interview. The metaphors need to be fitted to the children's cognitive levels (Whitt *et al.*, 1979).

The content of the interview can focus on the children's and parents' resources as well as the problems which they have. Only through finding out about the resources can these be enhanced and their relevance to the problem in hand made clear. This aspect of the interview gives it a role in preventive medicine, so that the child and his parents are better equipped to deal with the next episode. Additionally the family's sense of effectiveness in tackling difficulties is enhanced – a basic premise for increasing health behaviour. Through building on their current decision-making skills they are helped to refine their consultation behaviour.

Decision-making is dependent on noting differences in appearance and behaviour, both qualitative and quantitative. Parents know their children best and are in the best position to note deviations from the normal. The problems are greatest when finding out about insidious changes, and parents do not always have knowledge about the relevant points of view from which to evaluate the nature of their children's complaints. The interview in a consultation concerning a child has to respect and explore these factors. It was seen in chapter 8 that some people seem to have poor knowledge of their internal states, so that differences in these will be of little importance to them when deciding about their state of illness. It was suggested that this could have arisen through the ways in which changes in internal states were talked about, responded to and became salient. A helpful consultation should aim to facilitate the illness dialects which children have available so that their abilities to share their diverse internal states are fostered without their developing any simple somatic fixation.

It may appear that I am over-emphasising the psychological dimension because I am preoccupied with it as a child psychiatrist, but I would like to challenge that interpretation by looking at the frequency of psychological complaints in 'run of the mill' referrals to general practitioners (GPs) in England. Problems are rarely solely physical or psychological. Bailey, Graham & Boniface (1978) found that in about 25% of the referrals psychological factors were seen by the GPs as important. Garralda & Bailey (1986*a*, *b*, *c*) found a very similar incidence of psychiatric disorder (23%) in 7–12-year-old children taken to GPs in Manchester, England, but interestingly there was a variation between the GPs from 2% to 48%, independent of city area. Most disturbed children presented with somatic and not behavioural and emotional complaints. Interestingly, in the light of the previous discussion of social class differences, the GPs noted a relatively greater rate of surgery attendance of psychologically disturbed children from the more socially advantaged areas. When psychological problems in other family members were taken into consideration these factors played a part in about half of all the consultations concerning children (Bailey *et al.*, 1978), and these are the evaluations of GPs who are not particularly orientated towards psychology. A specific factor noted by Garralda & Bailey (1986*a*) was the increase in family arguments prior to the referral of the child with a somatic complaint.

The observations of Howie & Bigg from Aberdeen (1980) show some of the complicated interrelations between psychological states in the mother and physical complaints in the child – in their study the incidence of infections requiring antibiotic treatment. Amongst the mothers who had been taking antidepressants over a long period there was a significantly increased chance that their children would require antibiotics during the periods when they themselves were not taking the antidepressants. The associations between maternal medication and children's somatic complaints being presented in a consultation are more wide-ranging. Garralda & Bailey (1986c) reported that 43% of the mothers of children taken to GPs with somatic problems and where psychological problems were seen as contributing to the child's state, were taking a variety of medications, whereas only 16% of the mothers of children without psychological difficulties were taking medication. Interviews must be wide-ranging enough to encompass such issues (see for example the 'cultural hermeneutic model' of Good & Good, 1981).

A consultant tends to move on to examinations and investigations in order to clarify distinctions between signs and symptoms, and to plan treatment. Rather than discuss the necessity of those investigations, I want to point out that what is decisive for the children is how they interpret these investigations. Even the laying on of the stethoscope can have mystical significance as part of a treatment ritual ('to take the germs out' one 3-year-old said) or be seen as checking whether one has a heart (Bibace & Walsh, 1980). All too often explanatory words fail to accompany the examination, so that fantasy has to take over. Whilst palpating the body there is an excellent opportunity to explain to the child about his body so that the touch and pummelling makes sense to him. Without that sense, flights of fantasy create highly durable pictures which can hinder subsequent efforts at explanation. Our investigations become a pantomime created for the child, which he then uses to deduce our premises. In that connection repeat physical examinations may be actively harmful as they perpetuate uncertainty and magnify the physical aspects out of proportion (Apley, 1975 p. 103; van Eijk *et al.*, 1983).

Investigations are sometimes carried out on the principle that if one excludes physical illness then there is either no problem or a psychological one. It is better to come to a positive diagnosis of health or psychological difficulties. It is important to be able to describe a particular child's language for sharing his discomforts, and through a knowledge of the child's world and signs of illness avoid using investigations liberally. They are not without effect on the child's developing illness behaviour.

Equally important decisions concerning the investigations for learning that language and distinguishing pragmatic elements in the presentation involve choosing whom to meet for the consultation interview. Should the child be seen just with the mother, with all the adults living at home, or with his sibling? Should a meeting be set up with staff from school? The choices must depend on available knowledge of the child, his family and his school, as well as the pattern of the illness complaint which has been revealed. Is the presentation of the child hypochondriacal behaviour on the part of the parent who brings him (Pilowsky *et al.* 1982)? Is the mother depressed? Should the family stresses be investigated and incorporated in the treatment plan? These factors all fit in with children's grasp of the world of illness and they will not be surprised if they are introduced with understanding of the child's world of illness. Howie & Bigg (1980) concluded that 'in the long run more time might be saved by treating the cause of the consultation rather than the complaint offered'. Shapiro (1983) reported the usual tendency as being over-treatment of the child and undertreatment of the family. She went on to say that the 'mother's reaction to the illness is the most important aetiological factor in any subsequent behavioural disturbance in the child'.

What is more threatening is when the professional tries to elucidate problems concerning 'manipulation' of others through illness, as this introduces issues of approved behaviour and overt moral judgements, although these feelings are inherent in the concepts of illness as a liberator and as a destroyer. Duff & Hollingshead (1968) estimated that illness was used as a manipulator of the family in 33% of their cases, whereas in 29% of the families it was used to manipulate the patient. The predominant 'manipulators' in each case were the women. As was seen in chapter 8 concerning pretence, the critical factor in the analysis involves the attribution of the intention to manipulate, which is often negatively connotated. Whether the attributed intention and the perpetrators' meaning were the same remains unclear.

It is 'magic' if the consultant knows the problem without it being shared. If the child has not been able to share the problem in his own language so that it can become effective in a consultation, we do the child a lasting disservice.

### Explanations

*'Man can live the most amazing things if they make sense to him. But the difficulty is to create that sense.' C.G. Jung (Storr, 1983 p. 90)*

Although I have, for the purpose of analysis, separated interviewing and explanation, I hope it has become clear that they cannot be distinct. The questions asked are already setting the context for the explanations which will unify the otherwise diverse strands, and which will use the child's and family's languages as far as possible. The dialogue must make some sense to them in order for the interview to proceed. Thus explanatory statements will have sewn together the various elements, as a kind of punctuation throughout the interview. It is the more global explanations, the ones which necessarily incorporate as many as possible of the child's and family's premises, which will mean either that the child assimilates the explanation, or perhaps has to attempt over time to accommodate it through some basic modification of his premises. With this groundwork the recommendations for management become self-evident. Here I move in the direction of prescriptions for practice on the basis of my observations and a model of development of communication.

We have seen that theories of cause are central in children's and adults' constructions of illness models. Yet there are several different theories of cause which emphasise respectively the environmental factors, infectious agents and states of the individual, both genetic and immunological, to differing degrees. The models held by the social class IV and V mothers in Blaxter's (1983) sample were very complex and involved all these factors. Causal agents, for example, require precipitating factors and initial susceptibility before they could take effect. It was this complexity which made it difficult for the women to present all the factors they thought appropriate in an interview.

I have presented here the ways in which children of all ages also have a familiarity with several complex models of causality. Unless the diagnosis makes sense in terms of the patient's models it will not be accepted and they will tend to consult again and again until they know the cause (Blaxter, 1983). The favoured doctor in Koos's (1954 p. 58) community study in the United States showed a 'willingness to fit the diagnosis and treatement to the expectations of his patients'. There is an important distinction here between a diagnosis and a formulation. The latter can respond more adequately to this wish for complexity from the patient, and approaches Koos's use of 'diagnosis'. Recommendations for action follow naturally from a formulation but not from a diagnosis.

The theories of causality to be taken account of in the explanation can enable the child and family to deduce why the illness or complaint came when it did, and how it came. Yet some things can usefully be understated. The family members know what stresses they have been under, what precautionary habits they have bypassed, whom they have been in contact with and so on (all obviously from the points of view which they regard as relevant). This very detailed knowledge about the connections between events and symptoms is the family's own and they resent it if doctors attempt to impose their assumptions about these factors without being fully aware of their circumstances (Blaxter, 1983). By starting with the patients' points of view one can extend their vocabulary and facilitate their taking responsibility for their condition in alternative ways; only occasionally should it be necessary to challenge directly the patient's points of view with extended explanations in order to further accommodation rather than assimilation. People tend to eliminate those premises which are no longer required by themselves, but this takes time. By explaining in terms of how the illness affects the future, rather than being bound to how things were in past, one facilitates development, and alternative strategies for accounting for one's future state.

An adult is accountable for his own state but children only gradually achieve this personal responsibility. The nurturing of personal responsibility through the web of snares one is expected to avoid in order to remain healthy is a complicated business. It is only too easy to end up feeling either overawed by the task or not bothering about it because it makes no difference.

Children do not start with simple models of linear causality, where one thing leads to another. It would seem that doctors' explanations should take note of the multifactorial construction of their world of illness, where there is a balance between the differing elements. If the argument which appears logical to the consultant does not appear to be persuasive, the chances are that the patient has alternative premises to his logic. Until these are discovered an extended 'logical approach' will not succeed. A 'well-informed' child is not necessarily coping well. The giving of more information does not necessarily lead to greater cooperation; the timing and the way the information is given are all-important (Brewster, 1982; Kalnins & Love, 1982). Cooperation is more dependent on the social network.

One problem which arises in the giving of information is in the use of quantifiers such as 'highly probable', 'often' and 'seldom'. These mean different things to different people depending on their perspective. Doctors believe that it is more helpful to use common words and expressions rather than percentages, whereas the lay populations investigated prefer percentages (Brun & Teigen, 1986). Children's preferences have not been recorded.

In a consultation with a child a parent is usually present. The doctor can then present the explanation in various ways. On the thesis presented here about illness languages, I would sugggest that a helpful way of making certain that the child understands is first to explain to one of the adults and then encourage the adult to explain to the child in front of the consultant. In this way the child hears from the person who will be with him subsequently, using illness terms he is familiar with, but integrated with information from the consultant. At the same time the consultant can facilitate the parent's task as well as checking that the key information is conveyed. By addressing the communication between parent and child he carries out a health promotion role, at the same time as making certain that the explanation 'fits' (see also Whitt *et al.*, 1979).

The consultant's facilitation of the parents is through helping them with the translation between children's understandings and those of adults – much as the consultant has had to translate between the lay and professional languages. A consultant must be multilingual: he helps the parents find the metaphors which seem to fit their child's world and also make sense to them. In this way he may have to include metaphors from the school setting with which the parents are not familiar. As noted earlier, children tend not to have the same views on illness as their parents, but they do have the same views as those found in their local community. Metaphors are understood more literally by younger children and parents may need help to appreciate what this means in practice. However as the children's constructs tend to be looser than those of adults they can also move on from this stage of literal understanding without much difficulty.

This coordination of viewpoints is of the same type as that found to be of importance in predicting which families would engage best in a treatment programme in psychiatry. It was found that families which had a 'tendency to integrate individual members' ideas into a common solution and to synchronise their efforts to obtain information and test hypotheses' alone predicted engagement, as well as a higher level of ability to judge the motives of others (Costell *et al.*, 1981).

Some parents need help in appreciating the value of their myths, as many believe that all explanations must be couched in scientific language. It is here that the general factors about the development of children's communication presented in chapter 2 are useful. I believe that courses in the development of communication should be part of the training for all professionals working with children.

On occasion other children can do an excellent job of explaining to their peers, especially as their language is often similar to that of the patient and they can thus more easily establish a dialogue. Kendrick *et al.*, (1986) described how 9-year-old children on an oncology ward could provide very helpful explanations about treatment and investigations for the newcomers, and support them through their first courses of treatment. Interestingly, these children were not seeking to find out why the illness had happened to them (although the question was constantly being asked by the parents) and did not seem to attribute blame to anything or anybody. This contrasts with some of the earlier observations reported above, but is coherent with the thesis I have presented that such responses depend on the moral order of the setting and the forms of dialogue established. I am encouraged that the latest research seems to report a more helpful emotional climate, and the hope must be that changes in hospitals for children have led to these developments.

An important observation of Kendrick *et al.* (1986) was that after their initial talk with the child and parents concerning the diagnosis, the children entered a particularly receptive state for taking in further information. They described the children making 'very rapid developmental advances' in some areas, such as a surprisingly mature grasp of difficult cause and effect concepts, although there was regression in other areas, such as social functioning. Demystification of the illness plays an important role here.

The explanation needs to address the functional effects of the illness as well as provide factual information building on the children's constructs. The impact of illness on the family must be woven carefully into the treatment in a way that makes sense for the family. It is this coupling between the child and his environment which ensures his viability.

If one encounters a model of illness similar to that of illness as either a destroyer or a liberator it is necessary to find out how that perception could have arisen. Paradoxically, it may be pressure from parents to avoid the set of premises associated with the particular model (tables 3.1 and 3.2) which leads the child to that set of values. The same can happen with professionals; many doctors have a belief in illness as a destroyer, and avoid being off work ill themselves at almost any cost. They can have a more critical view of illness as a liberator, which can lead to their relationship with a person who holds such a view becoming tinged with their covert criticism; a less helpful moral order will have been established, and the patient will need his illness in other spheres to obtain the support he has failed to obtain in the consultation. A balanced view of the possibilities is required, with a finely tuned understanding of the psychosocial dimension as well as the physical.

I have not discussed aids to explanation such as books, games, computers and videos, which, if used, must also fit with the family's style. The pacing of the explanation is important and this in some ways is easier to achieve when aids are not used. In a dialogue the consultant gets continuous feedback about how the explanation is being digested, which bits need elaborating and which bits necessitate more support for the patient. The continuous monitoring of the conversation is an aspect of the skill required for maintaining intersubjectivity, and provided the consultant reacts helpfully to what he observes, the child's trust in him will be strengthened.

### Recommendations and treatment

The preparatory stages in the consultation pave the way for relevant recommendations (from the by-now shared perspectives of child, parents and doctor). Treatment is initiated in a context of maximal care for the child, with maximal support for those who will provide that care.

When presenting the recommendations the consultant must work hard at maintaining that trust so carefully nurtured in the consultation so far. The respect shown for the child's own world of illness will facilitate this, so that recommendations are placed in context. In this regard doctors fail all too often to acknowledge the limits which family circumstances such as poverty can impose. If this aspect of the family's constraints is forgotten the advice can be impossible to follow and lead to the undermining of the parents' esteem. Some parents are also liable to blame themselves for the illness if the recommendations include strategies which they had not previously used. But it does not mean that a lack of application of that strategy up to now was the cause of the problem. These strategies are for the future;

they do not account for the past. Respect for the strategies which had been used sets the new suggestions in context, hopefully as a natural development.

The parents will remember best what is told to them first and what they consider most important. Moderately anxious patients recall more of what they are told than highly anxious patients and those who are not anxious (Ley & Spelman, 1967 p. 89). Through monitoring the patient's state whilst the recommendations are being discussed (and, when the patient is a child, those of the accompanying parent also) it is possible for the consultant to pitch the advice at the most helpful emotional level. Poor interview techniques can lead to instructions not being followed. From the literature on adults it is known that cooperation is greatest with open communication and that this leads to better therapeutic results (Twaddle, 1981). The danger with children is that compliance can be achieved at the cost of the child's sense of mastery; the aim is maximalising cooperation and minimising compliance. To this end the consultant's recommendations can be arrived at by making decisions *with* the child and his family rather than *for* them.

The recommendations at the end of the consultation should leave everyone able to cope. As mentioned above, extending the explanation will not necessarily lead to better coping. I have referred throughout to Shapiro's (1983) review 'Family reactions and coping strategies' which gives a very useful overview of this area. One additional factor arises because of the responses which the child and his family have obtained from those with whom they have discussed the problem prior to the consultation. These will have moulded their anxieties. This will on occasion lead the consultant to adapt the support given so that the anxieties conferred on the problem by the helpers are also addressed.

The distinction between assurance and reassurance is relevant here. Assurance should be given with appropriate support, but if this is not effective, doing it once more (reassurance) will not help unless the premises to the form of the assurance and the support given are further examined. It is very important for all those working with children to be familiar with all the different sorts of support which may be required and the sorts of premises which children have concerning the world of illness.

A difficulty shared by parents and doctor is how to know what support to give when this does not involve direct action such as giving medication. The information presented here about the child's world should enable responses which minimise the child's vulnerabilities and maximise the security of their attachments. Prior to the development of modern medicines the great advances in ways of caring had already brought about radical changes in the prognosis of many ailments. Care facilitates cure. The failure of modern medicine is that it cures disease without healing illness (Good & Good, 1981 p. 101).

Children and parents who have a sense of mastery of their situation should be the goal of the treatment strategy. This can be achieved by paying attention to how daily routines can be maintained, friendships retained and needs for privacy recognised. The timing of return to nursery or school is important in this connection. Self-efficacy and mastery (Bandura, 1977) are the keys to growing up through the illness experience. This is aided by adequate explanation and demystification, although this should not be equated with attempting to eliminate myths. Parental resources are built upon where possible, and parents are aided in their decision-making in case there should be a next time, so that other relevant points of view are woven into their strategies. It is not immediately necessary to go over to quantifying signs from these points of view as this process in itself also alters illness behaviour. Each consultation becomes an exercise in health promotion as well as prevention (see also Bruvik *et al.*, 1986).

Coping is a central concept here and it refers not just to coping with the illness but with life. 'Illness can offer escape from difficult situations and thus soften the edges of a harsh world. To remove this freedom from individuals without having any better alternatives to put in its place is a brutal act' (Strong, 1979 p. 221). This is the illness as a liberator concept. Respect for the origins of this need enables helpful recommendations to be discussed and placed in the context of the child's social world.

The recommendation that a medicine should be used is based on the expertise of the consultant, although the child and parents often have clear expectations about the place of medicines in the treatment plan. At the time of this research the child would interpret the prescription of pills as a sign of the greater seriousness of his complaint compared with a prescription for a syrup, unless there was an accompanying explanation. With their growing awareness of the dangers of all things sweet, they could develop the alternative view that syrups were dangerous and doctors did not know about health matters (in a way analogous to what had happened with the sugar lumps used for their polio immunisations)! The advice given may have to challenge the nursery school literature about the necessity of obtaining prescriptions for the majority of ailments. The use of medicines in children has been increasing and in the last twenty years the average use of medicines by children in Scandinavia has doubled. What this will mean for their future expectations about adequate treatment is unknown.

The advantages of the placebo response must not be forgotten. This very real possibility for effective treatment free from side effects has rarely been harnessed effectively, yet recent research suggests that this should be possible to a greater extent (Kaada, 1986). There are observable biochemical changes elicited by Pavlovian conditioned reflexes. The expectation of effective treatment of pain leads to biochemical changes commensurate with effective treatment. The doctor's stance when discussing his recommendations must not minimise these therapeutic possibilities; a consultant must use the powers of suggestion responsibly whilst maximising the child's mastery of a difficult situation. A patient's expectations about the medication, confidence in those prescribing it and emotional state determine both the psychological and physiological response, even to the point of reversing the pharmacological actions of the drug (Strelnick & Massad, 1986). Children can so easily learn 'pharmacological coping'. One effective treatment can establish the criteria for subsequent successful treatment. If the use of 'doctor' as a drug is effective (Balint, 1964), so also can be the use of 'parent' or 'friend'. Consultants have a choice about what type of effective treatment they will facilitate.

The consultation cannot always lead to an answer to the problem, and in this situation further requests for assistance are required. In order to enable the next consultation to proceed it is helpful if the patient's problems are referred in the context of a provisional formulation rather than the diagnosis, on the basis of our Western medical system which is predominantly personalistic. Alternatively joint discussion of the problem can take place between the consultants. When a liaison service was established between paediatrics and child psychiatry in Oregon, USA, the need for psychiatric assistance in diagnostic dilemmas became more apparent (Sack & Blocker, 1978–9). It is this same focus on help with problems of decision-making which I believe can usefully be more central in consultations with parents and children.

These recommendations are multifaceted. By initiating action along several dimensions at once there will be a greater chance for change than if recommendations are introduced sequentially.

## Responsibility

The forms of responsibility given to children have changed over the years and in different cultures (Ariès, 1960). The ages at which children are assumed to have the same responsibilities as adults for their health have also changed. In the consultation the consultant operates with assumptions about what form of responsibility should be taken by the child for his own condition. In some cultures the child of 15 can give valid consent as regards undergoing medical procedures, whereas in others he cannot. But this involves placing responsibility within a tight legal framework rather than respecting the various understandings and positions of children. These problems are emphasised in connection with the delegation of responsibility to mentally handicapped adolescents and adults. The society's construction of childhood will affect how responsibility for a consultation is construed, and thus the ethical framework which plays its part in establishing the moral order of the consultation. I would expect this to affect further the child's developing illness behaviour at varying ages.

The consultant has responsibility for establishing the most helpful setting and for providing treatment and advice where asked for and required. The content and form to the subsequent consultation is then up to the participants. But the situation is different for children as they are seen as having diminished responsibilities. Recognising this extra responsibility placed on the consultant, Apley (1980) considered that if a child became distressed in a consultation the doctor should always regard it as his fault. Through the consultant's stance and the degree of child-centredness of the setting something of the expectations about the form of responsibility to be taken by the child for differing elements of the consultation are conveyed.

In a consultation with adults doctors aim to show respect for the patient's autonomy and ultimate responsibility for decision-making. Autonomy and reflexivity (the capacity to bring lower-order motivations under motivations and principles of a higher order) are the two basic moral principles necessary for grounding people's psychosociological capabilities (Harré, 1979 p. 387). But how do children learn to take responsibility and begin to delegate it and what can lead them to avoid taking it? What happens to responsibility when people are helped with their decision-making? Who is then responsible for what, and what effect will this have on illness behaviour? What kind and degree of choice can be handed over to the child? It is quite possible for conflicts to arise here between the consultant's view of what responsibility it is possible to transfer and the parents' views. Many people hold a theory of illness which they feel permits them to compete with the physician as the definer of appropriate illness behaviour (Berkanovic, 1972). Conflict arises when each parent feels he or she can define what is appropriate, as well as the child – and the doctor.

What happens to responsibility in the consultation is flavoured by what has happened before the consultation. Not all people come because they mean that it is really necessary for them to come with their child. They have not taken responsibility for the referral; instead this continues to lie with those who 'suggested' referral (see also Selvini-Palazzoli *et al.*, 1980*b*). In this situation it will not be possible to facilitate the family and child taking responsibility for what happens. Only through addressing the decision to take up the 'suggestion' can this be achieved. Within the lay network this can often mean looking at the role of women, as they play a central role in persuading mothers to take their children to the doctor (or the mother persuading the father) (Graham, 1984). When this female role is perceived by the patient as control rather than care – for example by the male adolescent whose mother tells him to arrange an appointment – it can be counter-productive for facilitating transfer of responsibility for the problem.

When screening is carried out routinely, the initiative for the consultation becomes anonymous. Depending on personality factors screening can be perceived either as control and checking – a kind of moral evaluation – or as a reassuring contact which is prearranged and so independent of any prevailing crises, and neutral to the possibility that those stresses have caused any problems. Its routine nature lessens anxieties which can be present. Screening procedures in Britain are carried out pre-school and by the school health service. Parents in Glasgow have a poor knowledge of the school health services and believe that they are not encouraged to attend. Parents described an uncritical appreciation of the service (Macaskill & MacDonald, 1982 p. 67–9). Preventive measures can be seen to be the responsibility of others rather than the family with the support of professionals. I do not know whether the situation is different in France and New Zealand where parents are encouraged to keep their children's developmental and health records.

In Lewis *et al.*'s (1977) investigation of children's self-initiated referrals within school, children who used the system placed greater emphasis on their own responsibilities for maintaining their health. But changes in their beliefs did not lead to them altering their utilisation of the service. The relationship between beliefs, illness behaviour and personal responsibility remains unclear. The researchers concluded that 'until we accept the fact that each future adult must be responsible for his own health and treat them accordingly, we shall always be looking to others for that which can only come from within'. My uses of the terms illness behaviour and sick role have made use of this distinction, but as we have seen, personal responsibility for one's illness behaviour can only artifically be divorced from social pressures as illness language is employed in interpersonal situations.

Campbell (1978) looked at the factors influencing children's willingness to define themselves as ill – what he termed 'initiating sick-role identification' – in a group of hospitalised children (aged 6–13) in Washington, USA. The children were more likely to claim they were ill if their mothers valued self-direction (cf. conformity to authority) and also valued attentiveness to others (cf. self-assertion). The boys said they would more often do this than the girls, who preferred to wait until the parents noticed their state. Those with less extensive prior illness experience also took more initiative, but it is inadvisable to generalise from this sample of hospitalised children.

I will now consider responsibilities in the later stages of the consultation. If the recommendations to the patient and his parents are based on the diagnosis given to them, rather than on a formulation, the result can be that the family is overwhelmed by a sense of helplessness because of what that diagnosis means for them. It can minimise their sense of being able to make connections between their daily world and the state of illness, with all that implies for care and treatment – connections which need to be made in order to enable them to feel that they can take responsibility for parts of the treatment (Carey & Sibinga, 1972). When mothers participated in the care of their children it facilitated resolution of their frequently occurring feelings of guilt that they had been in some way responsible. They had a reduced tendency to cope by denying (Shapiro, 1983), and gained in confidence and satisfaction (Shrand, 1965).

The consultation is to help people manage their areas of responsibility successfully. This is facilitated if in the consultation not all authority is transferred to the consultant. The child is the child of the parents and not of the medical staff, even when the child is in hospital without the parents present.

Does treatment occur only within 'treatment sessions', or between appointments depending on what the child and family do? The former strategy could be expected to minimise the child and family's sense of personal effectiveness in bringing about improvement. One aspect of the 'illness as an occupation' construct was that people were expected to play an active part in getting well again. Personal effectiveness is fostered provided that the responsibilities are made manageable. This will mean a formulation including the resources available to be built on, which occurs if there is sufficient attention to the psychosocial aspects of the formulation (for example Rolland, 1984). As consultations are often initiated when the support provided by the social network ceases to cope, it is necessary for the functioning of the support network to be addressed in each consultation.

Where required the social support network must be offered a useful role through the way in which the problem is formulated. If this dimension is not looked at it will be necessary for the responsibility for the problem to be passed up the hierarchy of expertise as lay people feel disqualified from helping.

By supporting the coping strategies of the parents they are able to manage their responsibilities. The characteristics of families which are able to cope and make good adjustments to family crises such as illness have been reported in Shapiro (1983). These families have a special sort of functioning characterised by clear separation of the generations, flexibility of family members to adjust or shift roles when necessary, a tolerance for individuality which permits the children room to change as they grow older and mature, free-flowing and easy communication amongst all members, and the ability to support each member's self-esteem. Common coping strategies of parents include seeking information, but parents' formal knowledge does not correlate with a score of their coping, at least when their children have asthma and allergy (Vassend, 1984). Other coping strategies noted in parents of children with cancer involve 'searching for a meaning of the disease (which can lead to a religious quest), increased motor activity, communication, avoiding visits to the patient, seeking support and comfort, and the use of defence mechanisms including isolation of affect, rationalizing and denial' (Van Dongen-Melman & Sanders-Woudstra, 1986). Regrettably in their crisis parents often forget to give adequate information to the siblings of patients, who must develop ways of coping on their own.

A growing area of discussion in Britain involves who should keep medical notes and who should have access to the notes if they are kept by professionals within the National Health Service (see for example two contrasting editorials in the *British Medical Journal* of 1 March 1986). Symbolically the person who keeps the notes is the one who is responsible for reminding others of the relevant medical history. In some countries, Brazil for example, patients have been encouraged to keep their own records in a folder which they take to any medical centre they attend. I am not aware of how parents transfer the responsibility for those notes to their children and what impact the differing strategies have on their children. A comprehensive project is needed in order to identify any changes in people's responsibility for their condition dependent on differing forms of access to, and responsibility for, their medical records. It would be important to control for the ways in which parents transferred the responsibility for those notes to their children. In Norway, where patients have a right to know the content of their medical records, it remains unclear how this right is handled in relation to adolescents and what role it plays in facilitating the patient's growing responsibility for his own treatment.

An associated issue is responsibility for keeping charge of the child's medication. How is this responsibility transferred? What sense of personal responsibility is fostered in children (of differing ages) if those with chronic conditions have their medication controlled by the hospital staff during admissions, in spite of managing their own medication when at school? Which ways of discussing management of medication lead to what sorts of responses in children of differing personalities? Who 'owns' the illness and its treatment? Regrettably the questions are endless. It would seem natural that there could helpfully be room for discussion of such issues with the majority of children, perhaps down to those of 5 years, on condition that people have learnt adequate skills for such communication with young children. Shared written instructions based on the outcome to such discussion can have their place in helping the child take an active role in curing his own illness and participating in his own care. His sense of helplessness is minimised, and he is no mere receptacle for a passing pill.

A different type of responsibility must be discussed in connection with the medical role in helping parents refine their decision-making skills. What sort of responsibility has the doctor for the way in which his advice to the third party, the parents, is used? A litigation-conscious society could well develop a requirement for such advice to be written down, and so make accountability clearer. But this would miss the point that the decision-making strategies which are applicable will vary over time and in different contexts. Flexibility and sensitivity must be fostered so that people are not rule-bound. Trust is the cornerstone of the treatment alliance.

The issues involve the delegation of responsibility. The same dilemmas are faced by parents of adolescents when they try to facilitate their children's abilities to decide on their own conditions. The moral considerations presented in chapter 8 make themselves felt again in this process, where there tends to be a special awareness of the possibilities of illness as a liberator from the increasing responsibilities that an adolescent must otherwise be undertaking.

Consultations also occur within the medical hierarchy of expertise. What effect does delegation of out-patient follow-up by the specialist to the GP and on down the line to the patient have, compared with repeat out-patient follow-ups without delegation? In principle, delegation as soon as the task becomes manageable by the next down the line – rather than when treatment is no longer required – seems desirable.

Finally yet more questions must be asked about where the responsibility lies for facilitating health promotion and illness prevention. Is it with those responsible for the child daily (direct prevention), or with those responsible for the local services, or those responsible for the national budget (indirect prevention)? The Royal College of General Practitioners (1981) observed that 'the promotion of health is the part of preventive work furthest from most doctors' habits of thought and action. It entails helping people to learn and to accept responsibility for their own well-being'. Doctors have an important role beside that of investigating illness, and that is confirming health. Treatment involves building health upon the resources available rather than concentrating uniquely on the problems. 'Illness as an occupation' could arise on those premises. Resilience in children does not lie in an avoidance of stress, but rather in encountering stress at a time and in a way that allows self-confidence and social competence to increase through mastery and appropriate responsibility (Rutter, 1985).

## The relationship between the physical and the psychological

I have postulated that there is an interaction between the way in which a child is handled, the language he develops and his sense of personal effectiveness. Young children appear to ask questions in two different ways depending on whether they are trying to find out facts about their world (the mathetic) or whether they are exploring the functional facets of their interactions with others (the pragmatic). For adults these aspects are intertwined into the ideational and interpersonal aspects of their communication. Throughout the consultation children are preoccupied with the same distinctions, and the forms of questioning to which they are exposed will confirm or deny their hypotheses about covert purposes to the consultation. Their 'techniques' for reaching their conclusions will depend on what has been helpful and appropriate in their other microsystems. A consultation must allow for such processes as well as the consultant's need to explore types of 'pretence' when investigating the veracity of a symptom.

Although in theory these differing aspects can be distinguished, in practice they are intimately bound together in a complementary way (the Piagetian viewpoint is the same: see Piaget & Inhelder, 1966 p. 21). In a consultation there will of necessity be a stream of misinterpretations as the interactants grapple with trying to understand what is going on. How these misinterpretations are handled will add to the construction of the total situation. As tensions rise and fall so also will symptoms which are linked to functioning of the autonomic nervous system, the states of arousal which can have diverse expression depending on their recognition and the languages developed to share them (Schacter & Singer, 1962).

My thesis is that the child learns an illness vocabulary and grammar dependent on how he has been responded to when suffering various types of discomfort. There is an interpersonal element here, the way in which the child has been responded to, as well as the child's state of discomfort, the mathetic. The consultation aims to address the child's state on the understanding that physical treatment must primarily be focussed on the child. But the consultation must constantly interpret the symptoms presented in order to deduce the signs which point to the child's state. As noted, the symptoms represent the child's and family's language of discomfort. The consultation must therefore include the evolution of the family's language so that accurate interpretations can be made.

At the same time the process of the consultation itself is just another factor in that continual evolution of the child's language of discomfort. A communication model suggests that how things are talked about alters children's states and the nature of their discomforts. As Brewster (1982) pointed out, a change in family interactional patterns, rather than continual re-education, was probably of greatest help to children who were doing poorly. Depending on the conversational skills of the consultant, this will predispose to the application of alternative vocabularies for describing discomforts. As was shown in chapter 8 moral codes are also transmitted in this process.

With a careful recognition of this dual process a consultation is maximally helpful. The problem for consultants in the medical professions is that the dual process has often been taught as if it were two separate processes. Diseases are learnt about as though they corresponded to the ideational elements, whereas it is illness which patients present. It is in illness that the effects of discomforts are reflected in the effects on people's relationships – the interpersonal. Psychiatry has traditionally been the discipline which has looked at how people talk about their states, and has been involved in teaching communication skills to those working in other branches of medicine. Just as the ideational and the interpersonal cannot be divorced from one another, so it is also with psychiatry and internal medicine. But what is the nature of that relationship? One can describe it as complementary, but that does not express the way in which the two elements coevolve. I would like to suggest that psychiatry is in a metaposition (see below) to that of internal medicine in relation to the patient.

I have not concentrated on sickness, which is society's concept in the terminology adopted here. The language of sickness is at yet another metalevel to that of the languages of illness and disease.

To return to the model of development, it was seen that as the child developed a sense of self he also developed an ability to reflect on the interactions in which he was participating. He developed the ability to function in two modes: that of primary intersubjectivity and also that of a metaposition in relation to the interactions in which he was engaged, from which he could evaluate and reflect on his part in those interactions. This is diagrammatically represented in fig. 9.1, where S represents the subject and O the object.

Consultants all need to develop techniques (built up through supervision and 'consultation') which enable them to do the same in a consultation, so that they begin by attaining that necessary primary engagement (O–S) but then also positions O' and S'. It is from these positions that interpretations about diseases are made from the illness discussion which has been the focus of the primary engagement. From the figure it becomes clearer that if a consultation begins with people trying to relate as O'–S or O–S', i.e. before primary engagement is established, then the interactions in the consultation will be hard to interpret. The flavour of the consultation will be of observation and control rather than cooperation. To reformulate Apley's (1980) maxim (see p. 212), just as a consultant is aware that he is evaluating the interaction and the patient (from position O') so also the patient has available position S' from which he can evaluate the consultant. If people try to start with O'–S' they will be in the position of wrestlers before the competition starts, circling round each other but not quite certain how to get started. Positions O' and S' are metapositions to O and S,

Fig. 9.1. Participation and observation. See text for explanation.

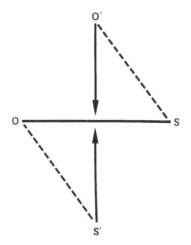

and vice versa. A brief return to the research method shows how these processes are reflected there. In the beginning was the interview, with respect for the primary place of intersubjectivity (O–S); after that came the analysis (from O').

I believe that an understanding of communication enables psychiatrists to play an important role in medicine through which the relation between the illness models which patients bring with them and the disease processes to which professionals direct their treatment can be elaborated. Others have said that the failure of modern medicine is that it can cure disease without curing illness. A cooperative venture is required so that psychiatry and medicine evolve in harness, and one avoids the alternative failure, also noted, that psychiatrists attempt to cure illness without addressing disease processes. By looking at the nature of decision-making and the effects of the different strategies available, the interpretative steps which make the links between symptoms offered and underlying body states are refined. My hope is that through an understanding of the development of communication and the child's world of illness that the foundation can be laid for more cooperation between psychiatry and psychology and other branches of medicine, rather than the climate of mutual suspicion and competition which exists in some places today. Psychiatry, psychology and medicine are so intertwined that the social constructions of the divisions of the territory must be expected to change with the years and public opinion; it is essential that these swings in opinion are not to the detriment of the care provided.

# 10

# Health education and health promotion

*'Carrots are good for your eyes – you never see rabbits with glasses.'*
*(Playground joke)*

The research presented has not involved efforts to change the views of the children or their behaviour. To use Bronfenbrenner's (1979, p. 41) terminology there have been no 'transforming experiments'. Such experiments would have highlighted the resistances to change and the stabilising homeostatic factors in the children's world. Nevertheless I feel that the applications of an understanding of the child's world of illness for health education and promotion must be explored. The necessary reservation is that the suggestions here need further evaluation – but they can form the bases for future research. I am not aiming to cover health education for adults, although the adult-orientated strategies in society will also influence the children.

Illness beliefs and behaviours are the natural target of health education rather than disease and sickness models, yet it has often been the latter that have attracted attention. It is through our understanding of illness that the information is meaningful to us; 'diseases' are less salient if they have not made a difference to our lives through being linked to the subjective elements inherent in illness concepts. Through discussing the causes of diseases some links can be made to illness models. Unless health education is presented in a relevant way and people have the competences to use it, it will not make a difference to people's ways of life.

There are, therefore, two aspects to health education. The first must be the creation of a structure in society, schools and families which facilitates child development, so that children's competences are maximised and they develop a constructive sense of their own efficacy. Healthy ways of showing and getting respect are developed; responsibility for their own condition and the condition of others evolves. Responsibility is not something forced onto another as in the classic paradox 'Be responsible' – a sort of parental shorthand for 'Do as I say'. Only on this basis can the other elements in health education and promotion, the factual information, be useful.

The Black Report of 1980 (Townsend & Davidson, 1982) identified clear links between poverty, social class effects and ill health. It spent less time exploring the marked differences in the health of the sexes, although it identified these. Health education needs to have clear goals so that the information and its presentation is as focused as possible. Males from social class V could be a priority target, on the basis of current morbidity statistics. The report presented clear recommendations about how some of the inequalities in health in Britain could be reduced, especially through looking at what restructuring could be done with legislation and alternative funding patterns.

The most notable thing which happened in response to the report was that the British Government effectively shelved it. It appears to be a case of giving information relevant for health which made no difference to the politicians with their own set of priorities and their own constraints. We must not be surprised when the same response is obtained among families and children who are given information but do not use it. They also have their own sets of priorities, and many important things constrain them which are certain to remain unknown. Several of the recommendations in the Black Report will be referred to in this chapter. One of the premises for the report was that 'early childhood is the period of life at which intervention could most hopefully weaken the continuing association bet-ween health and class' (see also the similar recommendations of the Euro-pean Health Committee, 1985 p. 97).

Before health education presenting information on special conditions is seen as relevant, it is essential that people perceive themselves as susceptible to the conditions being referred to. This could not have been the reason why the Black Report was shelved, because Britain has some of the highest rates of death, disease and handicap in the developed world. For example deaths from heart disease are not falling in Britain as they are in other countries, and the UK has the highest death rate from this cause in the world. Also the expectation of further life at the age of 45 in the UK is among the worst in the developed world (*British Medical Journal*, 5 July 1986, p. 56).

Illness models have as their basis an understanding of how illness affects children's senses of being themselves, and hence convey more relevance than disease models. The basic premises are that the children know where they stand through their interactions with others, and through changes in their relationships they experience many of the discomforts of illness. In relation to others they develop their language of discomfort. In this chapter I will not be looking at the ways in which the health education the children have received so far has affected their developing health and illness behaviour; instead I will present some of the implications as I see them for future developments in health education.

The differing elements in health education will mean that both those who administrate, including politicians at local and national levels, and those who have direct contact with children will need to investigate their policies to see in what ways they influence the development of health and illness behaviour in children. Health is not promoted solely through the work of health experts or teachers, but by all who have anything to do with people. I will first look at health education and promotion in schools and nursery schools as it is easier to define a role for education within the education system. Several of the approaches which I will mention can easily be translated to similar areas of relevance in the family and for the medical profession and I leave these to the reader's ingenuity.

## The education system

In 1986 the Department of Education and Science (England) produced the paper 'Health Education from 5 to 16' (HMI, 1986) which sets out a framework within which each school might develop its own health education programme. The discussion document is introduced with a statement which echoes the impression I have formed:

Education for health begins in the home where patterns of behaviour and attitudes influence health for good or ill throughout life and will be well established before the child is five. The tasks for the schools are to support and promote attitudes, practices and understanding conducive to good health'. (section 1; see also Graham, 1985)

The document stresses the need for the whole school environment to be health orientated, including the rules and regulations in force, staff behaviour and the content of the curriculum. Nevertheless, clashes between what the school teaches and what the school practises are commonly found; for example, teaching about nutrition and the content of school meals (Williams & Woesler de Panafieu, 1985 p. 64). Children will try to make sense of these apparent paradoxes and in so doing may distinguish between knowledge which is given in the classroom and that which is applicable in daily life.

The primary target of health education for 5–7-year-olds is seen as providing a secure environment in which self-confidence, self-knowledge, self-esteem, ability to share and cooperate and respect for others is built up (section 6). This is the primary aspect of health education which I pointed to in the introduction. The interdependence of man and other living things is included (section 19), but again the children may have problems making sense of that from their experiences in the school, where the interdependence of all that happens may not be clear. Respect for others may be lacking.

These themes are relevant for all levels of school provision. Children are always trying to integrate the different bits of information which they have received and it is this which poses problems for them (Tizard & Hughes, 1984 p. 99). It will be useful to begin with the children's personal experience and build on that (Davies *et al.*, 1982). The children find this easier if the above-mentioned aspects of health education and promotion are successful. As the varied approaches to school health education in Europe suggest, the aim should be to 'start where the people are and involve them' (Williams & Woesler de Panafieu, 1985 p. 83). There is no evidence that correct knowledge is related to the ultimate adoption of health behaviours among children (Kalnins & Love, 1982). Amongst other things the knowledge must be information which makes sense from their personal perspectives. Illness is what the children have experienced, whereas knowledge about diseases may have been what teaching concentrated on.

*Nursery school*

The descriptions of nursery school routines earlier should give plenty of scope for staff to create a nursery school environment which is as health-orientated as possible. Through inspecting the routines for their potential effect on the development of health and illness behaviour the staff would be addressing the primary structure of rules and regulations which moulds the developing child's secondary structure and which forms the basis for what he carries with him throughout life.

The nursery school environment is important for the development of certain behaviours which have a strong bearing on health. Recent research from the United States compared the long-term outcome of matched groups of deprived pre-school children who were randomly allocated to three different forms of pre-school provision (Schweinhart, Weikart & Larner, 1986). Remembering the gloomy morbidity and mortality statistics associated with social class V, it is reasonable to assume that these children would be very vulnerable. The two programmes which allowed the children to initiate activities produced adolescents 10 years later (aged 15 years) who were less delinquent and more committed to school and community. They also sought help more easily from others with their problems. I suggest that nursery school routines can facilitate varying degrees of cooperation with others and self-efficacy in the pupils, qualities which we have seen are necessary at so many crisis points in their lives, including illness. So far the effects of such routines on adolescents' subsequent illness careers is unknown. The important key is maximising of competence, and especially a *sense* of their own competence. Through that sense their performance is more likely to match their potential. These are potentially the resilient children of the future (Sylva, 1986).

An orientation to health education is necessary at so many different levels – not just amongst the nursery school staff who determine the ways in which the initiatives of the children can be nurtured, but also amongst education department officials who determine the budget allocation to the different areas and the priorities for further training. The above research provides additional support for recommendation 12 in the Black Report:

A statutory obligation should be placed on local authorities to ensure adequate day care in their area for children under 5, and that a minimum number of places (the number being raised after regular intervals) should be laid down centrally. Further steps should be taken to reorganize day nurseries and nursery schools so that both meet the need of children for education and care.   (Townsend & Davidson, 1982 p. 211)

Health education must be directed to the groups which can mould society's way of accounting for the values of nursery education. Nursery schools are not dumping grounds for the children of working mothers, or IQ boosters for the 'at risk'. The population needs to be made aware that it is not warranted to interpret uses of nursery schools in this way. The research has pointed throughout to the risks faced by children who have depressed parents, especially mothers. Provisions which can reduce depression in parents are beneficial for the health of their children. Otherwise these children are at risk of more illness, and a view of themselves as sickly. Their sense of having health resources would be expected to be lower than average. Providing nursery school places can amongst other things make it easier for mothers to work. Working mothers tend to have less depression (Brown, Bhrolchain & Harris, 1975). Provided that the nursery school routines foster the child's initiatives, there are then two factors which can work in harness to facilitate the development of self-concepts which are beneficial for health.

One of the especially vulnerable groups of mothers is composed of those who are of low income and non-working. They tend to have very small social networks (Hammer, 1983). If, however, their child can attend nursery it begins to increase their social network and introduce potential health benefits indirectly (see also Haggerty, 1980).

*The child's world of illness*

Presenting this information to politicians and the popular media will be unlikely to change their views, on the analogy that presenting information to children and parents does not necessarily lead to their altering their views or coping more adequately. Research is first needed which shows which premises they adopt to support their current views (but that is beyond my remit here). It is my impression that current lay views are not encouraging for nursery school provision and its long-term advantages. Although further research is required there is enough evidence already to support the case made in the Black Report (recommendation 12).

In the above I have emphasised the general values of particular sorts of nursery school. Within the schools other additional factors are important for health education and promotion. The general tenor of the observations which have been made suggest the strong need to build up understanding and respect between parents and staff, which can lead further to interpretations of the children's elementary languages of discomfort that are as accurate as possible. Using technical language, mesosystems must function facilitatively for children to integrate the education they receive. When they are acquainted with the local culture the staff will know what range of views the children bring, but knowing the views of the parents will not necessarily help them to know the premises held by the child of those parents (chapter 3).

Dental Health Weeks have had a big impact on the Edinburgh children. There is proven potential for specific initiatives directed at children of this age. At present dental education in Edinburgh is well advanced, to the detriment of other aspects of their health education. I hope that school health services will react to this as soon as possible and integrate their programme with that of the dentists. The sex of the personnel carrying out the programmes is very important for the children's views of what roles the different sexes have in health care and cure. The classical family divisions of expertise are not necessarily the best, and the effects of being exposed to alternative sex models should be monitored.

France is one of the few countries which has developed specific health educational materials for 3–5-year-olds. Perhaps rather than concentrating first on such ventures in other countries, it could be useful to review what is already in use. For example the literature to which the children are exposed could be assessed for its health-promoting potential, especially the health and illness habits covered. The Health Education Council could then allocate a 'seal of approval', visible on the spine of the book, in order to help hard-pressed staff when they make their purchases.

## *School*

Health education in schools must begin at the point the children have reached in their understanding of illness. Their view of illness is based on the effect of what has been labelled illness has on their relationships. This suggests that education should begin with an understanding of relationships, or at least that teaching should make sense through linking the content of the teaching to the effects which ensue for the children's relationships. For this an understanding of the child's world of illness is required. It will help if teaching is related to the status of particular conditions in the local community. In principle this is the reverse order to that which has been suggested (HMI 1986, section 30). Changing the order round has several advantages. It will place information on the common topics of health education in schools, hygiene, alcohol, sex and smoking, in the context of the children's personal relationships and their ways of coping and making decisions about their own health. Information is placed in a social context.

It is not my aim to discuss the distinction between teaching and education in detail, but it is necessary to underline that one of the aims in health education is to foster autonomy, that is 'the capacity to act independently of any given influence, whether external or internal' (Harré, 1979 p. 387). Autonomy tends to grow through education whereas teaching has the danger that it can reduce children's sense of autonomy as they are 'told' to a greater extent than they 'find out'.

Children attempt to find out the difference beteen pragmatic and mathetic information. They try to find out when they are, in their view, being manipulated rather than being provided with relevant factual information. If that information on health and illness matters is presented with an understanding of how it affects the children's relationships it will make it easier for them to distinguish between different types of information. Quite appropriately the Department of Education and Science (DES) recommends that children be taught the skills of 'how to distinguish between fact, promotion and polemic, and how to weigh and interpret information' (HMI, 1986 section 25). It is more difficult for teachers to develop the group leadership skills to facilitate discussion amongst the pupils (see section 29) so that the pupils can evaluate the information given to them in the school about health and illness matters; but it is the active applied use of such evaluation techniques which fixes the information in the children's vocabularies and would help them to make sense of health education in school. Through such discussion some of the problems with 'questioning' can be avoided and with skill the most vulnerable sections of the class can be helped.

The differing responses which children have to being questioned by teachers have already been mentioned. Children from different social backgrounds react differently to alternative teaching styles, although they have similar abilities to question and actively explore at home. It is important for children to be able to find out what sorts of question they are being asked. Are they 'felicitous'(see Leech, 1981, and chapter 9)? Through the sorts of question adults ask, children are introduced to different moral orders, which are more or less facilitative for their developing sense of personal effectiveness, as well as introducing them to alternative points of view. Differing styles of questioning and discussion will be required for children of differing backgrounds and differing developing personalities in order to facilitate their health-orientated development. As these styles will also differ day by day depending on the states of the children, no simple guidelines can be offered and it is not relevant simply to split classes into different groups. Instead a flexibility in the teachers and an understanding of relationships in the class will facilitate them establishing the most helpful moral order in the class.

When teachers are doing most of the questioning they have the initiative. Yet we have noted that to increase the child's sense of personal efficacy, education needs to build contingently on the initiatives of the pupils. Self-efficacy and personal competence prepare people for mastering the crises of their lives which will include illness. When encouraged at the same time as cooperation, self-efficacy is not at the expense of someone else's reduced self-efficacy. 'Cooperation' and learnt helpfulness are other important ingredients in the teaching programme, and prepare the pupils for constructive use of social networks – another basic resource for use in both reducing the likelihood of illness and aiding recovery when one is ill. A problem in schools is obtaining the most helpful balance between the needs for compliance by the pupils; and facilitating the pupils' senses of autonomy, abilities to cooperate and respect for others. The balance will have to adjust to the adolescents' individuation and thrust for autonomy.

Predictability and routine are necessary parts of daily life both at home and at school. Yet it is difficult to build on the pupils' initiatives in a teaching programme which is very structured. One interesting way that this has been done in Hungary is through using the routine event of the school medical to act as a trigger for more informal discussion. The district paediatrician and the GP join in taking group consultations on health education in connection with school medicals. The doctors, who have all had obligatory health education as part of their medical training, act as consultative members of the teaching staff and can come to take over the class at the request of the teacher (Williams & Woesler de Panafieu, 1985 p. 32).

Through the school ethos and milieu the effectiveness of particular interpersonal strategies and resources in the pupils are built up (Rutter *et al.*, 1979). These will include the strategies which are effective in convincing others of one's discomforts, such as in illness, although these remain to be investigated. Differing coping strategies will be more or less effective. At the same time a value system is transmitted through the introduction of relevant points of view about how these pupils can do things to prevent illness or promote health. Through the questions asked these views convey alternatives to those the children will have experienced before. Unless the questions are asked with an understanding of the limitations of personal strategies for maintaining health the points of view run the risk of exaggerating the pupils' sense of helplessness, rather than suggesting things which they can do to help themselves. For example, if a pupil is asked how much exercise he has taken, and he lives in one of the more deprived inner city areas in Britain, he may well be made aware of the lack of possibilities in his environment rather than what he could do. Poverty, religious beliefs and racial discrimination can all set different sorts of limits.

In this connection it is useful to be reminded of the complex models of causality held by children and their parents. These include environmental and personal factors, things which have been inherited, as well as the place of allergies and infective agents. By focusing on the importance of the interplay of these factors it is possible for people to feel responsible for parts of the problem but not the whole (see also Pill & Stott, 1982); the responsibility is made manageable. At the same time it is possible to differentiate between responsibility for the problem and responsibility for helping put it right. Complex models of causality enable each person to take a part in a complicated process where cooperation between people is important. The value of cooperation is again emphasised.

Much of current health education in schools in Britain is on topics which are associated with particular moral points of view: sex, smoking and alcohol. Teaching on hygiene orientates the pupils to the 'best' way to run their daily lives; it provides the rationales for their personal and household routines (HMI, 1986 sections 44–9 and 51–5). The risk is that the pupils will regard the school as the purveyor of the moral good, that they must comply with. This can be interpreted by some adolescents as losing their identity by adopting the values of others rather than building their own autonomy and ability to choose a healthy life style. The adolescent's need for respect from his peers may lead him to adopt what he knows is unhealthy in order to belong to the group. As breaking of hygiene taboos often has no immediate repercussions, other than perhaps cementing membership of an adolescent peer group by creating one's reputation; it is particularly easy to avoid following the rituals. It is not easy to give people the sense that they can make informed choices. The exploration of decision-making can be relevant here.

Child development – social, physical and psychological – could usefully be a central part of health education. The child's developing relationships are important factors in his development of psychosocial and biological maturity. A stage model of development can introduce unhelpful limitations to this part of the curriculum. The core concept is intersubjectivity. Concepts concerning health and illness fit in naturally as they are noted through their effects on relationships. The values of attachments show respect for the important peer attachments and group pressures, as well as presenting a helpful model for the parenting skills which may be required in the future. Cooperation is placed in a developmental context. Through looking at child development rather than their own development, possibilities are opened up for the children for doing things differently in the future. The information at one step removed from themselves may be more digestible. At the same time respect must be shown for the range of possibilities and the restraints of circumstance as otherwise helplessness will be fostered. Their own development is placed in a historical perspective and so respect shown for those factors which limited what it was possible for their parents to accomplish. The 'interdependence of man and other living things' as one curriculum element (HMI, 1986 section 19) fits in naturally here. If the interdependence between people and things at school is not clear because of the way the school is ordered, this part of health education is unlikely to make sense.

Teaching about child development will naturally include parenting effects. As part of looking at what parents do the children can usefully explore decision-making strategies concerning health in others, as well as through group discussion look at their own decision-making strategies. The decisions people make depend on the consequences for themselves and others. It is necessary to include at the same time teaching about coping strategies, as the ways of coping available to people also affect their decisions. Coping strategies in turn will be dependent on both personal and environmental factors. A range of cognitive, affective and behavioural coping strategies are available (Shapiro, 1983). The values of support networks and how they can be used to foster health and aid recovery will be a natural part of this teaching.

Some ways of coping, for example the use of cigarettes and alcohol, will be more dangerous for health than others. By placing the teaching on these subjects in the context of coping mechanisms, they can be approached in alternative ways. Rightly the DES (HMI, 1986 section 53) is concerned that teaching about drugs and solvents could lead to experimentation. Children are exposed to conflicting information in relation to drugs. There is a positive correlation between the use of psychotropic drugs and increasing age yet the focus of intervention is mainly on adolescents (Strelnick & Massad, 1986). With such models from society available to the children the information on drugs can well be interpreted pragmatically – 'an adult strategy to control adolescents'.

An increasing problem for some children is to integrate the information they get at school with what is happening at home. If they rely on the information about the health-damaging effects of smoking at school, yet return home to parents who are smoking, they can come to be anxious about their parents' condition. Although parents are known to have stopped smoking in response to pressure from their children this is not an approach to be advocated. Instead an understanding that some people develop certain habits in particular circumstances and that it is not easy to change habits, can make discussion of smoking at home easier and more constructive. Drug abuse is found more often in families with particular structures (Strelnick & Massad, 1986). Through including parenting and division of responsibility and authority in families as part of the curriculum, prevention of drug and solvent abuse is indirectly addressed.

When children evaluate the consequences for them of a particular condition, for example cancer, their beliefs about their own susceptibility, as well as the benefits for them of taking action, affect what action they take. Information on smoking will make no difference to those who believe either that they cannot take any useful action, that they are not susceptible to the effects of smoking, or that their children could not be susceptible to their smoking. It would be expected to find these characteristics in those sections of the community most at risk, those with least sense that their own actions can rescue them from difficulties. In a small sample of children in the United States Michielutte & Diseker (1982) found that children viewed themselves as more highly susceptible to cancer than heart disease, but believed there were fewer benefits to treating cancer. The few perceived benefits of treatment of cancer create a barrier to effective health education which begins with a disease model, e.g. teaching about cancer.

One of the tragedies of schooling today is that it is having to prepare many pupils for a time of unemployment. The connections between illness and unemployment suggest that health education in schools should include educating pupils in how to cope when they are unemployed. Much more research is needed here before it is clear which ways of coping are most beneficial for adolescents. Provisional coping strategies which maintain the pupils' self-efficacy and self-respect, as well as facilitating their social functioning so that they obtain the benefits of an appropriate social network, will be expected to offer the best health-promoting possibilities during their unemployment. Whilst they feel that there is nothing they can do to help themselves they will be most vulnerable.

Coping strategies are needed in a wide range of differing situations. Haggerty (1980) has pointed out their direct relevance to promoting children's health. Among the relevant strategies can be teaching the skills of relaxation, and some have suggested the skills of self-hypnosis. Teachers are not always interested or able to teach relaxation, or other relevant social skills. Yet Botvin, Eng & Williams (1980) used social modelling techniques to show pupils how they could cope with situations where they were offered cigarettes, or were being teased for being unadventurous. This led to one quarter the rate of smoking in the group given social modelling compared with a control group. Conversely boys are more likely to smoke if the male teachers smoke (Bewley, 1979). Psychologists attached to the school health service could have a useful function in assisting with this teaching.

If teachers feel unqualified to move into this field it may help to look at some of the skills they might need. Wood (1982) reports that people can, with training, change their styles of interaction with children at will, so I hope teachers will not feel helpless to try. I am venturing out of my own area if I discuss teaching skills in general, so instead will quote Bandura's (1977) summary of the key points in helping people develop self-efficacy:

> Generalized, lasting changes in self-efficacy and behavior can be best achieved by participant methods using powerful induction procedures initially to develop capabilities, then removing external aids to verify personal efficacy, then finally using self-directed mastery to strengthen and generalize expectations of personal efficacy.

Unfortunately participant methods tend not to feature prominently in the classroom. The size of the class introduces important limitations.

Generalised instruction is the least effective way of influencing knowledge, attitudes or behaviour compared with individual or small-group learning (Williams, 1984). Although people tend to avoid conflict situations it must be remembered that ideas develop in them. Through facilitating discussion of the different points of view in the group, at the same time as creating a climate in which it is easy to change one's point of view through supporting face saving manoeuvres, the pupils can learn that they have a lot to offer each other. They can build on their previous points of view, build on their intuitions and begin to be able to rely on them and the advantages of discussing their intuitions with peers. They discover that they knew more than they thought they did. Their own points of view are expanded upon. Advanced intuition and social competence are fostered. With the feedback available their ability for self-reflection grows alongside their autonomy.

Some special programmes have been devised which try to include the above principles. In California, Lewis's 'Action for Health' programme for schools is made up of four units which cover 'decision-making', 'self-reliance' 'body cues' and 'balanced living'. The philosophy behind the programme is that 'the children must be actively involved in decision making training that will prepare them for future responsibilities related to their own health care as adults' (Lewis & Lewis, 1974). A British programme for 9–13-year-olds is called 'Think Well' (Schools Council, 1977), and it includes similar elements: decision-making, health careers and self-concepts. These programmes come with a variety of teaching aids, reflecting a recognition of the critical importance of the way in which these topics are taught. In the future more refined video games and other aids can be expected to brighten up health education in schools. When people come to the limits of what they know and can manage with help, they need to know where to turn next, and an important additional topic to include is how to use the health service. This makes a natural bridge to the contribution of the school health service, which could have a useful role here.

### School health personnel

In spite of not having observed the functioning of the school health service there appear to be consequences of my observations which can facilitate its health educatory potential.

At the moment the service is organised as a 'check-up' type service, where medical staff are perceived as initiating the consultations. The children are vulnerable to perceiving it as part of the school authority's long arm of control rather than a support service. The children regard it as irrelevant, or as they put it 'it's a waste of time'. The current evidence

suggests that if children's initiatives are built upon, their sense of competence to handle illness and health matters can be increased. At the moment
it is the welfare assistant/school secretary who is in a position to capitalise
on an actual illness episode once the child has left the class, and not the
school health service.

The walk-in school clinic in California referred to ealier (Lewis *et al.*,
1977) provides an alternative model for capitalising on children's own
requests for a consultation. In Norway there is no equivalent of the welfare
assistant/school secretary. Children make their own decisions about their
states of health to a much greater degree than in Britian. They also have
possibilities for initiating their own referrals to a school nurse and to the
school dental service. In France and Ireland the parents can take the
initiative to request a medical examination of their child by the school
medical staff. There is a great need to compare the effects which such
alternative routines have on the social construction of the role of the school
health service, and the ways in which the children are enabled to take
responsibility for their own decisions and learn about health and illness.

There appears to be scope for a revitalisation of the British school medical
service, its integration with the other provisions in the school, as well as
a role in health education (for one possibility see p. 244 above). The Black
Report suggested linking school health care with general practice. The
important element is the connections of the service with both the worlds
of school and family health. It can on occasion be a helpful bridge between
them, and facilitate schools' and families' understanding of the languages
which children use to share their discomforts. In order to do so they need
an understanding of how the functioning of schools and families can affect
the illness languages available to the pupils, how the pupils keep face with
each other and how families make their health and illness decisions and
communicate these to the school. The model provided for microsystems
and mesosystems can help them put their role in context.

The current monitoring role of the school health service must not come
out of the blue, but be part of the offer to children to help them take
better care of themselves. Children's initiatives can be built upon through
open meetings with doctors and visits to health service resources. This
should be done when the children are well and before the additional
anxieties of illness play on their other uncertainties when they are first
referred to hospital. The problems become those of creating enough flexibility in the service so that the timing of particular initiatives can foster
the children's senses of competence. Each contact with a professional is
an opportunity to learn. Hopefully the children's views on illness as pre-

sented here will help people to find out what stage the children have reached so that learning builds on what the children already know. Doctors' pedagogic skills need to be improved so that styles of teaching are as creative and applicable as possible to maximise education.

Another possibility for the school health service was tried out in Finland (Puska, 1982). As part of the school medical check-ups a group of 13–15-year-old children had a biochemical work-up which included measurement of serum cholesterol. Their health habits and current health status were also monitored and then the whole picture was fed back to each child. In addition they received health education in school. Two years later those who got the full medical work-up and analysis of their health habits had half the increase in smoking noted amongst the controls, and the girls had a significantly lower serum cholesterol level.

The value of feedback is important in all learning. Yet it is not often afforded its special place in schools. The value of keeping his own health records can play a role in increasing the feedback which each pupil gets about his health, depending on the content of the health record. Biofeedback techniques may have a special role in increasing pupils' understanding of how their bodies function. In a learning situation pupils could use biofeedback to increase their own ability to alter at will various bodily functions which normally remain beyond their immediate awareness. It would be expected to help those who had little faith in their ability to control their own bodily functions – those who are hypothesised to have a predominantly external locus of control and who are most vulnerable to developing a somatic language of discomfort without any sense that they could do anything about it. Through biofeedback one could also make connections to relaxation techniques and other coping strategies. The place of psychologists in the service should be reviewed in connection with these possibilities.

An additional type of useful feedback is the prevalence of particular disorders in the local community, so that the pupils' field of relevance is extended from what they have encountered in their families. These local data are required before the introduction of national data, as local data are more salient.

The DES (HMI, 1986) does not suggest that doctors participate in health education in schools, laying most emphasis on the role of the health visitors. This may reflect the reality that doctors in Britain do not get taught pedagogy, and that they have difficulties giving priority to such work. If health education is to get the status it requires and deserves then high-status medical staff are going to have to get involved as they have done in other

European countries (Williams & Woesler de Panafieu, 1985), at least whilst the curriculum is under development and respect for the subject is rudimentary. Through outside experts coming in, the subject can more easily be seen as not being presented in order for the teachers to impose their standards on the children; the aim must be for the subject to be integrated into the school, with the skills for its presentation being held by all in the school – the problem being to establish it and respect its importance.

In this regard it is as well to remember the Minneapolis Children's Hospital's 'ecology programme' (Wallinga, 1982), which appeared to be successful through creating an environment where everyone shared basic knowledge about children and their ways of communicating and understanding about illness. It is my belief that similar initiatives should occur in schools under the joint supervision of the school medical service and psychology service. In this way children's illness language as it develops in the school will also evolve as helpfully as possible. Although the need for coordinators for school health education is acknowledged by the DES (HMI, 1986) they offer no concrete suggestions for their work. There were, though, already health education coordinators in two-thirds of secondary schools in England in 1983. It may be that health education officers will also fit into the evolving school health service (interestingly the title 'officer', in line with the warfare metaphors discussed earlier, has been chosen rather than consultant).

One possibility is that the current school health care system will change in line with the recommendation in the Black Report (recommendation 13: Townsend & Davidson, 1982 p. 211), although this now seems unlikely. There it was suggested that it be linked to general practice and that there would be 'intensified surveillance and follow-up both in areas of special need and for certain types of family'. The problems posed by the initiative lying with the service are not adequately addressed, but the need for special priorities in the work of the school health service in relation to the prevailing vulnerabilities in society means that some way must be found to help children avoid developing the patterns of illness of their parents.

There is a fine balance to be achieved between making children aware of what they can do for change without making the responsibilities to use those skills overwhelming. The balance between the different factors is important – the exogenous and the endogenous. Encouraging people to take responsibility does not mean that they will or can do it. The sex of the school health personnel who are in contact with the children is important for the models of expertise which they provide for the children. Males and females take responsibility for their health in different ways and have different patterns of consultation. There is not yet enough information to say how important differences in the sexes can best be used to promote health and health education. When choosing the staff who will make interventions in schools these factors need to be considered. Sexual politics cannot be avoided.

The possibilities for change are altering all the time. Towards the end of 1986 the British Government announced that the Health Education Council (England) would be replaced by a special health authority. It would seem beneficial for school health service revitalisation to be considered in the light of the possibilities created for an amalgamation into the new health authority. In Edinburgh the very active and successful dental health unit appeared not to have coordinated its work with that of the school health service. Under the aegis of a special health authority there is room for more coordination as well as monitoring of the effects of the differing initiatives which combine to affect the child's world of illness. The evidence from the success of the dental programme suggests that the school health personnel can be active with children as young as 3 years old. To do so they need to develop the skills of communicating with young children and to understand their world of illness. Their contacts with nursery schools can increase. I hope that the new health authority will explore these issues.

School health education may turn out to have some of the most profound effects of all learning achieved in school. It has the potential to alter a pupil's life span and the quality of his life. In addition it will alter the lives of the others in his family – spouse and children. It should at least be on a par with the three 'R's, and a case can be made for putting it first of all. The school health service has an important role which deserves to develop rapidly. With enterprising changes in their roles and relations to schools and families, school health personnel can come to stand in the centre of the health education and promotion services.

## The family

*'The best doctor for a child is an old woman'*
*(old folk saying.)*

The different ways which are used to evaluate the condition of children at home and at school do not disturb them. Nevertheless they are helped to make sense of the different approaches if there is good communication between home and school, with respect for the differing languages used and the limitations posed by the differing settings. Families and schools will need to know each other moderately well, with parents being as free to question the staff as the staff are to question the parents. The timings of parent/teacher meetings are important, otherwise working fathers and mothers can easily be discriminated against. It helps if their ranges of relevant points of view on health and illness matters are compatible. Some families will feel on more of an equal footing with teachers than others and so find it easier to establish a dialogue which approaches the ideal. In these circumstances it is easier to coordinate support for a child. The different relationships found between home and school will lead to differences in the forms of the children's mesosystems, and will indirectly lead to differences in the children's abilities to integrate the differing worlds of school and home and to the effectiveness of their illness behaviour.

I will not explore this aspect of the family's effect on health education and promotion further. Instead I will look at family functioning, which is relevant for the health of the children, and some ways it can be maximised. This will as much emphasise the role of others as of family members. Through pointing out recurring themes it will be possible for others to devise more concrete health-promoting responses. A natural point to begin is with the birth of the child.

Earlier I pointed out that the development of communication has its basis in the early interaction patterns eastablished from birth onwards. Children's subsequent competences can be affected by how their different states are responded to. The physical state of the child will affect how easy it is for parents to establish the early preverbal 'dialogue' with their child – what type of 'dance' they take up together. The states of the parents alter their availability for the child. Parents' expectations of the forms of distress which their child can experience will affect the languages of discomfort to which they introduce their child, through the points of view which they use for evaluating their child's condition. These will either be more or less health promoting. On the basis of this early experience some of the foundations for the child's subsequent health and illness behaviour will be built. Through school teaching on parenting and child development these issues will already have been raised, but there is still scope for an important role for both health professionals, such as midwives, and other parents, in further health promotion. Through their support for mothers and their contact with their children they re-emphasise the importance of those interactions. The coping techniques which can have been learnt at school include relaxation techniques which can used again by the midwives in preparation of the mothers for labour. At the same time mothers and fathers can be reminded of the benefits of relaxation as a way of coping which is applicable in other situations.

In a survey in Birmingham, England, it was found that only 1 in 5 GPs provided classes for parents. The majority were either unsure how to or felt that they lacked the skills for providing such a service (*Health Education News* no. 59, July/August 1986). It is a sad situation if everyone feels unskilled, both parents and professionals. Although other health workers, or other parents, could potentially provide the classes, I find it telling that such basic human skills as caring for children and facilitating these skills in others are not necessarily part of an average doctor's repertoire. In such circumstances it will be difficult for the doctor to support parents in their tasks with ill children and, I would hypothesise, make it easier for him to 'medicalise' children's problems. Doctors feel uncertain about how to take groups – the same problem referred to above for teachers (see Heap, 1985, for assistance).

The security of the attachments formed in early life are important for the child's later self-esteem and adaptive social functioning (Wolkind & Rutter, 1985), which are themselves important factors in relation to the child's subsequent health. They will be related to the types of interaction established in early life. At the same time the strategies developed in families to cope with a variety of situations can respect the child's attachment needs to varying degrees. In the preceding chapters it was seen that children could feel vulnerable when they went to sleep and when mothers were away. In illness closeness to the parents is seen by the child as an important part of the 'cure'.

I mentioned above that parents could lead the parent groups. What I was trying to suggest was a way in which parents could be reminded that they have the basic competences,and that not all the expertise which they will develop during the time of parenting is to be learnt from professional 'experts'. It is potentially more applicable for a doctor to have the skills to facilitate parents leading such groups, and to be available for consultation for them, than for the doctor to aim to lead the group himself. The skills of communication and knowledge of group function must be integrated with a GP's factual knowledge about health and illness states so that the local lay potential to support vulnerable people is maximised. Expertise is simultaneously created and released in the group.

A group contact enables mothers and fathers to receive confirmation that their actions are leading to desirable or anticipated consequences (see also Hammer, 1983, for similar social network effects). There is a protective effect of such contact on their children's health (Haggerty, 1980). Spencer (1984) also suggests the value of mothers' groups for providing the responsibility of confirming some areas of their performance, as well as of learning of other possibilities through shared experiences. To return to the functioning of one of the children's mesosystems, in their contact with school mothers can either get these necessary confirmations or be denied them.

Pregnant mothers have been described as being most responsive to personally transmitted information on the dangers of smoking, that is the information which they get from family and friends, rather than any pre-packaged health-orientated information (Graham, 1976). It is as though they rely on the experiences of known others to a greater extent than expert-prepared information. Such groups as I have suggested above could maximise the giving and taking of 'valid' information to which mothers appear to be receptive. Through confirming what they thought they knew it would maximise their sense of competence, as well as open up other relevant points of view through building on what they know.

This value of personal knowledge was evident in Blaxter & Paterson's (1982*a*,*b*) observations of Scottish mothers. They had found that the role of the mothers' mothers in their survey were most notable where preventive health was concerned. This should not be surprising as family rituals and routines are established for their protective effects, and it would be expected that these are transmitted to the children independently of the family's actual views on illness.

Without family routines it will be difficult for parents to notice differences in their children's states using the common strategies referred to in chapter 4. Yet our routines are often based on rationales which we find difficult to defend in the face of the persistent questioning of childhood. Often we do things because they were done with us when we were children and are part of our basic 'structure'. The ways in which families defend their routines are important for introducing children to the family's set of values. The routines in relation to the management of dirt are amongst those which establish particular moral orders in the home. My belief is that homes need such order, but that the ways in which the order is defended are also important. Routines also introduce predictability, which plays a role in reducing the effects of stress.

Breslow & Enstrom (1980) looked at the prognostic implications of health habits in a large cohort of adults in the United States. In relation to the routines described in the preceding chapters it is interesting to note that they included regular physical activity, 7–8 hours sleep each night, eating breakfast and not eating between meals. In addition they included no smoking, moderate or no use of alcohol and maintenance of appropriate body weight. After 9 years the mortality of those with all seven habits was 28% lower than for those with three or fewer.

But in contrast when Boyce *et al.* (1977) looked at respiratory infections in children they found that family routines could contribute to the severity of illness in the presence of high stress. A routine is a complicated concept which is hard to describe and monitor. It can be more or less fixed, and there can be varying rules for altering routines in the face of illness. Routines can be inflexible or not; they can take care of children's attachment needs or not. At present it is inappropriate to assert simply that routines in themselves are enough to promote health.

Our routines are often based on premises related to relics of our child-hood. These relics can have the status of myths. The family 'myths' about illness prevention are complex but coherent with views on the complex nature of causality of illness. When families are being formed the respective myths are moulded into a new whole in relation to how the parents bring up their children and establish their family's life style. The degree of integration will correspond to the ease with which the family routines make sense to the child, and in that way play their part in health promotion.

Group discussion themes are likely to include family routines and myths. If respect is shown for all kinds of myth it will make it easier for parents to participate as otherwise forms of contempt in the group can establish a climate which makes it difficult for the most vulnerable parents to obtain any benefit, or even bother to come back after a first try. Group classes on parenting run the risk of enabling only those already parenting at full throttle.

The suggestion is that those mothers with an internal locus of control seek out more health-related information than others. It may turn out to be those mothers who can use their own mothers for advice on preventive health measures. In childhood our sense of mastery of our environment, our loci of control and our sense of an ability to be helpful are being established. Some people start as parents with very poorly established senses that they can do anything to improve their lot or that of their child. Their attributions and their points of view reinforce their helplessness in the face of what is often to them a hostile environment. Shapiro (1983), in summarising the research in the field, was of the opinion that mothers with an active interventionist approach to health care, who attributed good health and low illness susceptibility to their children, were high users of preventive services and generated few illness/accident visits. By contrast mothers with a more passive attitude, who perceived their children to be in poor health and susceptible to illness generated fewer well-child and more illness visits. Throughout, parents need to be responding to their children so that the children's sense of coping and mastery are maximised, with a sense of the value of learnt helpfulness.

A person's predominant locus of control plays a role in the way in which significance is attributed to the signals received in different body states. Bandura (1977) pointed out another factor influencing the interpretation of internal cues; 'the same source of physiological arousal may be interpreted differently in ambiguous situations depending on the emotional reactions of others in the same setting'. The half-ill states when children are 'under the weather' are ambiguous. The reactions of the parents will influence the child's understanding of the changes in his body states. If the parents are prone to ascribe the changes to internal events rather than things happening in the child's environment this can result in reciprocally escalating distress and arousal. The situation becomes unmanageable and has no connection with the child's world. The words used to describe the children's states and their origins are of importance for the connections they make to things with which the child is familiar. Putting a name on something unknown may be the first step to helping the child master it. In consultations parental vocabularies are enlarged.

The media, both television and the printed word, may work to minimise parental expertise and introduce them to additional vocabularies of spuriously relevant events. The information is necessarily disease rather than illness orientated and although there is no direct dialogue with media their potential for influence through suggestion is large. Most television watching happens at home; the images provided and the methods of presentation have profound effects on children and the statements made tend to be uncritically received, especially amongst children from the lower social classes. The effects of television need to be closely monitored, but are likely to be hard to discern from the effects of the multiple influences on children's lives. It will be easy for media people to demand that there is a greater degree of certainty about the effects of their programmes before they are forced to alter their style, but if they asked 'Would it be helpful if . . . ?' there is already enough evidence to suggest that other approaches deserve a trial.

In addition to the information which children believe they are getting from television, it is necessary to note that television has an effect on other aspects of their developing personality which can be detrimental to the development of their health and illness behaviour (see also chapter 5). Cooperative social behaviour plays a protective role in ameliorating illness, and yet there are suggestions (Gadow & Sprafkin, 1986) that television watching, regardless of content, leads to higher levels of negativistic interpersonal interaction. Television watching becomes established as part of a life style through its place in both the home and school.

In the family various elements in the children's life style become established. Their life styles are either more or less healthy. Their skills and their awareness of them are built up, and used further in their health careers. The family interactions around illnesss plays an important role in health promotion and illness prevention. In adolescents varying degrees of individuation will occur; they will be more or less autonomous and able to evaluate realistically the information subsequently provided in the light of new developments, such as AIDS. The forms of discussion they have been exposed to and participated in will affect their understanding of the nuances of illness and the ways in which they negotiate with illness.

The politics of the family has not always addressed the effect it has on the developing health and illness behaviour of the children, or its effect on health promotion in the children. Indirect factors acting on the health of the child, such as unemployment of the parents – exosystem effects – are also important. The ways in which work-places and families negotiate their respective requirements for adults' time can usefully include the effect on the health of the children. I believe that employers need to be encouraged through legislation to make it easy for parents – fathers as well as mothers – to meet the needs of their children in illness. Males are most at risk of a premature death, and I believe there is already enough evidence to encourage men to take a more caring role to help establish a useful model for their growing children. Further research may suggest that the advantages to be gained from encouraging workers to take time off when their spouses are under treatment for a variety of conditions warrant legislation to make it easier for this to happen. For example maternal depression affects the health of the children. If legislation was such that men could be encouraged to participate in the treatment of their wives' depression it may have marked effect on the illness behaviour and health of the next generation at the work-place.

In this section I have noted some of the important things occurring in families which can be built upon in health promotion programmes. In addition many of the points raised in connection with the education system are also relevant, but I leave it to the reader to translate these to his or her own particular areas of interest.

## The Government and the community

Families and schools function within the rules and regulations of the community and tend to follow the cultural norms of the macrosystem. At the same time they play their own role in the further evolution of the community in a transactional process. A characteristic of transactional relationships is that change can be initiated at any point, but the resistance to change of the larger institutions means that some of the most creative initiatives can only be fostered by changes at the highest administrative levels in society. The Black Report, through its analysis of the origins of health inequalities, identified two potential ways of altering the health of the British people. First, it emphasised the potential for Government to alter the structure moulding people's daily lives. The second way was for people to develop alternative health behaviours, but this was felt to be too dependent on the first way for it to be given priority (Townsend & Davidson, 1982).

The Government's ability to alter society's structure of rules and regulations through legal and fiscal measures is open to public inspection. Through such measures the wearing of seat belts in cars has increased, and increased taxation of alcoholic drinks has been shown to be an effective brake on otherwise increasing consumption. Such factors affect the child's environment in important ways and, as the Black Report pointed out, administrations have the power to create health-facilitating environments for children.

I have emphasised that children's views coevolve with those of the community. The rules and regulations used when deciding about children's states are modified in line with the ways in which those states are presented, and vice versa. The research reported suggests that certain family structures can be more conducive than others to health in children. In order to maximise children's health this knowledge must be made available to those who make the administrative decisions which can make it more or less easy to adopt these ways of living. The Government's family policies can be either more or less health orientated. But as Sir Richard Doll (1983) points out 'new ways need to be found for providing government with authoritative scientific opinion that can be seen to be independent of the interests affected' – a general point, not limited to family politics. But it was unlikely to be this which made the Black Report difficult to use.

Besides these new ways of providing scientific opinion, there also need to be new ways of ensuring that central and local authorities do not violate the rights of children. It is this function which ombudsmen cover. A powerful and respected health ombudsman could free doctors from having to be ambassadors on behalf of their child patients in the political arena.

Additional information is required by Government on the values of exercise and diet etc., so that the balance between the advantages and disadvantages of fostering different programmes can be assessed. The speciality of public health used to have the standing and respect to provide what has been termed type 3 health education (Draper, *et al.*, 1980). (Type 1 health education was seen as education about the body and how to look after it; type 2 was seen as education about available services and the 'sensible' use of health care resources.) But like others who have tried to give and expected a consequent change they have not always perceived themselves as effective. In type 3 health education one has to inform those who determine policy on food and transport etc. so that the easiest choices for people to make become the healthiest choices. This can be coupled with what Draper *et al.* (1980) termed the community development approach to health education: 'The essence of this approach is that health educators enter into a dialogue with the community, encouraging its members to articulate their needs, and conveying skills and information to help them take action to overcome health and related social problems'. They believe that because public health is a social change movement, there always being room for improvement in health, it tends to be opposed by all of the essentially conservative forces in society.

Doctors have often shied away from the political implications of their work. The effects of parents' unemployment on children's health is detrimental, independent of social class effects (Brennan & Lancashire, 1978). It appears to be largely with the recent increase in unemployment that doctors in Britain are realising they are one of the important groups in society which can point out some of the health and illness consequences of unemployment. There is a distinction between those who are responsible for formulating the solutions to the problems and those who, like the doctors and social scientists, can identify the areas for appropriate action. Unemployment, though, must be seen in the context of its effect on health, and tackling unemployment can be seen as part of the Government's health promotion effort. These problems place doctors in the centre of the political arena as important sources of information, without having to find solutions to the unemployment problem.

Government programmes have often appeared to focus on detailed concrete plans, such as screening programmes and regulations about where people can smoke, rather than on what can be done to help people make use of health resources already available. It is the facilitative nature of the primary structure which needs to be the priority in relation to health promotion (see the preceding section 'The education system'). If people have not grown up with the idea of respect for and cooperation with others being important, it seems quite pointless laying down rules about 'smoking areas' because no one will pay any attention to them.

Through policies it is possible both to show the importance of the support available in the social network and enable it to function maximally. Some suggestions about employment regulations and how it could be made easier for workers to be with their families and children at times of illness were raised earlier. Several possibilites seem to founder over the issue of trust – will the opportunities be abused? An essential part of arrangements must be flexibility so that people can react quickly. If economic criteria are to be used for policy decisions then it needs to be known whether it is cheaper for a worker to go home to support a family with a sick child, where otherwise that child might have to be hospitalised, than to stay at work. Additional longer-term benefits of such maximising of the home resources may follow and need to be worked out. If everything is done on the assumption that it is not possible to trust, there will be no trust. Without basic trust further development is hindered (Erikson, 1965).

I do not want to rule out regulations on smoking or screening programmes. But there is a price to be paid for compulsory screening which is hard to quantify. Compulsory screening can put the person performing it in a controlling relation to the person being checked (see also chapter 9). For example, the first contact which immigrants have with the health service is when they are checked by a medical representative of the 'authorities'. The medical service is not seen as an understanding support with which they could establish a useful relation, or a setting in which consultations can approach the 'ideal speech act'. It is part of an initiation ritual which emphasises the conformity required of the subject rather than respect for his individuality and does not build up his feelings of self-esteem and efficacy which are important for the whole of his future health career. Screening must make sense to the recipients and be seen as an offer of help, part of a partnership they can establish with health personnel (see also the importance of the climate of trust: section 276, European Health Committee, 1985 p. 98); much more time and care needs to be given to establishing this first contact with the health service. It is undesirable that immigration checks become the shop window for a country's health service, especially for a section of that community which is likely to be especially vulnerable and in need of that service.

Screening facilities amongst adults are more often directed to women than to men, and yet it is the men who are most vulnerable to early death. Because cervical cancer and breast cancer can be screened for, the view can be portrayed that women are still the more vulnerable sex (the belief found amongst children). Male 'toughness' can hide a multitude of problems, and one of these is that it makes them resistant to health education initiatives as they are not sensitive to the information about their special vulnerabilities. The 'tough man' syndrome starts early in childhood in the ways in which masculinity and feminity are construed. Whilst those who govern are predominantly men there is a danger that the male myths, balanced by corresponding female myths, will continue unless they receive understandable health education.

The media propagates several images which can make it hard to initiate changes. The images of men and women, and pseudo-health information (commercially sponsored educational material) often run counter to what is health promoting. The media provide points of view which appear to make things intelligible, but to a smaller degree does it look at whether it is warranted to account for things in the way it does? Reports are often unbalanced; there appears to be a tendency to reinforce existing beliefs rather than explore change. There also appears to be more focusing on what is dangerous than what can build up health. The latter, especially the undramatic, appears less newsworthy. I am not suggesting government intervention in the media, but those with access to health-promoting information need to make as much use of the media as possible. The ways in which the media construe health issues lead to either more or less health promotion. The questions asked by reporters can either open up possibilities available to people, such as when they explore the social aspects and how people can use their social networks, or reduce them when medical expertise and technological revolutions are emphasised. Suggesting hope for a cure through technological developments is not enough without at the same time building up people's sense of personal competence to look after themselves.

The medical profession is a potential bridge between the individual who is suffering and the community to which both the doctor and the patient belong. Just as the medical person must be able to translate the individual's different languages of discomfort so also he must be able to make these comprehensible to politicians and administrators. He is bound by the rules and regulations established by his paymaster and to an extent is also their agent, but he must also play his part in developing these rules so that his health-promoting potential is maximised.

## The medical profession

The potential for health education is present in every consultation. As the European Health Committee (1985 p. 95) put it, 'Every member of the health professions should consider that his work encompasses "activities which increase health consciousness and responsibility and people's ability to take informed decisions affecting their personal, family and community well-being'". The value of the health education component is determined by the form of communication skills used. These lie in a different plane to the general factual information which provides the basis of a doctor's training, but they can never be divorced from the application of this knowledge. Some of the communication aspects of consulting were covered in the preceding chapter for their effects on health promotion.

Rather than look again at the health-promoting potential of consultations I will discuss here a few ways in which the controlling authorities could facilitate a health-promoting orientation. One of these can be through reviewing medical training for its health-promoting potential.

In order to respect the complex interaction of the two facets to communication with patients, the pragmatic and the mathetic, it would seem appropriate that training also integrates them. Child development in all its facets and the development of communication are important basic knowledge for medical personnel. Medical education will need to include more than just teaching about these. Group work and experiential approaches will need a large place if the information being provided is to be made use of. It may require the reorganisation of the curriculum so that basic interpersonal understanding is the core onto which an understanding of the pathological is built. An understanding of healthy relations can be the starting point. The problem is similar to that pointed out in relation to the school curricula, where study of relationships currently comes in last rather than first. Yet the intersubjective basis to human development must be respected. The definition of illness I proposed is based on the effect which illness has on relationships. It seems medical education, after familiarising students with health, should first move on to the illness, before disease and the social forces which mould sickness are included.

Medical personnel have as great a need for health education as other people, and it could usefully start at the beginning of their training. Throughout we have seen that families influence the illness behaviour developed and children's resources for coping with illness in the future as well as the course of each illness episode, yet medical education pays little attention to family processes. If doctors were taught more about child development the family approach may make more sense to them. If male doctors were seen to respect the importance of their own potential roles as fathers and husbands for their own health and that of their families they could be setting a good example for health education. They urgently need to learn about better ways of coping with a stressful profession. Doctors in England are liable to develop alcoholism (there were four times the expected deaths of doctors over 65 years from cirrhosis of the liver in 1980) and are twice as likely to commit suicide in the age range 25–34. The curriculum suggested for use in schools could well be adapted for medical schools.

Throughout the training a particular sort of moral order will be established; this needs to be as helpful as possible for assisting the doctor create health-promoting moral orders in his own consultations and when he partakes in health education. The styles of communication established in medical schools need to be monitored for the health-promoting models they provide. Just as health coordinators have been appointed to schools, there may well be a place for them in medical schools also.

Examinations could, for example, still consist of the current written answers and clinical examinations; but instead of these being marked solely for their factual content, they could be reassessed for the degree to which the replies showed an awareness of health-promoting potential – one answer, two different marks (but inapplicable to the multiple choice format). Medical training must put future doctors in the position where they can translate between disease and illness models, and do it in ways which maximise the health of the individual and the population.

It is possible that the same constructs of locus of control and sense of self-efficacy are important in why doctors tend to adopt their classical approaches. It could be that doctors who believe that internal factors and disease agents are the most important are reflecting their own personalities and upbringing. This may be associated with missing out on the balance between endogenous and exogenous factors in illness causality. It may be that they will be more likely to view illness as a destroyer because of their own active life styles. Through an awareness of the development of views on illness they may gain an understanding of how other people could have alternative views on illness, and so find it easier to establish helpful contact with them.

Although some of these recommendations may be due to the bias of a child psychiatrist, I hope that through the preceding illustration of the child's world of illness the relevance of the emphasis on child development and communication will be intelligible. Further research is still needed to explore the degree to which it is warranted.

## Summary

The aim of health education in all its aspects can be the building up of a sense in each person that they have a resource of health which is in equilibrium with constraints imposed by their local environment. People will have a sense of their own strength to tackle difficult situations, a trust that people will help them, and an ability to cooperate in getting themselves well again. They will be able to search out relevant information, asking questions of whoever can help. They will be able to make informed choices based on points of view which are both intelligible and warranted. On these criteria health education and promotion can only be either more or less helpful, rather than more or less effective. This is because responsibility for health resides with all different levels in a society, which must all take responsibility for their own part in creating a climate of health in which the easiest choices are the healthiest choices.

I will quote Winnicott again on one way to use the media, where he avoided the problems of propaganda. He advised attempting 'to get hold of the ordinary things that people do, and to help them understand why they do them . . . What people do like is to be given an understanding of the problems they are tackling, and they like to be made aware of the things that they do intuitively. They feel unsafe when left to their own hunches, to the sort of things that come to them at the critical moment, when they are not thinking things out' (Davis & Wallbridge, 1983 p. 160). In the circumstances of the moment parents must react intuitively, taking as much account as they are able of the immediate constraints. I hope that my presentation of the world of childhood, and how we come to develop our varying languages for sharing discomforts, will enable people to understand how they come to do and say the things which they do. At the same time I hope that it opens up possibilities for change. Our past is not our prison, but a foundation on which we can build provided we have that vital sense that we can do something about our state. I hope that the results which have been presented can be used to foster trusting and caring relationships with children through which they can grow even in illness.

# Appendix 1 Themes for the family interviews

1. Experience of illness within the family
2. Words used to describe illness
3. Experience of accidents within the family
4. How it is suspected that the child is ill, together with how the child lets the parents know.
5. When decision-making is difficult, how the uncertainty is resolved
6. How the child's attendance at nursery/school is decided if the child is a little unwell
7. Allocation of the role of health expert between the parents
8. Who the best worrier is about illness in the family
9. The child's 'attachment person' when ill
10. The things done in the family to 'make things better'
11. Experience of various kinds of health workers
12. Things the family does to keep as healthy as possible
13. The family's view on the causes of illness and the nature of germs
14. The place of cautionary tales
15. Tooth fairies
16. How illness in one family member affects how everyone else gets on together
17. Any other comments

# Appendix 2 Open-ended questionnaire

When I am ill, I . . .
I became ill because . . .
If I am ill, I am supposed to . . .
Germs are . . .
I feel sick when . . .
The best thing my father does when I am ill . . .
Hospitals . . .
* People get food poisoning because . . .
If I am ill I miss . . .
Doctors . . .
If you are mad . . .
* I know when I am tired but not ill because . . .
People who are handicapped . . .
When I am ill I like my mother to . . .
I pretend to be ill by . . .
* When people are allergic they . . .
I know when I am starting to be ill because . . .
Illness . . .
If I am ill it is wrong to . . .
The best thing about being ill is . . .
If a close friend is ill I . . .
* Vitamins are . . .
My illness is serious if . . .
I feel sick when . . .
In order to keep healthy I . . .
These questions are . . .
The best way of pretending to be ill is . . .
If my friend said I was more often ill than other children I would . . .
I would pretend to be ill if . . .
The worst illness I've had . . .
The illness I fear most is . . .

* These questions were introduced for the secondary school children on the
basis of the primary school children's responses.

# Appendix 3 Themes for the group discussions

1. The range of illnesses which the children have experienced
2. Decision-making about illness:
    Parents of children
    Teachers/welfare assistants of children
    Children of peers/parents
3. Responses to being seen as ill:
    Boys cf. girls
    Mothers cf. fathers
    Home cf. school
    Aimed at care
    Aimed at cure
    The role of a medical consultation
    The roles of special foods, medicines, bandages etc.
4. Causes of illness, including the importance of germs/bugs/viruses and allergy
5. Things which are done to keep healthy
6. The sources of the children's information
7. Experience of games involving illness themes
8. What makes two of the following alike and different from the third one: feeling 'tired', 'ill' and 'fed up'?
9. Tooth fairies
10. Anthing else which the children wanted to talk about

# References

Abramson, L.Y., Seligman, M.E.P. & Teasdale, J.D. (1978). Learned helplessness in humans: critique and reformulation. *Journal of Abnormal Psychology*, **87**(1), 49–74.

American Psychiatric Association, Committee on Nomenclature and Statistics (1980). *Diagnostic and Statistical Manual of Mental Disorders III*. Washington, DC: American Psychiatric Association.

Anastas, J.W. & Reinherz, H. (1984). Gender differences in learning and adjustment problems in school. *American Journal of Orthopsychiatry*, **54**, 110–22.

Apley, J. (1975). *The Child with Abdominal Pains*. Oxford: Blackwell Scientific.

Apley, J. (1980). Listening and talking to patients. V. Communicating with children. *British Medical Journal*, **281**, 1116–17.

Apple, D. (1960). How laymen define illness. *Journal of Health and Human Behaviour*, **1**(3), 219–25.

Ariès, P. (1960). *Centuries of Childhood*. (English edn 1979. Harmondsworth: Penguin.)

Ariès, P. (1977). *The Hour of our Death*. (English edn 1983. Harmondsworth: Penguin.)

Avorn, J., Chen, M. & Hartley, R. (1982). Scientific vs commercial forces of influence on the prescribing behaviour of physicians. *American Journal of Medicine*, **73**, 4–8.

Bailey, V., Graham, P. & Boniface, D. (1978). How much child psychiatry does a general practitioner do? *Journal of the Royal College of General Practitioners*, **28**, 621–6.

Balint, M. (1964). *The Doctor, His Patient and the Illness*, 2nd edn. London: Pitman.

Bandura, A. (1977). Self-efficacy: toward a unifying theory of behavioural change. *Psychological Review*, **84**, 191–215.

Bannister, D. & Fransella, F. (1980). *Inquiring Man*, 2nd edn. Harmondsworth: Penguin.

Bateson, G. (1955). A theory of play and fantasy. In *Play: Its Role in Development and Evolution*, ed. J.S. Bruner, A. Jolly & K. Sylva, pp. 119–29. Harmondsworth: Penguin (1976).

Becker, E. (1971). *The Birth and Death of Meaning*, 2nd edn. Harmondsworth: Penguin.

Berger, P. & Luckmann, T. (1966). *The Social Construction of Reality*. Harmondsworth: Penguin (1980).

Berkanovic, E. (1972). Lay conceptions of the sick role. *Social Forces*, **51**, 53–64.

Bettelheim, B. (1976). *The Uses of Enchantment: The Meaning and Importance of Fairy Tales*. Harmondsworth: Penguin (1978).

Bewley, B.R. (1979). Teachers' smoking. *British Journal of Preventive and Social Medicine*, **33**, 219–22.

Bibace, R. & Walsh, M.E. (1980). Development of children's concepts of illness. *Pediatrics*, **66**(6), 912–17.

Black, D. (1985). Adolescent soma and psyche. *British Medical Journal*, **291**, 1523–4.

Blaxter, M. (1983). The causes of disease: women talking. *Social Science and Medicine*, **17**, 59–69.

Blaxter, M. (1984). Equity and consultation rates in general practice. *British Medical Journal*, **288**, 1963–7.

Blaxter, M. & Paterson, E. (1982*a*). Family attitudes to health and health services. *Social Work Today*, **13**(35), 10–14.

Blaxter, M. & Paterson, E. (1982*b*). *Mothers and Daughters: A Three Generational Study of Health Attitudes and Behaviour*. London: Heinemann.

Bloor, M. & Horobin, G. (1975). Conflict and conflict resolution in doctor/patient interactions. In *A Sociology of Medical Practice*, ed. C. Cox & A. Mead, pp. 271–84. London: Collier-Macmillan.

Bohman, M., Cloninger, R.C., von Knorring, A.L. & Sigvardsson, S. (1984). An adoption study of somatoform disorders. III. Cross fostering analysis and genetic relationship to alcoholism and criminality. *Archives of General Psychiatry*, **41**, 872–8.

Botvin, G.J., Eng, A. & Williams, C.L. (1980). Preventing the onset of cigarette smoking through life-skills training. *Preventive Medicine*, **9**, 135–43.

Bowlby, J. (1969). *Attachment and Loss, vol. 1, Attachment*. Harmondsworth: Penguin (1971).

Boyce, W.T., Jensen, E.W., Cassel, J.C., Collier, A.M., Smith, A.H. & Ramey, C.T. (1977). Influences of life events and family routines on childhood respiratory illness. *Pediatrics*, **60**, 609–15.

Brennan, M.G. & Lancashire, R. (1978). Association of childhood mortality with housing status and unemployment. *Journal of Epidemiology and Community Health*, **32**, 147–54.

Breslow, L. & Enstrom, J.E. (1980). Persistence of health habits and their relation to mortality. *Preventive Medicine*, **9**, 469–83.

Brewster, A.B. (1982). Chronically ill hospitalized children's concepts of their illness. *Pediatrics*, **69**, 355–62.

Brodie, B. (1974). Views of healthy children toward illness. *American Journal of Public Health*, **64**(12), 1156–9.

Bronfenbrenner, U. (1979). *The Ecology of Human Development*. Cambridge, Mass.: Harvard University Press.

Brown, G., Bhrolchain, M.N. & Harris, T. (1975). Social class and psychiatric disturbance among women in an urban population. *Sociology*, **9**, 225–54.

Brown, G.W., Craig, T.K.J. & Harris, T.O. (1985). Depression: distress or disease? Some epidemiological considerations. *British Journal of Psychiatry*, **147**, 612–22.

Brun, W. & Teigen, K.H. (1986). Språk og sannsynligheter. (Do we understand each other's probabilities?) *Tidsskrift for Den Norske Lægeforening*, **106**, 1967–8.

Bruvik, T., Raundalen, M., Moelv, R. & Ramsdal, G.H. (1986). Mestringsstrategier hos familier med kronisk syke barn. (Ways of coping in the families of chronically sick children.) *Tidsskrift for Norsk Psykologforening*, **23**, 63–73.

Burck, C. (1978). A study of family's expectations and experiences of a child guidance clinic. *British Journal of Social Work*, **8**(2), 145–58.

Burns, R.C. & Kaufman, S.H. (1971). *Kinetic Family Drawings*. London: Constable.

Burton, L. (1975). *The Family Life of Sick Children*. London: Routledge and Kegan Paul.

Caldwell, S.M. & Pickert, J.W. (1985). Systems theory applied to families with a diabetic child. *Family Systems Medicine,* **3,** 34–44.

Calnan, M. (1983). Social networks and patterns of help-seeking behaviour. *Social Science and Medicine,* **17,** 25–8.

Campbell, E.J.M., Scadding, J.G. & Roberts, R.S. (1979). The concept of disease. *British Medical Journal,* **279,** 757–62.

Campbell, J.D. (1975). Illness is a point of view: the development of children's concepts of illness. *Child Development,* **46,** 92–100.

Campbell, J.D. (1978). The child in the sick role: contributions of age, sex, parental status, and parental values. *Journal of Health and Social Behaviour,* **19,** 35–51.

Campion, P.D. & Gabriel, J. (1984). Child consultation patterns in general practice comparing 'high' and 'low' consulting families. *British Medical Journal,* **288,** 1426–8.

Campion, P.D. & Gabriel, J. (1985). Illness behaviour in mothers with young children. *Social Science and Medicine,* **20,** 325–30.

Cantwell, D.P. (1972). Psychiatric illness in the families of hyperactive children. *Archives of General Psychiatry,* **27,** 414–17.

Carandang, M.L.A., Folkins, C.H., Hines, P.A. & Steward, M.S. (1979). The role of cognitive level and sibling illness in children's conceptualisations of illness. *American Journal of Orthopsychiatry,* **49**(3), 474–81.

Carey, W.B. & Sibinga, M.S. (1972). Avoiding pediatric pathogenesis in the management of acute minor illness. *Pediatrics,* **49,** 553–62.

Carlson, B.E. (1984). The father's contribution to child care: effects on children's perceptions of parental roles. *American Journal of Orthopsychiatry,* **54,** 123–36.

Cazden, C.B. (1973). Play with language and meta-linguistic awareness: one dimension of language experience. In *Play,* ed. J.S. Bruner, A. Jolly & K. Sylva, pp. 603–8. Harmondsworth: Penguin (1976).

Chapman, C.M. (1986). More action for community nurses. *British Medical Journal,* **293,** 289–90.

Chen, E. & Cobb, S. (1960). Family structure in relation to health and disease. *Journal of Chronic Diseases,* **12,** 544–67.

Cline, T. (1985). Clinical judgement in context: a review of situational factors in person perception during clinical interviews. *Journal of Child Psychology and Psychiatry,* **26,** 369–80.

Cloninger, C.R., Sigvardsson, S., von Knorring, A.-L. & Bohman, M. (1984). An adoption study of somatoform disorders. II. Identification of two discrete somatoform disorders. *Archives of General Psychiatry,* **41,** 863–71.

Coddington, R. (1972). The significance of life events as etiologic factors in the disease of children. *Journal of Psychosomatic Research,* **16,** 205–13.

Cogill, S.R., Caplan, H.L., Alexandra, H., Robson, K.M. & Kumar, R. (1986). Impact of maternal postnatal depression on cognitive development of young children. *British Medical Journal,* **292,** 1165–7.

Committee on Medical Aspects of Food Policy (1984). *Diet and Cardiovascular Disease.* London: Department of Health and Social Security.

Condon, W.S. & Sanders, L.W. (1974). Neonate movement is synchronised with adult speech: interactional participation and language acquisition. *Science,* **183,** 99–101.

Cosminsky, S. (1977). The impact of methods on the analysis of illness concepts in a Guatemalan community. *Social Science and Medicine,* **11,** 325–32.

Costell, R., Reiss, D., Berkman, H. & Jones, C. (1981). The family meets the hospital: predicting the family's perception of the treatment program from its problem solving style. *Archives of General Psychiatry,* **38,** 569–77.

Cox, J.L., Connor, Y. & Kendell, R.E. (1982). Prospective study of the psychiatric disorders of childbirth. *British Journal of Psychiatry*, **140**, 111–17.

Craft, A.W., Lawson, G.R., Williams, H. & Sibert, J.R. (1984). Accidental childhood poisoning with household products. *British Medical Journal*, **288**, 682.

Craig, K.D. (1978). Social modeling influences on pain. In *The Psychology of Pain*, ed. R.A. Sternbach, pp. 73–109. New York: Raven Press.

Crain, A., Sussman, M. & Weil, W. (1966). Family interaction, diabetes and sibling relationships. *International Journal of Social Psychiatry*, **12**, 35–43.

Cullen, J. & Connolly, J.A. (1982). Infants under stress: tomorrow's adults. In *The Child in his Family, vol. 7, Children in Turmoil: Tomorrow's Parents*, ed. E.J. Anthony & C. Chiland, pp. 43–68. New York: Wiley.

Dare, C. & Lindsey, C. (1979). Children in family therapy. *Journal of Family Therapy*, **1**, 253–69.

Davidoff, L. (1976). Rationalization of housework. In *Dependence and Exploitation in Work and Marriage*, ed. D.L. Baker & S. Allen, pp. 121–151. Harlow: Longman.

Davies, J., Prendergast, S., Prout, A. & Tuckett, D. (1982). The Final Report of the Schools' Education Project: Health Knowledge of School Children, their Parents and Teachers. Health Education Council internal document.

Davis, M. & Wallbridge, D. (1983). *Boundary and Space: An Introduction to the Work of D.W. Winnicott*. Harmondsworth: Penguin.

Davison, I.S., Faull, C. & Nicol, A.R. (1986). Research note: temperament and behaviour in six-year-olds with recurrent abdominal pain: a follow up. *Journal of Child Psychology and Psychiatry*, **27**, 539–44.

Dielman, T.E., Leech, F.L., Becker, M.H., Rosenstock, I.M., Horvath, W.J. & Radius, S.M. (1980). Dimensions of children's health beliefs. *Health Education Quarterly*, **7**(3), 219–38.

Doll, R. (1983). Prospects for prevention. *British Medical Journal*, **286**, 445–53.

Donaldson, M. (1978). *Children's Minds*. London: Fontana.

Donaldson, M. & McGarrigle, J. (1974). Some clues to the nature of semantic development. *Journal of Child Language*, **1**, 185–94.

Donohue, T.R. & Meyer, T.P. (1984). Children's understanding of television commercials. In *Competence in Communication*, ed. R.N. Bostrom, pp. 129–49. London: Sage.

Douglas, M. (1966). *Purity and Danger: An Analysis of Concepts of Pollution and Taboo*. London: Routledge and Kegan Paul.

Drake, D.P. (1980). Acute abdominal pain in children. *Journal of the Royal Society of Medicine*, **73**, 641–5.

Draper, P., Griffiths, J., Dennis, J. & Popay, J. (1980). Three types of health education. *British Medical Journal*, **281**, 493–5.

Duff, R.S. & Hollingshead, A.B. (1968). *Sickness and Society*. New York: Harper & Row.

Dunn, J.B. (1977). *Distress and Comfort*. London: Fontana.

Dunn, J. (1984). *Sisters and Brothers*. London: Fontana.

Dunn, J., Wooding, C. & Hermann, J. (1977). Mothers' speech to young children: variation in context. *Developmental Medicine and Child Neurology*, **19**, 629–38.

Eiser, C. (1984). Communicating with sick and hospitalised children. *Journal of Child Psychology and Psychiatry*, **25**, 181–9.

Eiser, C. Patterson, D. & Eiser, R. (1983). Children's knowledge of health and illness: implications for health education. *Child: Care, Health and Development*, **9**, 285–92.

Eiser, C., Patterson, D. & Tripp, J.H. (1984). Illness experience and children's concepts of health and illness. *Child: Care, Health and Development*, **10**, 157–62.

Elmer, E. & Gregg, G.S. (1967). Developmental characteristics of abused children. *Pediatrics*, **40**, 596–602.

Erikson, E.M. (1965). *Childhood and Society*, 2nd edn. London: Granada (1977).

European Health Committee (1985). *Child Health Surveillance*. Strasbourg: Council of Europe.

Farr, R.M. (1977). Heider, Harré and Herzlich on health and illness: some observations on the structure of 'representations collectives'. *European Journal of Social Psychology*, **7**(4), 491–504.

Faull, C. & Nicoll, A.R. (1986). Abdominal pain in six year olds: an epidemiological study in a new town. *Journal of Child Psychology and Psychiatry*, **27**, 251–60.

Feinstein, A.R. (1967). *Clinical Judgements*. Baltimore: Williams and Wilkins.

Ferrari, M. (1984). Chronic illness: psychosocial effects on siblings. I. Chronically ill boys. *Journal of Child Psychology and Psychiatry*, **25**, 459–76.

Ford, F. (1983). Rules: the invisible family. *Family Process*, **22**, 135–45.

Foster, G.M. (1976). Disease etiologies in non-western medical systems. *American Anthropology*, **78**, 773–82.

Fraser, W.I. & Grieve, R. (1979). The work of a communications research project. *Health Bulletin*, **37**, 135–40.

Freer, C.B. (1980). Health diaries: a method of collecting health information. *Journal of the Royal College of General Practitioners*, **30**, 279–82.

Freidson, E. (1960). Client control and medical practice. *American Journal of Sociology*, **65**, 374–82.

Freidson, E. (1961). *Patients' Views of Medical Practice*. New York: Russell Sage Foundation.

Freidson, E. (1970). *Profession of Medicine: A Study of the Sociology of Applied Knowledge*. New York: Dodd, Mead & Co.

Frueh, T. & McGhee, P.E. (1975). Traditional sex role development and amount of time spent watching television. *Developmental Psychology*, **11**, 109.

Gadow, K.D. & Sprafkin, J. (1986). Television violence and childhood aggression: the field experiments. Paper presented to the annual meeting of the Royal College of Psychiatrists, Southampton.

Garralda, M.E. & Bailey, D. (1986*a*). Psychological deviance in children attending general practice. *Psychological Medicine*, **16**, 423–9.

Garralda, M.E. & Bailey, D. (1986*b*). Children with psychiatric disorders in primary care. *Journal of Child Psychology and Psychiatry*, **27**, 611–24.

Garralda, M.E. & Bailey, D. (1986*c*). The contribution of psychological factors to children's consultations in primary care: doctors' views. Paper presented to the International Association for Child and Adolescent Psychiatry, Paris.

Garvey, C. (1984). *Children's Talk*. London: Fontana.

Gentry, W., Shows, W. & Thomas, N. (1974). Chronic low back pain : a psychological profile. *Psychosomatics*, **15**, 174–7.

Gillon, R. (1985). 'It's all too subjective': scepticism about the possibility or use of philosophical medical ethics. *British Medical Journal*, **290**, 1574–5.

Gillon, R. (1986). On sickness and health. *British Medical Journal*, **292**, 318–20.

Gochman, D.S. (1970). Children's perceptions of vulnerability to illness and accidents. *Public Health Reports*, **85**(1), 69–73.

Gochman, D.S. (1971*a*). Some correlates of children's health beliefs and potential health behaviour. *Journal of Health and Social Behaviour*, **12**, 148–54.

Gochman, D.S. (1971*b*). Some steps towards a psychological matrix for health behaviour. *Canadian Journal of Behavioural Science*, **3**(1), 88–101.

Goffman, E. (1955). On face-work. In *Interaction Ritual*, E. Goffman (1967), pp. 5–46. Harmondsworth: Penguin (1972).

Goffman, E. (1961). *Encounters*. Harmondsworth: Penguin (1972).

Good, B.J. & Good, M.J.D. (1981). The meaning of symptoms: a cultural hermeneutic model for clinical practice. In *The Relevance of Social Science for Medicine*, ed. L. Eisenberg & A. Kleinman, pp. 165–96. Dordrecht: Reidel.

Gottschalk, L.A. (1976). Children's speech as a source of data toward the measurement of psychological states. *Journal of Youth and Adolescence*, 5, 11–36.

Graham, H. (1976). Smoking in pregnancy: the attitudes of expectant mothers. *Social Science and Medicine*, 10, 399–405.

Graham, H. (1984). *Women, Health and the Family*. Brighton: Harvester Press.

Graham, P. (1985). Psychology and the health of children. *Journal of Child Psychology and Psychiatry*, 26, 333–47.

Granger, R.H., Mayes, L.C., Fearn, K.A. & Stone, E.L. (1986). Early intervention: the pediatric role defined. Paper presented to the International Association for Child and Adolescent Psychiatry, Paris.

Greene, G.J. & Sattin, D.B. (1985). A paradoxical treatment format for anxiety-related somatic complaints. *Family Systems Medicine*, 3, 197–204.

HM Inspectorate (DES) (1986). *Health Education from 5 to 16*. London: Her Majesty's Stationery Office.

Haggerty, R.J. (1980). Life stress, illness and social supports. *Developmental Medicine and Child Neurology*, 22, 392–400.

Haley, J. (1976). *Problem Solving Therapy*. San Francisco: Jossey-Bass.

Halliday, M.A.K. (1973). *Explorations in the Function of Language*. London: Edward Arnold.

Halliday, M.A.K. (1975). *Learning How to Mean: Exploration in the Development of Language*. London: Edward Arnold.

Hamilton, M. (1983). On informed consent. *British Journal of Psychiatry*, 143, 416–18.

Hammer, M. (1983). 'Core' and 'extended' social networks in relation to health and illness. *Social Science and Medicine*, 17, 405–11.

Hansson, I. (1985). A Danish view. *British Medical Journal*, 290, 436–8.

Harré, R. (1977). The ethogenic approach: theory and practice. In *Advances in Experimental Social Psychology*, ed. L. Berkowitz, pp. 283–314. New York and London: Academic Press.

Harré, R. (1979). *Social Being*. Oxford: Basil Blackwell.

Harré, R. (1983). *Personal Being*. Oxford: Basil Blackwell.

Harris, R., Linn, M.W. & Pollack, L. (1984). Relationships between health beliefs and psychological variables in diabetic patients. *British Journal of Medical Psychology*, 57, 253–9.

Hartvig, P. & Sterner, G. (1985). Childhood psychologic environmental exposure in women with diagnosed somatoform disorder. *Scandinavian Journal of Social Medicine*, 13, 153–7.

Health Education Studies Unit (HESU). (1982). *The Patient Project: Final Report*. London: Health Education Council.

Heap, K. (1985). *The Practice of Social Work with Groups: a Systematic Approach*. London: George Allen & Unwin.

Heider, F. (1958). *The Psychology of Interpersonal Relations*. New York: Wiley.

Helman, C.G. (1978). 'Feed a cold, starve a fever': folk models of infection in an English suburban community, and their relation to medical treatment. *Culture, Medicine and Psychiatry*, 2, 107–37.

Herzlich, C. (1973). *Health and Illness*. New York: Academic Press.

Hill, P. (1985). The diagnostic interview with the individual child. In *Child and Adolescent Psychiatry: Modern Approaches*, 2nd edn, ed. M. Rutter & L. Hersov, pp. 249–63. Oxford: Blackwell Scientific.

Hinde, R.A. (1982). *Ethology*. London: Fontana.

Hobson, R.P. (1980). The question of egocentrism: the young child's competence in the coordination of perspectives. *Journal of Child Psychology and Psychiatry*, **21**, 325–31.

Hobson, R.P. (1982). The question of childhood egocentrism: the coordination of perspectives in relation to operational thinking. *Journal of Child Psychology and Psychiatry*, **23**, 43–60.

Hodges, K., Kline, J.J., Barbero, G. & Flanery, R. (1985). Depressive symptoms in children with recurrent abdominal pain and in their families. *Journal of Pediatrics*, **107**, 622–6.

Hodgkin, P. (1985). Medicine is war: and other medical metaphors. *British Medical Journal*, **291**, 1820–1.

Hoffman, L. (1974). Effects of maternal employment on the child: a review of the research. *Developmental Psychology*, **10**, 204–28.

Hopkins, B. (1983). The development of early non-verbal communication: an evaluation of its meaning. *Journal of Child Psychology and Psychiatry*, **24**(1), 131–44.

Horder, J., Bosanquet, N. & Stocking, B. (1986). Ways of influencing the behaviour of general practitioners. *Journal of the Royal College of General Practitioners*, **36**, 517–21.

Horwitz, A. (1977). The pathways into psychiatric treatment: some differences between men and women. *Journal of Health and Social Behaviour*, **18**, 169–78.

Howie, J.G.R. & Bigg, A.R. (1980). Family trends in psychotropic and antibiotic prescribing in general practice. *British Medical Journal*, **280**, 836–8.

Huttenlocher, J., Eisenberg, K. & Strauss, S. (1968). Comprehension relation between perceived actor and logical subject. *Journal of Verbal Learning and Verbal Behaviour*, **7**, 527–30.

Hwang, C.P. & Danielsson, B. (1985). Dicyclomine hydrochloride in infantile colic. *British Medical Journal*, **291**, 1014.

Jago, J.D. (1975). 'Hal' – old word, new task: reflections on the words 'health' and 'medical'. *Social Science and Medicine*, **9**, 1–6.

James, A. (1979). Confections, concoctions and conceptions. *Anthropological Society of Oxford Journal*, **10**, 83–95.

Jemmott, J.B., Borysenko, M., Chapman, R., Borysenko, J.Z., McClelland, D.C., Meyer, D. & Benson, H. (1983). Academic stress, power motivation, and decrease in secretion rate of salivary secretory immunoglobulin A. *Lancet*, **I**, 1400–2.

Jenkins, R. & Clare, A.W. (1985). Women and mental illness. *British Medical Journal*, **291**, 1521–2.

Jones, P.F. (1969). Acute abdominal pain in childhood, with special reference to cases not due to acute appendicitis. *British Medical Journal*, **i**, 284–6.

Kaada, B. (1986). Placebo-gåten mot sin løsning? (The mystery of the placebo. A Pavlovian reflex for activation of self-healing mechanisms.) *Tidsskrift for Den Norske Lægeforening*, **106**, 635–41.

Kagan, J. (1982). The emergence of self. *Journal of Child Psychology and Psychiatry*, **23**(4), 363–81.

Kalnins, I. & Love, R. (1982). Children's concepts of health and illness–and implications for health education: an overview. *Health Education Quarterly*, **9**, 104–15.

Kasl, S.V. & Cobb, S. (1966). Health behaviour, illness behaviour and sick role behaviour: I and II. *Archives of Environmental Health*, **12**, 246–66 and 531–41.

Kasl, S.V., Evans, A.S. & Neiderman, J.C. (1979). Psychosocial risk factors in the development of infectious mononucleosis. *Psychosomatic Medicine*, 41, 445–66.

Kendrick, C., Culling, J., Oakhill, T. & Mott, M. (1986). Children's understanding of their illness and its treatment within a paediatric oncology unit. *Association for Child Psychology and Psychiatry Newsletter*, 8, 16–20.

Kenny, A. (1975). *Wittgenstein*. Harmondsworth: Penguin.

Kister, M.C. & Patterson, C.J. (1980). Children's conceptions of the causes of illness: understanding of contagion and use of immanent justice. *Child Development*, 51, 839–46.

Kleinman, A. (1978). Concepts and a model for the comparison of medical systems as cultural systems. *Social Science and Medicine*, 12, 85–93.

Kolvin, I., Berney, T.P. & Bhate, S.R. (1984). Classification and diagnosis of depression in school phobia. *British Journal of Psychiatry*, 145, 347–57.

Koos, E.L. (1954). *The Health of Regionville: What the People Thought and Did About It*. New York: University of Columbia Press.

Kuhn, D., Nash, S.C. & Brucken, L. (1978). Sex role concepts of two- and three-year-olds. *Child Development*, 49, 445–51.

Kumar, A. & Vaidya, A.K. (1986). Locus of control in short and long sleepers. *British Journal of Psychiatry*, 148, 739–40.

Kvideland, R. (1979). Verbal transmission in the process of enculturation. *Ethnologica Scandinavica*, 9, 36–48.

Lacan, J. (1968). The mirror-phase as formative of the function of the I. *New Left Review*, 71–7.

Langford, W.S. (1948). Physical illness and convalescence: their meaning to the child. *Journal of Paediatrics*, 33, 242–50.

Laver, J. (1980). *The Phonetic Description of Voice Quality*. Cambridge: Cambridge University Press.

Leech, G. (1981). *Semantics: The Study of Meaning*, 2nd edn. Harmondsworth: Penguin.

Lefcourt, H.M. (1966). Internal versus external control of reinforcement: a review. *Psychological Bulletin*, 65, 206–20.

Levenson, H. (1973). Multidimensional locus of control in psychiatric patients. *Journal of Consulting and Clinical Psychology*, 41, 397–404.

Lewis, C.E. & Lewis, M.A. (1974). The impact of television commercials on health-related beliefs and behaviour of children. *Pediatrics*, 53, 431–5.

Lewis, C.E., Lewis, M.A., Lorimer, M.P.H. & Palmer, B.P. (1977). Child initiated care: the use of school nursing services by children in an 'adult-free' system. *Pediatrics*, 60, 499–507.

Lewis, G. (1976). A view of sickness in New Guinea. In *Social Anthropology and Medicine*, ed. J, Loudon, pp. 49–103. New York and London: Academic Press.

Lewis, G. (1980). Cultural blocks between doctors and patients. *MIMS Magazine*, (1 May), 51–7.

Ley, P. & Spelman, M.S. (1967). *Communicating with the Patient*. London: Staples Press.

Livingston, R. & Martin-Cannici, C. (1985). Multiple somatic complaints and possible somatization disorder in prepubertal children. *Journal of the American Academy of Child Psychiatry*, 24, 603–7.

Locker, D. (1981). *Symptoms and Illness*. London: Tavistock.

Loudon, J.B. (1976). Introduction. In *Social Anthropology and Medicine*, ed. J. Loudon, pp. 1–48. New York and London: Academic Press.

McCarthy, T.A. (1973). A theory of communicative competence. In *Critical Sociology*, ed. P. Connerton, pp. 470–97. Harmondsworth: Penguin.

Macaskill, S. & MacDonald, M.B. (1982). *Childhood 5–10: An Exploratory Study of Parental Experience*. Research Report of Department of Marketing: University of Strathclyde, Glasgow.

Maccoby, E.E. & Jacklin, C.N. (1980). Psychological sex differences. In *Scientific Foundations of Developmental Psychiatry*. ed. M. Rutter, pp. 92–100. London: Heinemann.

Mackie, J.E. (1980). The development of the child's concept of illness: a Piagetian framework. BA Psychology Thesis, University of Strathclyde, Glasgow.

McKinlay, J.B. (1981). Social network influences on morbid episodes and the career of help seeking. In *The Relevance of Social Science for Medicine*, ed. L. Eisenberg & A. Kleinman, pp. 77–107. Dordrecht Reidel.

McLaughlin, J.A. & Sims, A. (1984). Co-existence of the Capgras and Ekbom syndromes. *British Journal of Psychiatry*, **145**, 439–41.

Madanes, C. (1980). Protection, paradox, and pretending. *Family Process*, **19**, 73–85.

Maguire, P., Fairbairn, S. & Fletcher, C. (1986). Consultation skills of young doctors. I. Benefits of feedback training in interviewing as students persist. *British Medical Journal*, **292**, 1573–6.

Manning, M. & Hermann, J. (1981). The relationships of problem children in nursery schools. In *Personal Relationships in Disorder*, ed. R. Gilmour & S. Duck, pp. 143–67. New York and London: Academic Press.

Manning, M., Heron, J. & Marshall, T. (1978). Styles of hostility and social interactions at nursery, at school and at home. In *Aggression and Anti-social Behaviour in Childhood and Adolescence*, ed. L. Hersov, M. Berger & D. Shaffer, pp. 29–58. Oxford: Pergamon.

Mannoni, M. (1973). *The Child, his 'Illness', and the Others*. Harmondsworth: Penguin.

Mattsson, A. & Weisberg, I. (1970). Behavioral reactions to minor illness in preschool children. *Pediatrics*, **46**(4), 604–10.

Mayall, B. (1986). *Keeping Children Healthy*. London: Allen & Unwin.

Mayer, J.E. & Timms, N. (1969). Clash in perspective between worker and client. In *Basic Readings in Medical Sociology*, ed. D. Tuckett & J.M. Kaufert, (1978) pp. 98–104, London: Tavistock.

Mead, G.H. (1934). *Mind, Self and Society*. Chicago: University of Chicago Press (1962).

Mearns, C. & Kay, B. (1985). Referred but not seen. *Association for Child Psychology and Psychiatry Newsletter*, **7**(3), 16–18.

Mechanic, D. (1962). The concept of illness behaviour. *Journal of Chronic Diseases*, **15**, 189–94.

Mechanic, D. (1964). The influence of mothers on their children's health attitudes and behaviour. *Pediatrics*, **33**, 444–53.

Meyer, R.J. & Haggerty, R.J. (1963). Streptococcal infections in families. *Pediatrics*, **29**, 539–49.

Michielutte, R. & Diseker, R.A. (1982). Children's perceptions of cancer in comparison to other chronic illnesses. *Journal of Chronic Diseases*, **35**, 843–52.

Miller, B.D., Hollingsworth, E. & Sander, L.W. (1985). Assessment of infant-caregiver interaction using cardiac, respiratory, and behavioural monitoring: conceptual and technical issues in a new methodology. *Journal of the American Academy of Child Psychiatry*, **24**, 286–97.

Miller, C.J. (1980). *Faith-healers in the Himalayas*. Nepal: Tribhuvan University Press.

Millstein, S.G., Adler, N.E. & Irwin, C.E. (1981). Conceptions of illness in young adolescents. *Pediatrics*, **68**, 834–9.

Minuchin, S. (1974). *Families and Family Therapy*. London: Tavistock.

Moss, H.A. (1967). Sex, age and state as determinants of mother–infant interaction. *Merrill-Palmer Quarterly*, **13**, 19–36.

Nagy, M.H. (1951). Children's ideas of the origin of illness. *Health Education Journal*, **9**, 6–12.

Nagy, M.H. (1953). The representation of 'germs' by children. *Journal of Genetic Psychology*, **83**, 227–40.

Needham, R. (1962). *Structure and Sentiment: A Test Case in Social Anthropology*. Chicago: University of Chicago Press.

Neuhauser, C., Amsterdam, B., Hines, P. & Steward, M. (1978). Children's concepts of healing: cognitive development and locus of control factors. *American Journal of Orthopsychiatry*, **48**(2), 335–41.

Newson, J. & Newson, E. (1963). *Patterns of Infant Care in an Urban Community*. Harmondsworth: Penguin (1965).

Newson, J. & Newson, E. (1976). *Seven Years Old in the Home Environment*. Harmondsworth: Penguin.

Nightingale, F. (1860). *Notes on Nursing: What It Is, And What It Is Not*. London: Harrison.

Opie, I. & Opie, P. (1969). *Children's Games in Street and Playground*. Oxford: Oxford University Press (1970).

Oswald, I. (1986). Drugs for poor sleepers (editorial). *British Medical Journal*, **292**, 715.

Ounstead, C., Gordon, M., Roberts, J. & Milligan, B. (1982). The fourth goal of perinatal medicine. *British Medical Journal*, **284**, 879–82.

Oxman, T.E., Rosenberg, S.D., Schnurr, P.P. & Tucker, G.J. (1985). Linguistic dimensions of affect and thought in somatization disorder. *American Journal of Psychiatry*, **142**, 1150–5.

Papousek, H. & Papousek, M. (1983). Biological basis of social interactions: implications of research for an understanding of behavioural deviance. *Journal of Child Psychology and Psychiatry*, **24**(1), 117–29.

Paterson, F. (1986). Truancy: explorations in social cartography. PhD Thesis, University of Edinburgh.

Pattison, C.J., Drinkwater, C.K. & Downham, M.A.P.S. (1982). Mothers' appreciation of their children's symptoms. *Journal of the Royal College of General Practitioners*, **32**, 149–62.

Pearson, D.J. (1986). Pseudo food allergy. *British Medical Journal*, **292**, 221–2.

Perrin, E.C. & Gerrity, P.S. (1981). There's a demon in your belly: children's understanding of illness. *Pediatrics*, **67**, 841–49.

Peters, B.M. (1978). School-aged children's beliefs about causality of illness: a review of the literature. *Maternal–Child Nursing Journal*, **7**, 143–54.

Piaget, J. (1926). *The Language and Thought of the Child*. London: Routledge and Kegan Paul.

Piaget, J. (1932). *The Moral Judgement of the Child*. Harmondsworth: Penguin (1977).

Piaget, J. (1946). *Play, Dreams and Imitation in Childhood*. London: Routledge and Kegan Paul.

Piaget, J. (1970). *Psychology and Epistemology: Towards a Theory of Knowledge*. Harmondsworth: Penguin (1972).

Piaget, J. & Inhelder, B. (1966). *The Psychology of the Child*. London: Routledge and Kegan Paul (1973).

Pill, R. & Stott, N.C.H. (1982). Concepts of illness causation and responsibility: some preliminary data from a sample of working class mothers. *Social Science and Medicine*, 16, 43–52.

Pill, R. & Stott, N.C.H. (1985) Choice or chance: further evidence on ideas of illness and responsibility for health. *Social Science and Medicine*, 20, 981–91.

Pilowsky, I., Bassett, D.L., Begg, M.W. & Thomas, P.G. (1982). Childhood hospitalization and chronic intractable pain in adults: a controlled retrospective study. *International Journal of Psychiatry in Medicine*, 12, 75–84

Posner, T.R. (1980). Ritual in the surgery. *MIMS Magazine*, (1 August), 41–8.

Postman, N. (1985). *Amusing Ourselves to Death: Public Discourse in the Age of Show Business*. New York: Elisabeth Sifton/Viking.

Pratt, L. (1972). Conjugal organization and health. *Journal of Marriage and the Family*, 2, 85–95.

Prout, A. (1986). 'Wet children' and 'little actresses': going sick in primary school. *Sociology of Health and Illness*. 8, 111–36.

Puska, P. (1982). The North Karelia youth project. *Preventive Medicine*, 11, 550–70.

Rashkis, S.R. (1965). Child's understanding of health. *Archives of General Psychiatry*, 12, 10–17.

Richman, N., Stevenson, J. & Graham, P. (1982). *Pre-School to School: A Behavioural Study*. New York and London: Academic Press.

Rix, K.J.B., Pearson, D.J. & Bentley, S.J. (1984). A psychiatric study of patients with supposed food allergy. *British Journal of Psychiatry*, 145, 121–6.

Roghmann, K.J. & Haggerty, R.J. (1973). Daily stress, illness and use of health services in young families. *Paediatric Research*, 7, 520–6.

Rolland, J.S. (1984). Toward a psychosocial typology of chronic and life-threatening illness. *Family Systems Medicine*, 2, 245–62.

Rosenstock, I.M. (1966). Why people use health services. *Millbank Memorial Fund Quarterly*, 44, 94–127.

Royal College of General Practitioners (1981). *Health and Prevention in Primary Care*. London: Royal College of General Practitioners.

Ruberman, W., Weinblatt, E., Goldberg, J.D. & Chaudhary, B.S. (1984). Psychosocial influences on mortality after myocardial infarction. *New England Journal of Medicine*, 311, 552–9.

Rutter, M. (1980). Attachment and the development of social relationships. In *Scientific Foundations of Developmental Psychiatry*, ed. M. Rutter, pp. 267–79. London: Heinemann.

Rutter, M. (1985). Resilience in the face of adversity. *British Journal of Psychiatry*, 147, 598–611.

Rutter, M. & Graham, P. (1966). Psychiatric disorder in ten and eleven year old children. *Proceedings of the Royal Society of Medicine*, 59, 382–7.

Rutter, M., Maughan, B., Mortimore, P. & Ouston, J. (1979). *Fifteen Thousand Hours: Secondary Schools and their Effects on Children*. London: Open Books.

Sack, W.H. & Blocker, D.L. (1978–9). Who gets referred? Child psychiatric consultations in a pediatric hospital. *International Journal of Psychiatry in Medicine*, 9,(3&4), 329–37.

Samuel, J. & Bryant, P. (1984). Asking only one question in the conservation experiment. *Journal of Child Psychology and Psychiatry*, 25, 315–18.

Schacter, S. & Singer, J.E. (1962). Cognitive, social and physiological determinants of emotional state. *Psychological Review*, 69, 379–99.

Schools Council. (1977). *Think Well*. London: Nelson.

Schweinhart, L.J., Weikart, D.P. & Larner, M.B. (1986). Consequences of three pre-school curriculum models through age 15. *Early Childhood Research Quarterly*, 1, 15–45.

*Science* News and Comments (1984). Studying learning in the womb. *Science*, 225, 302–3.

Seltzer, W.J. (1985*a*). Conversion disorder in childhood and adolescence. I. A familial/cultural approach. *Family Systems Medicine*, 3, 261–80.

Seltzer, W.J. (1985*b*). Conversion disorder in childhood and adolescence. II. Therapeutic issues. *Family Systems Medicine*, 3, 397–416.

Selvini-Palazzoli, M., Cecchin, G., Prata, G. & Boscolo, L. (1978). *Paradox and Counter Paradox*. New York: Aronson.

Selvini-Palazzoli, M., Boscolo, L., Cecchin, G. & Prata, G. (1980*a*). Hypothesising – circularity – neutrality: three guidelines for the conductor of the session. *Family Process*, 19, 3–12.

Selvini-Palazzoli, M., Boscolo, L., Cecchin, G. & Prata, G. (1980*b*). The problem of the referring person. *Journal of Marital and Family Therapy*, 6, 3–9.

Shapiro, E.G. & Rosenfeld, A.A. (1987). *The Somatizing Child: Diagnosis and Treatment of Conversion and Somatization Disorders*. New York: Springer-Verlag.

Shapiro, J. (1983). Family reactions and coping strategies in response to the physically ill or handicapped child: a review. *Social Science and Medicine*, 17, 913–31.

Shrand, H. (1965). Behaviour changes in sick children nursed at home. *Pediatrics*, 36, 604–7.

Sigvardsson, S., von Knorring, A.L., Bohman, M. & Cloninger, R.C. (1984). An adoption study of somatoform disorders. I. The relationship of somatization to psychiatric disability. *Archives of General Psychiatry*, 41, 853–9.

Simeonsson, R.J., Buckley, L. & Monson, L. (1979). Conceptions of illness causality in hospitalized children. *Journal of Pediatric Psychology*, 4, 77–84.

Sluckin, A. (1981). *Growing up in the Playground*. London: Routledge and Kegan Paul.

Sontag, S. (1979). *Disease as metaphor*. New York: Vintage.

Spencer, N.J. (1984). Parents' recognition of the ill child. In *Progress in Child Health*, vol. 1, ed. J.A. McFarlane, pp. 100–12. Edinburgh: Churchill Livingstone.

Stacey, M. (1980). Sociological and anthropological perspectives of health and disease: their contribution to historical analysis. Paper presented to the Social Science Research Council Sheffield Symposium.

Stein, M., Keller, S.E. & Schleifer, J. (1985). Stress and immunomodulation: the role of depression and neuroendocrine function. *Journal of Immunology*, 135, 827–33.

Steward, M. & Regalbuto, G. (1975). Do doctors know what children know? *American Journal of Orthopsychiatry*, 45(1), 146–49.

Stimson, G.V. & Webb, B. (1975). *Going to See the Doctor*. London: Routledge and Kegan Paul.

Stoeckle, J.D., Zola, I.K. & Davidson, G.E. (1963). On going to see the doctor: the contributions of the patient to seek medical aid. *Journal of Chronic Disease*, 16, 975–89.

Storr, A. (ed.) (1983). *Jung: Selected Writings*. London: Fontana.

Storr, A. (1985). Isaac Newton. *British Medical Journal*, 291, 1779–84.

Strelnick, A.H. & Massad, R.J. (1986). Preventing drug habits by changing physicians habits: obstacles and opportunities. *Family Systems Medicine*, 4, 51–71.

Strohner, H. & Nelson, K.E. (1974). The young child's development of sentence comprehension. *Child Development*, 45, 567–76.

Strong, P.M. (1979). *The Ceremonial Order of the Clinic: Parents, Doctors and Medical Bureaucracies*. London: Routledge and Kegan Paul.

Sylva, K. (1986). Hard choices in the nursery. Paper presented to the annual meeting of the Association of Child Psychology and Psychiatry, London.

Tatam, J. (1974). *The Effects of an Inappropriate Partner on Infant Sociability.* MA Thesis, University of Edinburgh.

Taylor, F.K. (1979). *The Concepts of Illness, Disease and Morbus.* Cambridge: Cambridge University Press.

Taylor, G.J. (1984). Alexithymia: concept, measurement, and implications for treatment. *American Journal of Psychiatry,* 141, 725–32.

Tizard, B. & Hughes, M. (1984). *Young Children Learning: Talking and Thinking at Home and at School.* London: Fontana.

Townsend, P. & Davidson, N. (eds.) (1982). *Inequalities in Health.* Harmondsworth; Penguin.

Trevarthen, C. (1974). Conversations with a two-month-old. *New Scientist,* (2 May), 230–5.

Trevarthen, C. (1980). The foundations of intersubjectivity: development of interpersonal and co-operative understanding in infants. In *The Social Foundations of Language and Thought: Essays in Honour of J.S. Bruner,* ed. D. Olsen, pp. 316–42. New York: Norton.

Trevarthen, C. (1982). The primary motives for cooperative understanding. In *Social Cognition: Studies of the Development of Understanding,* ed. G. Butterworth & P. Light, pp. 77–109. Brighton: Harvester Press.

Trevarthen, C. (1984). Emotions in infancy: regulators of contact and relationships with persons. In *Approaches to Emotion,* ed. K. Scherer & P. Ekman, pp. 129–57. Hillsdale, NJ: Erlbaum.

Trevarthen, C. (1985). Facial expressions of emotion in mother–infant interaction. *Human Neurobiology,* 4, 21–32.

Trevarthen, C. & Marwick, H. (1982). Co-operative understanding in infants. Project Report for the Spencer Foundation of Chicago. University of Edinburgh Department of Psychology.

Tuch, R.H. (1975). The relationship between a mother's menstrual status and her response to illness in her child. *Psychosomatic Medicine,* 37, 388–94.

Turkat, I.D., Kuczmierczyk, A.J. & Adams, H.E. (1984). An investigation of the aetiology of chronic headache: the role of headache models. *British Journal of Psychiatry,* 145, 665–6.

Twaddle, A.C. (1981). Sickness and the sickness career: some implications. In *The Relevance of Social Science for Medicine,* ed. L. Eisenberg & A. Kleinman, pp. 111–33. Dordrecht: Reidel.

Ullian, D. (1984). Why girls are good: a constructivist view. *American Journal of Orthopsychiatry,* 54(1), 71–82.

Van Dongen-Melman, J.E.W.M. & Sanders-Woudstra, J.A.R. (1986). Psychosocial aspects of childhood cancer: a review of the literature. *Journal of Child Psychology and Psychiatry,* 27, 145–80.

Van Eijk, J., Grol, R., Huygen, F., Mesker, P., Mesker-Niesten, G., van Mierlo, G., Mokkink, H. & Smits, A. (1983). The family doctor and the prevention of somatic fixation. *Family Systems Medicine,* 1(2), 5–15.

Vassend, O. (1984). Sykdom, familie og mestring. (Illness, family and coping.) *Fokus på Familien,* 12, 187–201.

Volkmar, F.R. & Siegel, A.E. (1979). Young children's responses to discrepant communications. *Journal of Child Psychology and Psychiatry,* 22, 139–49.

Wallinga, J.V. (1982). Human ecology: primary prevention in pediatrics. *American Journal of Orthopsychiatry,* 52, 141–5.

Wallston, B.D. & Wallston, K.A. (1978). Locus of control and health: a review of the literature. *Health Education Monographs*, **6**, 107–17.

Watzlawick, P., Beavin, J.H. & Jackson, D.D. (1967). *Pragmatics of Human Communication*. New York: Norton.

Watzlawick, P., Weakland, J. & Fisch, R. (1974). *Change: Principles of Problem Formation and Problem Resolution*. New York: Norton.

Whitt, J.K., Dykstra, W. & Taylor, C.A. (1979). Children's conceptions of illness and cognitive development. *Clinical Pediatrics*, **18**, 327–39.

Wilkinson, S.R. (1983). Talking with children. *Medical Teacher*, **5**, 11–15.

Wilkinson, S.R. (1984). Children's views on the causality of illness. MD Thesis, University of Cambridge.

Wilkinson, S. (1985). Drawing up boundaries: a technique. *Journal of Family Therapy*, **7**, 99–111.

Williams, B.T. (1984). Are public health education campaigns worthwhile? *British Medical Journal*, **288**, 170–1.

Williams, P.D. (1977). A comparison between concepts of body organs and illness of children from a laboratory school with an experimental curriculum to that of children from three public schools. *ANPHI Papers*, **12**, 2–12.

Williams, R.G.A. (1981). Logical analysis as a qualitative method. I: Themes in old age and chronic illness. II: Conflict of ideas and the topic of illness. *Sociology of Health and Illness*, **3**(2), 140–64 and 165–87.

Williams, T. & Woesler de Panafieu, C. (eds.) (1985). *School Health Education in Europe*. Southampton: Health Education Unit, University of Southampton.

Willis, D.J., Elliott, C.H. & Jay, S. (1982). Psychological effects of physical illness and its concomitants. In *Handbook for the Practice of Pediatric Psychology*, ed. J.M. Tuma, pp. 28–66. New York: Wiley.

Winkler, J.T. (1985). The COMA report: what it left out. *British Medical Journal*, **290**, 685–7.

Winnicott, D.W. (1967). Mirror-role of mother and family in child development. In *Playing and Reality*, D.W. Winnicott, pp. 130–8. Harmondsworth: Penguin (1980).

Winnicott, D.W. (1971). *Playing and Reality*. Harmondsworth: Penguin (1980).

Wolff, P.H., Waber, D., Bauermeister, M., Cohen, C. & Ferber, R. (1982). The neuropsychological status of adolescent delinquent boys. *Journal of Child Psychology and Psychiatry*, **23**, 267–79.

Wolff, S. (1981). *Children under Stress*. 2nd edn. Harmondsworth: Penguin.

Wolin, S.J. & Bennett, L.A. (1984). Family rituals. *Family Process*, **23**, 401–20.

Wolkind, S. (1985). Mothers' depression, and their children's attendance at medical facilities. *Journal of Psychosomatic Research*, **29**, 579–82.

Wolkind, S. & Rutter, M. (1985). Separation, loss and family relationships. In *Child and Adolescent Psychiatry: Modern Approaches*, 2nd edn, ed. M. Rutter & L. Hersov, pp. 34–57. Oxford: Blackwell Scientific.

Wood, D.J. (1982). Talking to young children. *Developmental Medicine and Child Neurology*, **24**, 856–9.

Wood, D., McMahon, L. & Cranston, Y. (1980). *Working with Under Fives*. London:Grant McIntyre.

Wright, P. & Treacher, A. (eds.) (1982). *The Problem of Medical Knowledge: Examining the Social Construction of Medicine*. Edinburgh: Edinburgh University Press.

Yudkin, S. (1961). Six children with coughs, the second diagnosis. *Lancet*, **II**, 561–3.

Zeanah, C.H., Keener, M.A., Stewart, L. & Anders, T.F. (1985). Prenatal perception of infant personality: a preliminary investigation. *Journal of the American Academy of Child Psychiatry*, **24**, 204–10.

Zeitlin, H. (1986). *The Natural History of Psychiatric Disorder in Children: A Study of Individuals Known to have Attended both Child and Adult Psychiatric Departments of the Same Hospital*. Maudsley Monographs 29. Oxford: Oxford University Press.

Zoccolillo, M. & Cloninger, C.R. (1985). Parental breakdown associated with somatisation disorder (hysteria). *British Journal of Psychiatry*, **147**, 443–6.

Zola, I.K. (1972). Medicine as an institution of social control. *Sociological Review*, **20**(4), 487–504.

Zola, I.K. (1973). Pathways to the doctor – from person to patient. *Social Science and Medicine*, **7**, 677–89.

Zola, I.K. (1975). Medicine as an institution of social control. In *A Sociology of medical Practice*, ed C. Cox & A. Mead, pp. 170–85, London: Collier-Macmillan.

# Index